Neonatology

A Practical Guide

4th Edition

Neonatology

A Practical Guide

Alistair G.S. Philip, MD (Edin), FRCP(E)

Professor of Pediatrics
Department of Pediatrics
Stanford University School of Medicine
Palo Alto, California
Medical Director, Neonatology Service
El Camino Hospital
Mountain View, California

W.B. SAUNDERS COMPANY
A Division of Harcourt Brace & Company
Philadelphia London Toronto Montreal Sydney Tokyo

W.B. SAUNDERS COMPANY
A Division of Harcourt Brace & Company

The Curtis Center
Independence Square West
Philadelphia, Pennsylvania 19106

Library of Congress Cataloging-in-Publication Data

Philip, Alistair G. S.
  Neonatology: a practical guide / Alistair G.S. Philip—4th ed.

  p. cm.

Includes bibliographical references and index.

ISBN 0–7216–4776–6

  1. Neonatology—Handbooks, manuals, etc.   I. Title.
  [DNLM: 1. Infant, Newborn, Diseases.   2. Infant,
  Newborn. WS 420 P549n 1996]

RJ251.P47   1996

618.92′01—dc20

DNLM/DLC   95–9516

NEONATOLOGY: A PRACTICAL GUIDE, Fourth Edition   ISBN 0–7216–4776–6

Printed in the United States of America.

Last digit is the print number: 9   8   7   6   5   4   3   2   1

PREFACE

In my preface to the third edition of this text, I apologized for the long gap between editions. Advancing years have not improved the situation, as the gap between the third and fourth editions has been even longer. While the basic problems encountered in neonatology remain much the same, in some cases our understanding of pathophysiology has improved and our ability to manage most of the problems has been refined. Consequently, I have incorporated as much new knowledge into this revision as I could, without deviating from my original intent to provide a concise understanding of neonatology.

This book is not intended to "provide all the answers," but it should provide the basic information needed to understand and evaluate the more common problems in neonatology. The bibliography for each topic should allow the interested reader to seek more detailed information from a medical library. If pertinent information is not provided in the text, I encourage readers to look at the bibliography for the topic, because I sometimes include references that deal with details that cannot be covered in this concise format.

Several new sections have been added, such as AIDS, Bilirubin and the Breast-Fed Infant, Cordocentesis, Dwarfism, Fever, Immunizations, Non-immune Hydrops, Positioning, and Pulse Oximetry. In addition, some subjects have been substantially modified, such as management of persistent pulmonary hypertension, use of surfactants for the respiratory distress syndrome, prevention of intraventricular hemorrhage, effects of cocaine, use of erythropoietin for anemia of prematurity, and many others. It is salutary to examine how many important changes have occurred in the last few years. Further evidence is provided in Chapter 23, Milestones in Neonatology, where once again I have tried to select events that have made an impact on those who practice neonatology.

As with previous editions, I have updated the references for almost every topic. Some earlier references that no longer seemed relevant have been eliminated, but I have tried to leave in some that deal with original reports or are clear reviews.

I have provided an entirely new multiple-choice quiz and hope that the answers continue to be correct over the next few years.

In the preface to the first edition of this book I stated that my intent was "to provide a practical approach to the assessment and management of the newborn infant" and that the book "is directed primarily to medical students, interns and residents, but it is hoped the the practicing pediatrician will also find some of these pages helpful." *Some* pediatricians have told me that it *has* helped them! In addition, it has proved to be well accepted and appreciated by neonatal nurses and neonatal nurse practitioners. I hope the present edition brings the readers up to date in neonatology and remains current for several years.

Alistair G.S. Philip, MD (Edin), FRCP(E)

ACKNOWLEDGMENTS

Although many individuals have helped me over the years, I would like to thank my neonatology colleagues at the Maine Medical Center who sustained me from 1987 through 1992.

In addition, I am grateful to Ms. Jodi Blanchard for her secretarial assistance in the preparation of this fourth edition.

CONTENTS

PART 1

GENERAL CONCEPTS AND COMMON PROBLEMS

 1. The Fetus Prior to Delivery 3
 2. The Delivery Room 13
 3. The Normal Newborn 19
 4. Routine Procedures 33
 5. Thermoregulation 44
 6. Assessment of Gestational Age 49
 7. Regionalized Care and Transport of the Sick Neonate 63
 8. Common Congenital Malformations 68
 9. Respiratory Problems 107
10. Bilirubin Metabolism and Jaundice 134
11. Feeding 152
12. Problems of Prematurity 163
13. Multiple Pregnancies 170
14. Parent-Infant Interaction 175
15. Neonatal Infection 182
16. Disordered Growth 204
17. Metabolic Disorders 214
18. Necrotizing Enterocolitis 228
19. Intracranial Hemorrhage 233
20. Blood Disorders 238
21. Drugs and the Fetus and Neonate 246
22. Neonatal and Perinatal Mortality 257
23. Milestones in Neonatology 264

PART 2

CLINICAL PRESENTATIONS AND THEIR ASSESSMENT

24. Neonatal Emergencies 281
25. Color Disorders 293
26. Respiratory Signs 298
27. Cardiac Signs 305
28. Abdominal Signs 309

ix

29. Neurologic Signs 319
30. Abnormalities of the Head and Neck 324
31. Abnormal Eye Examination 332
32. Skin Changes 336
33. Miscellaneous Presenting Signs 346
34. Interpreting Laboratory Tests and X-Ray Studies 357

PART 3
PROCEDURES

35. Diagnostic Techniques 365
36. Therapeutic Techniques 385
37. Mini-Pharmacopeia 397

PART 4
QUIZZES

38. Pictorial Quiz 407
39. Written Quiz 452

PART 5
APPENDICES

Appendix 1 Technique for Placement, Sampling, and Removal of
             Umbilical Artery Catheter 477
Appendix 2 Exchange Transfusion Technique 483
Appendix 3 Weight Conversion 484
Appendix 4 Acid-Base Nomogram 486
Appendix 5 Growth Record for Infants 487
Appendix 6 Blood Pressure in the Newborn 488
Appendix 7 "Fool's Guide" to Respirator Management of the
             Neonate 491
Appendix 8 Normal Values 492
Appendix 9 Neonatal Mortality 496
Appendix 10 Glucose Rate Calculator 500
Suggested Reading 501
Index 503

General Concepts and Common Problems

THE FETUS PRIOR TO DELIVERY

ASSESSMENT

A full account of the techniques available to the obstetrician interested in fetology is beyond the scope of this book. Nevertheless, a passing acquaintance with the more frequently used techniques is desirable.

ULTRASONOGRAPHY

Measurement of the fetal skull, usually the biparietal diameter, allows an estimate of fetal size and continuing growth. The presence of twins and some fetal abnormalities may also be detected. To obtain accurate estimates of gestational age, crown-rump length or biparietal diameter must be measured before 20 weeks' gestation. A single measurement is of limited value in most cases but may allow an estimate of maturity in the planning of an elective cesarean section (or induction). Measurements of fetal head to abdomen circumference ratio and estimates of total intrauterine volume have improved the accuracy of fetal weight prediction.

In recent years, more attention has been given to measurement of femoral length as an indicator of fetal maturity. Limits are narrow in early gestation but (like other measurements) broaden later. Confusion may also arise in cases of symmetric intrauterine growth retardation. Fetal well-being (see later) can also be assessed by using a biophysical profile, which incorporates ultrasonic estimation of fetal growth, activity, and breathing movements as well as amount of amniotic fluid present. An ultrasonographic appearance may even suggest imminent fetal death.

For many years, it was assumed that two ultrasonographic examinations during pregnancy, one early and one late, would provide optimal information about gestational age, multiple pregnancy, and major malformations. The practice of performing these prenatal ultrasonographic evaluations routinely has recently been called into question. Frequent prenatal ultrasonographic examinations were linked to an increase in low birth weight for gestational age, and routine testing did not improve outcome when compared with selective ultrasonography (based on medical indications).

With recent improvements in technology and in the skill of those interpreting the images, many congenital abnormalities can be detected before delivery.

This knowledge may enable planned delivery, which may minimize morbidity. For example, ventral wall defects (especially gastroschisis) require the services of a pediatric surgeon, who can plan to be available and schedule time in the operating room.

Another technical advance is the ability to predict fetal sex with a high degree of accuracy fairly early in gestation, but whether or not this information is accurate enough to enter into decisions concerning sex-linked genetic disorders remains to be elucidated.

AMNIOTIC FLUID STUDIES (AMNIOCENTESIS)

Early in pregnancy, various genetic abnormalities may be detected or virtually excluded. Techniques involve cell tissue culture for chromosomal analysis or for detection of hereditary biochemical disorders. The rate of chromosomal abnormalities rises with maternal age, being approximately 5, 15, and 50 per 1000 births at ages 35, 40, and 45, respectively. Use of amniotic fluid α-fetoprotein level may allow detection of open neural tube defects (open in this context means not covered by skin). Further refinement in detection has come from acetylcholinesterase studies, using a monoclonal antibody.

Later in pregnancy, bilirubin levels may be used in Rh-sensitized mothers and in those with other blood group incompatibilities. Fetal maturity may be assessed by creatinine level (kidney), fetal squames (skin), and, most important, lecithin to sphingomyelin (L:S) ratio or foam stability test (shake test) for determination of lung maturity. An L:S ratio of greater than 2:1 usually signifies mature lungs. More accurate predictive information may be derived from the individual lecithins. Presence of phosphatidylglycerol seems to be most important for the activity of surfactant.

CHORIONIC VILLUS SAMPLING

Because culturing cells from amniocentesis samples for chromosomal or hereditary disorders usually cannot be accomplished much before 16 to 18 weeks' gestation, considerable concern arises when termination of the pregnancy is being considered. The technique of chorionic villus sampling may allow much more time for discussion of such decisions. Cells may be obtained by direct needle aspiration (under ultrasonographic guidance), and cells can be grown for chromosomal analysis or DNA probes can be used to detect genetic disorders. Generally, the experience with this technique has been satisfactory, but a case of fetal exsanguination was recently reported, and chromosomal mosaicism is sometimes confusing (1 per 100 samples). Limb reduction defects have also been associated with the procedure.

FETAL HEART RATE MONITORING

Fetal heart rate monitoring assesses the fetal heart response to uterine contractions during labor. This monitoring is achieved via electronic monitoring, either with an external electrode or, more reliably, with an internal electrode (attached to the fetal scalp) and an intrauterine pressure transducer (probe). This technique is most valuable in high-risk patients. In some centers, it has been used on practically all patients, but the value of this approach is questionable. Patterns are variable but show three major types of disorganization:

1. *Early deceleration* in association with the height of uterine contractions, indicating head compression

2. *Late deceleration*, which occurs after the uterine contraction has subsided, indicating compromised fetal perfusion (most likely at a placental level)

3. *Variable deceleration*, in which bradycardia occurs randomly (during uterine contractions), most likely caused by cord compression (U or V patterns)

Loss of baseline or beat-to-beat variability may be of even more significance than either late or variable decelerations. However, loss of variability is more difficult to interpret in the preterm fetus. A sinusoidal pattern has been most frequently associated with fetal anemia.

FETAL SCALP SAMPLING

Much can be learned from fetal heart rate monitoring, but satisfactory assessment of fetal well-being also requires measurement of fetal pH (or lactic acid). This assessment may be performed by use of intermittent scalp blood samples. Although continuous recordings of fetal pH (through a probe incorporated into a scalp electrode) and transcutaneous pO_2 have been performed and have provided interesting information, these techniques have not yet been incorporated into routine clinical practice.

TESTS OF FETAL WELL-BEING

In the past few years, there has been a shift from stress tests, which usually incorporate oxytocin challenge or exercise to induce contractions, toward nonstress tests. The latter are usually directed toward the activity of the fetus. When fetal movement is well demonstrated, especially with increased fetal heart rate during movement, the nonstress test is considered reactive. One approach for stress tests is the use of nipple stimulation to induce contractions. Another approach to the study of fetal well-being is the biophysical profile. Recent studies suggest that the sleep state of the baby may be an important variable that needs to be considered in the assessment of fetal well-being.

AMNIOSCOPY

Examination of the color and consistency of amniotic fluid through intact fetal membranes is possible in many women late in pregnancy. The presence of meconium-stained amniotic fluid usually dictates delivery soon after detection.

Despite its simplicity, this technique does not seem to have gained widespread acceptance.

CORDOCENTESIS

In the past, fiberoptic systems were used to assess the fetus for congenital abnormalities and to sample pure fetal blood. This technique has largely been replaced by cordocentesis, in which the umbilical cord is punctured close to its insertion into the placenta. Cordocentesis, or percutaneous umbilical blood sampling, under ultrasonographic guidance has allowed fetal blood samples to be obtained primarily to detect fetal anemia, but also to assess thrombocytopenia and to evaluate for intrauterine infection, particularly toxoplasmosis. By use of the same technique, the fetus may undergo transfusion to correct anemia. More recently, information about compromise of the growth-retarded fetus has been obtained in this manner, possibly allowing therapeutic intervention (e.g., oxygen therapy).

FETAL BREATHING MOVEMENTS

Normal fetuses seem to "practice" breathing for a good part of the day, and gasping patterns have been associated with impending intrauterine death. Cyclic variations in the amount of fetal breathing movements complicate interpretation. However, assessment of fetal breathing movements may allow intelligent decisions to be made about the best time to deliver the compromised fetus, but this has not been widely applied to date.

MATERNAL SCREENING FOR FETAL DISORDERS

The use of maternal serum α-fetoprotein levels originated in Great Britain, where the prevalence of neural tube defects is high (see Chapter 8). Several states in the United States, including Maine, established maternal serum α-fetoprotein screening programs, with significantly increased levels suggesting neural tube defects, abdominal wall defects, twins, and high-risk pregnancy. Further differentiation among the various disorders came from acetylcholinesterase and pseudocholinesterase ratios performed on amniotic fluid samples, with additional information obtained from ultrasonographic evaluation of the fetus.

Subsequently, low levels of maternal serum α-fetoprotein were associated with chromosomal abnormalities, particularly Down's syndrome (trisomy 21). In recent years, additional diagnostic accuracy in Down's syndrome is provided by combining maternal serum α-fetoprotein with serum unconjugated estriol levels which are abnormally low, and chorionic gonadotropin levels, which are abnormally high (so-called triple testing), and taking maternal age into consideration.

MANAGEMENT

Several techniques that influence fetal development and directly bear on neonatal management have been added to the obstetrician's armamentarium. The most important of these are summarized here.

TREATMENT OF TOXEMIA

In most cases of toxemia, obstetrical intervention is dictated by fetal indications (see below), but occasionally, the obstetrician deems it necessary to deliver the fetus to correct a maternal problem. The most common maternal indication for intervention is pregnancy-induced hypertension, which may be associated with proteinuria, excessive edema, and hyperreflexia, features that constitute toxemia (or preeclampsia). In some cases, a syndrome consisting of hemolysis, elevated liver enzyme levels and low platelet counts (HELLP syndrome) develops. Occasionally, eclampsia with seizures may occur. Delivery of the fetus is indicated whenever moderate to severe toxemia occurs.

Toxemia's effects on the fetus are variable, but pregnancy-induced hypertension may be associated with decreased perfusion of the fetus and poor fetal growth, and both neutropenia and thrombocytopenia have been seen in neonates. Infants delivered to mothers with the syndrome of hemolysis, elevated liver enzyme levels, and low platelet counts are occasionally extremely sick. Another possible problem in the neonate is hypermagnesemia (see Chapter 17), particularly if intravenous magnesium sulfate has been given to the mother for more than 12 hours.

INFLUENCING FETAL GROWTH

Alterations in fetal growth at both extremes can now be modified under certain circumstances. Careful attention to regulation of blood sugar in diabetes mellitus has resulted in a decrease in the number of significantly large-for-gestational age babies born to diabetic mothers. This means that they may be allowed to approach term gestation before delivery is mandatory. In turn, there is greater likelihood of pulmonary maturation. In addition, tight prepregnancy control of diabetes may decrease fetal malformations. On the other hand, infants who begin to demonstrate intrauterine growth retardation (by ultrasound) may respond to either glucose infusions or lipid supplementation of the maternal diet. Other techniques have been used (e.g., intermittent abdominal decompression) or await further study (e.g., administration of drugs to improve placental perfusion).

STIMULATING PULMONARY MATURATION

The ability to prevent or alleviate the symptoms of the respiratory distress syndrome by prenatal administration of corticosteroids was first demonstrated by Liggins and Howie in 1972. Since that time, a considerable amount of evidence has accumulated to support their findings. To date, no evidence indicates that this artificial acceleration of pulmonary maturity adversely affects the human fetus, although theoretical objections have been raised. A slight increase in maternal morbidity (greater susceptibility to infection) may occur.

Despite the fact that other pharmacologic agents (e.g., heroin and aminophylline) can enhance pulmonary maturation, corticosteroids remain the most popular therapeutic agents for attempting to induce accelerated lung maturity. The infant who benefits most from this therapy seems to be a white female between 28 and 32 weeks' gestation, but less mature infants may also benefit. Little (if any) advantage to corticosteroid use seems to exist in women with prolonged rupture of membranes.

ARRESTING PREMATURE LABOR

Tocolytic agents (drugs that inhibit uterine contractions) are now widely used to suppress preterm labor. The most widely used group of drugs has been the β-sympathomimetic agents (e.g., ritodrine, terbutaline, and isoxsuprine), although more recently, their efficacy has been called in question. Use of magnesium sulfate as a tocolytic agent has increased, but high levels are needed, which can cause respiratory depression in the neonate and can suppress fetal breathing movements. Other tocolytic agents, such as indomethacin and nifedipine (a calcium-channel blocker), have been used successfully but require caution.

Most tocolytic agents are used for only 24 to 48 hours in the presence of ruptured membranes. Frequently, prenatal corticosteroids are administered when treatment with the tocolytic agent is begun. However, when corticosteroids are used in conjunction with a β-sympathomimetic agent, pulmonary edema may develop in the mother.

It may also be important to demonstrate that no obvious major congenital abnormality exists (by ultrasound or x-ray study) before attempting to suppress premature labor. Acute and chronic abnormalities of placental function should also be considered. In the presence of chorioamnionitis, suppressing labor may not be possible with tocolytics (increased levels of maternal C-reactive protein may indicate the nonresponders). If premature labor is arrested, the pregnancy may continue for an indefinite period. The chances of delivering a baby who is not of low birth weight (< 2500 g) certainly increases. As stated elsewhere (see Chapter 22), any decrease in low-birth-weight rate inevitably decreases both neonatal mortality and morbidity.

In addition to these important approaches, two other approaches to the treatment of the fetus have had a significant impact on neonatal morbidity. These are changes in the management of breech presentation and the prevention of postterm delivery (postmaturity and "postdatism"). The former has resulted in avoidance of trauma to the preterm infant (who is usually delivered by cesarean section), and the latter has decreased the frequency of asphyxia and meconium aspiration syndrome.

FETAL SURGERY

As a result of advances in ultrasonography and fetoscopy, several disorders that are potentially amenable to surgery can now be detected. These disorders include hydronephrosis, hydrocephalus, and diaphragmatic hernia, but questions about the efficacy and advisability of fetal surgery continue to be raised, although experience has expanded.

BIBLIOGRAPHY

Symposium on Early prenatal diagnosis. *Br. Med. Bull.* 1983, 39:301–408.

Ultrasonography

Hobbins, J. C.: Use of ultrasound in complicated pregnancies. *Clin. Perinatol.* 1980, 7:397–411.

O'Brien, G. D., Queenan, J. T., and Campbell, S.: Assessment of gestational age in the second trimester by real-time ultrasound measurement of the femur length. *Am. J. Obstet. Gynecol.* 1981, 139:540–545.

Hill, L. M., Breckle, R., Wolfgram, K. R., and O'Brien, P. C.: Oligohydramnios: Ultrasonically detected incidence and subsequent fetal outcome. *Am. J. Obstet. Gynecol.* 1983, 147:407–410.

Hobbins, J. C.: Determination of fetal sex in early pregnancy (Editorial). *N. Engl. J. Med.* 1983, 309:979–980.

Editorial: When ultrasound shows fetal abnormality. *Lancet* 1985, i:618–619.

Campbell, S., Warsof, S. L., Little, D., and Cooper, D. J.: Routine ultrasound screening for the prediction of gestational age. *Obstet. Gynecol.* 1985, 65:613–620.

Vintzileos, A. M., Fleming A. D., Scorza, W. E., et al.: Relationship between fetal biophysical activities and umbilical cord blood gas values. *Am. J. Obstet. Gynecol.* 1991, 165:707–713.

Nicolaides, K. H., Suijders, R. J. M., Gosden, C. M., et al.: Ultrasonographically detectable markers of fetal chromosomal abnormalities. *Lancet* 1992, 340:704–707.

Berkowitz, R. L.: Should every pregnant woman undergo ultrasonography? (Editorial) *N. Engl. J. Med.* 1993, 329:874–875.

D'Alton, M. E., and DeCherney, A. H.: Current concepts: Prenatal diagnosis. *N. Engl. J. Med.* 1993, 328:114–120.

Keirse, M. J. N. C.: Frequent prenatal ultrasound: Time to think again (Commentary). *Lancet* 1993, 342:878–879.

Amniotic Fluid Studies (Amniocentesis)

Golbus, M. S., Loughman, W. D., Epstein, C. J., et al.: Prenatal genetic diagnosis in 3,000 amniocenteses. *N. Engl. J. Med.* 1979, 300:157.

Hallman, M., and Teramo, K.: Measurement of the lecithin/sphingomyelin ratio and phosphatidylglycerol in amniotic fluid: An accurate method for the assessment of fetal lung maturity. *Br. J. Obstet. Gynaecol.* 1981, 88:806–813.

Yambao, T. J., Clark, D., Smith, C., and Aubry, R. H.: Amniotic fluid phosphatidylglycerol in stressed pregnancies. *Am. J. Obstet. Gynecol.* 1981, 141:191–194.

Hook, E. B., Cross, P. K., and Schreinemachers, D. M.: Chromosomal abnormality rates at amniocentesis and live-born infants. *J.A.M.A.* 1983, 249:2034–2038.

Brock, D. J. H., and Barron, L.: Prenatal diagnosis of neural-tube defects with a monoclonal antibody specific for acetylcholinesterase. *Lancet* 1985, i:5–8.

Haddow, J. E., Palomaki, G. E., Knight, G. J., et al.: Reducing the need for amniocentesis in women 35 years of age or older with serum markers for screening. *N. Engl. J. Med.* 1994, 330:1114–1118.

Chorionic Villus Sampling

Rodeck, C. H., and Morsman, J. M.: First trimester chorion biopsy. *Br. Med. Bull.* 1983, 39:338–342.

Schreck, R. R., Falik-Borenstein, Z., and Hirata, G.: Chromosomal mosaicism in chorionic villus sampling. *Clin. Perinatol.* 1990, 17:867–888.

Los, F. J., Jahoda, M. G. J., Wladimiroff, J. W., and Brezinka, C.: Fetal exsanguination by chorionic villus sampling. *Lancet* 1993, 342:1559.

Smidt-Jensen, S., Lundsteen, C., Lind, A. M., et al.: Transabdominal chorionic villus sampling in the second and third trimester of pregnancy: Chromosome quality, reporting time, and feto-maternal bleeding. *Prenat. Diagn.* 1993, 13:957–969.

Firth, H. V., Boyd, P. A., Chamberlain, P. F., et al.: Analysis of limb reduction defects in babies exposed to chorionic villus sampling. *Lancet* 1994, 343:1069–1071.

Fetal Heart Rate Monitoring

Westgren, M., Holmquist, P., Svenningsen, N. W., and Ingemarsson, I.: Intrapartum fetal monitoring in preterm deliveries: Prospective study. *Obstet. Gynecol.* 1982, 60:99–106.

Yen, S. Y., Diaz, F., and Paul, R. H.: Ten year experience of intrapartum fetal monitoring in Los Angeles County/University of Southern California Medical Center. *Am. J. Obstet. Gynecol.* 1982, 143:496–500.

Leveno, K. J., Williams, L., DePalma, R. T., and Whalley, P. J.: Perinatal outcome in the absence of antepartum fetal heart acceleration. *Obstet. Gynecol.* 1983, 61:347–355.

Neuman, M. R.: Electronic monitoring of the fetus. *Clin. Perinatol.* 1983, 10:237–252.

Dawes, G. S., Moulden, M., and Redman, C. W. G.: Short-term fetal heart rate variation, decelerations, and umbilical flow velocity waveforms before labor. *Obstet. Gynecol.* 1992, 80:673–678.

Morrison, J. C., Chez, B. F., Davis, I. D., et al.: Intrapartum fetal heart rate assessment: Monitoring by auscultation or electronic means. *Am. J. Obstet. Gynecol.* 1993, 168:63–66.

Fetal Scalp Sampling

Boenisch, H., and Saling, E.: The reliability of pH-values in fetal blood samples—A study of the second stage. *J. Perinat. Med.* 1976, 4:45.

Lauersen, N. H., Miller, F. C., and Paul, R. H.: Continuous intrapartum monitoring of fetal scalp pH. *Am. J. Obstet. Gynecol.* 1979, 133:44.

Lofgren, O.: Continuous transcutaneous oxygen monitoring in fetal surveillance during labor. *Am. J. Obstet. Gynecol.* 1981, 141:729–734.

Amnioscopy

Zabkar, J. H.: Evaluation of fetal maturity by amnioscope. *J. Perinat. Med.* 1975, 3:145.

Cordocentesis

Elias, S.: Fetoscopy in prenatal diagnosis. *Clin. Perinatol.* 1983, 10:357–367.

Bell, J. G., and Weiner, S.: Has percutaneous umbilical blood sampling improved the outcome of high-risk pregnancies? *Clin. Perinatol.* 1993, 20:61–80.

Snijders, R. J. M., Abbas, A., Melby, O., et al.: Fetal plasma erythropoietin concentration in severe growth retardation. *Am. J. Obstet. Gynecol.* 1993, 168:615–619.

Soothill, P. W.: Cordocentesis and fetuses that are small for gestational age (Editorial). *N. Engl. J. Med.* 1993, 328:728–729.

Fetal Breathing Movements

Castle, B. M., and Turnbull, A. C.: The presence or absence of fetal breathing movements predicts the outcome of preterm labour. *Lancet* 1983, ii:471–472.

Connors, G., Hunse, C., Carmichael, L., et al.: Control of fetal breathing in the human fetus between 24 and 34 weeks' gestation. *Am. J. Obstet. Gynecol.* 1989, 160:932–938.

Maternal Screening for Fetal Disorders

Brock, D. J. H., Barròn, L., Watt, M., et al.: Maternal plasma α-fetoprotein and low birth weight: A prospective study throughout pregnancy. *Br. J. Obstet. Gynaecol.* 1982, 89:348–351.

Goldfine, C., Miller, W. A., and Haddow, J. E.: Amniotic fluid gel cholinesterase density ratios in fetal open defects of the neural tube and ventral wall. *Br. J. Obstet. Gynaecol.* 1983, 90:238–240.

Haddow, J. E., Kloza, E. M., Smith, D. E., and Knight, G. J.: Data from an alpha-fetoprotein pilot screening program in Maine. *Obstet. Gynecol.* 1983, 62:556–560.

Persson, P. H., Kullander, S., Gennser, G., et al.: Screening for fetal malformations using ultrasound and measurements of α-fetoprotein in maternal serum. *B.M.J.* 1983, 286:747–749.

Haddow, J. E., Palomaki, G. E., Knight, G. J., et al.: Prenatal screening for Down's syndrome with use of maternal serum markers. *N. Engl. J. Med.* 1992, 327:588–593.

Treatment of Toxemia

Koenig, J. M., and Christensen, R. D.: Incidence, neutrophil kinetics and natural history of neonatal neutropenia associated with maternal hypertension. *N. Engl. J. Med.* 1989, 321:557–562.

Ruduicki, M., Frölich, A., Rasmussen, W. F., and McNair, P.: The effect of magnesium on maternal blood pressure in pregnancy-induced hypertension: A randomized double-blind placebo-controlled trial. *Acta Obstet. Gynecol. Scand.* 1991, 70:445–450.

Influencing Fetal Growth

Abell, D. A., Beischer, N. A., and Wood, C.: Routine testing for gestational diabetes, pregnancy hypoglycemia and fetal growth retardation and results of treatment. *J. Perinat. Med.* 1976, 4:197.

Rubaltelli, F. F., Enzi, G., De Biasi, F., et al.: Effect of lipid loading on fetal uptake of free fatty acids, glycerol and β-hydroxybutyrate. *Biol. Neonate* 1978, 33:320.

Adashi, E. Y., Pinto, H., and Tyson, J. E.: Impact of maternal euglycemia on fetal outcome in diabetic pregnancy. *Am. J. Obstet. Gynecol.* 1979, 132:268.

Uzan, S., Beaufils, M., Breart, G., et al.: Prevention of fetal growth retardation with low-dose aspirin: Findings of the EPREDA trial. *Lancet* 1991, 337:1427–1431.

Stimulating Pulmonary Maturation

MacArthur, B. A., Howie, R. N., Dezoete, J. A., and Elkins, J.: Cognitive and psychosocial development of 4-year-old children whose mothers were treated antenatally with betamethasone. *Pediatrics* 1981, 68:638–643.

Ward, R. M.: Pharmacologic enhancement of lung maturation. *Clin. Perinatol.* 1994, 21:523–542.

Arresting Premature Labor

Brazy, J. E., Little, V., Grimm, J., and Pupkin, M.: Risk benefit considerations for use of isoxsuprine in the treatment of premature labor. *Obstet. Gynecol.* 1981, 58:297–303.

Benedetti, T. J., Hargrove, J. C., and Rosene, K. A.: Maternal pulmonary edema during premature labor inhibition. *Obstet. Gynecol.* 1982, 59:33S–37S.

Peaceman, A. M., Meyer, B. A., Thorp, J. A., et al.: The effect of magnesium sulfate tocolysis on the fetal biophysical profile. *Am. J. Obstet. Gynecol.* 1989, 161:771–774.

Leonardi, M. R., and Hawkins, G. D. V.: What's new in tocolytics. *Clin. Perinatol.* 1992, 19:367–384.

Fetal Surgery

Redwine, F., and Petres, R. E.: Fetal surgery—past, present and future. *Clin. Perinatol.* 1983, 10:399–410.

Adzick, N. S., and Harrison, M. R.: Fetal surgical therapy. *Lancet* 1994, 343:897–902.

Other

Lauersen, N. H., Kurkulos, M., Graves, Z. R., and Lewin, K.: Reliability of antenatal testing: Estriol levels versus nonstress testing. *Obstet. Gynecol.* 1983, 62:11–16.

Main, D. M., Main, E. K., and Mauer, M. M.: Cesarean section versus vaginal delivery for the breech fetus weighing less than 1500 grams. *Am. J. Obstet. Gynecol.* 1983, 146:580–584.

Flamm, B. L., Newman, L. A., Thomas, S. J., et al.: Vaginal birth after cesarean delivery: Results of a 5 year multicenter collaborative study. *Obstet. Gynecol.* 1990, 76:750–754.

Thorpe-Beeston, J. G., Benfield, P. J., and Saunders, N. J. St. G.: Outcome of breech delivery at term. *B.M.J.* 1992, 305:746–747.

Votta, R. A., and Cibils, L. A.: Active management of prolonged pregnancy. *Am. J. Obstet. Gynecol.* 1993, 168:557–563.

2
THE DELIVERY ROOM

EVENTS OCCURRING AT DELIVERY

There seems little doubt that the adaptation required of the baby who is moving from fetal to neonatal life is greater than that demanded at any other time in its life. One can only wonder how so many infants make this transition without faltering.

The fetus, who has relied so much on the placenta to provide a stable environment, is suddenly separated from this faithful friend and asked to "go it alone."

Relative weightlessness succumbs to gravity; a warm, fluid environment (37°C) becomes a cool, breezy one (22°C); where the lungs were merely practicing they must now function efficiently. Sixty to 90 ml of blood is transfused in 60 to 90 seconds from the placenta to the baby, when the umbilical cord is left unclamped. An arterial pO_2 of 25 mm Hg rapidly becomes 80 to 90 mm Hg. The pulmonary resistance decreases, pulmonary blood flow increases, and pulmonary artery pressure rapidly drops below that of the aorta. The fetal right-to-left shunt of blood at the patent ductus arteriosus becomes the neonatal left-to-right shunt, and eventually the ductus arteriosus closes. Other structures vital to the fetus that no longer serve the neonate are the foramen ovale and ductus venosus.

Other organs not essential to survival of the fetus are also called into play. The gastrointestinal tract will soon be asked to digest food and supply nutrients to prevent breakdown and to build new body tissues. The kidneys now become essential in the regulation of body fluid and electrolytes and have a concomitant increase in blood flow.

Occasionally, the newborn continues to respond as a fetus, and what served the fetus well may serve the newborn poorly. The most striking example is that in response to asphyxia (hypoxia and acidosis), the fetus is well served by decreasing blood flow through the lungs, intestines, kidneys, and skin. The asphyxiated newborn is compromised by this response and benefits from good lung perfusion; he may have difficulty handling fluid loads and may be predisposed to ischemic enterocolitis.

Most newborns are able to adapt to their new circumstances remarkably well and seem to accept the vagaries of obstetric practice with equanimity. Delivering infants into warm water with a minimum of light and sound (the Leboyer technique) does not appear to have any advantage over gentle delivery and routine management.

13

RESUSCITATION IN THE DELIVERY ROOM

Anticipation of complications is most important. For complicated deliveries (e.g., emergency cesarean section or breech position) or when there is a good possibility that some difficulty may arise with the fetus (e.g., prematurity, fetal distress, dysmaturity), it is important that someone trained to resuscitate babies be available to accept care of the baby at delivery.

When called to the delivery room under these circumstances, it is important to check the resuscitation equipment. Such checks include making sure that sufficient oxygen is present in the cylinder; that the laryngoscope has adequate light; that a suitably sized endotracheal tube, suction equipment, and bag and mask are available; and that any injectable likely to be used (e.g., sodium bicarbonate) is also available.

When the newborn is evaluated in the delivery room, the Apgar scoring system has proved valuable (Table 2–1). Extremely preterm infants will have reduced muscle tone and responsiveness (reflex irritability) under the best of circumstances and inevitably have somewhat decreased Apgar scores.

Assessment is carried out within the first minute, and resuscitative efforts are made (if necessary) to improve the score by 5 minutes. If depression persists, a score at 10 minutes and beyond may be helpful in the evaluation. In general, a score of 0 to 3 indicates a need for endotracheal intubation, a score of 4 to 6 requires bag and mask assistance, and a score of 7 to 10 requires minimal interference.

Probably the most important feature to evaluate is respiratory effort (breathing). The reason for this is explained by the difference between primary and secondary apnea. When experimental animals (monkeys) are asphyxiated, an initial period of a few minutes of apnea (primary apnea) is followed by gasping respiration for a few minutes, with eventual cessation of breathing movements (secondary apnea). If this apnea is not relieved by resuscitation, the animal will die within several minutes. Consequently, the baby who is born without any respiratory effort requires immediate resuscitation and ventilation. Pressures

TABLE 2–1. THE APGAR SCORING SYSTEM

Sign	0	1	2	Score 1 min	Score 5 min
Heart rate	Absent	<100/min	>100/min		
Respiratory rate	Absent	Gasping or irregular respiration	Regular respiration or crying		
Muscle tone	Flaccid	Some flexion	Good flexion; active		
Reflex irritability	No response	Some motion (grimace)	Withdrawal; crying		
Color	Blue; pale	Blue hands and feet	Pink all over		
			Total		

required to open up uninflated alveoli may be 70 to 80 cm H_2O. If a baby is observed to be breathing, the necessity for speedy resuscitation is less, and the pressures needed to inflate the lungs are much less (30 to 40 cm H_2O). Some evidence suggests that in most infants, the pressures spontaneously generated are not of this magnitude, and this evidence also challenges the concept of elastic recoil of the thorax in lung inflation.

A paper published in 1975 suggested that if resuscitative efforts do not result in spontaneous respiration within 30 minutes, the prognosis is uniformly bad with respect to gross neurologic impairment. This finding has been confirmed by others. It is therefore entirely appropriate to discontinue active resuscitative efforts after 30 minutes if no spontaneous respiration has been observed, provided that the baby has been given intermittent opportunities to demonstrate spontaneous breathing.

Prevention (or minimization) of cooling may contribute greatly to ultimate survival (see Chapter 5).

The following steps are a guide to the appropriate actions to be taken in the delivery room. On receiving the baby, this sequence should be followed:

1. Place the baby under a radiant heat warmer, with the head slightly lower than the body and the body turned slightly to the right side (semilateral or oblique position).

2. Listen to the heart: (a) if there is no heartbeat, administer a few beats of external cardiac massage before going directly to endotracheal intubation; (b) if the heart rate is less than 60 beats/min, external cardiac massage may also be required (ratio: 3 beats to 1 breath), but perform step 3 first (see also p. 281).

3. Suction the oropharynx and both nostrils with a bulb syringe and/or a DeLee suction trap.

4. If the heart rate is over 100/min, stimulate the baby by flicking its heels. CAUTION: Do *not* stimulate the body when it is covered with meconium or meconium-stained amniotic fluid until the larynx has been visualized and any fluid has been suctioned.

5. If the baby is still unresponsive, place an oxygen source close to the baby's face and, if muscular tone is adequate, start bag-and-mask ventilation. If the baby is flaccid, it is probably best to go directly to visualization of the vocal cords (where mucus or blood may be seen and suctioned) and insertion of an endotracheal tube if spontaneous respiration has not started. The first few breaths are then given by bag-to-tube ventilation with 100% oxygen. (The bag should be hooked up to a manometer so that inflation pressure can be varied.)

6. If the baby is still unresponsive or appears rather pale (especially when preceded by fetal distress), sodium bicarbonate should be administered directly into the umbilical vein in a dosage of approximately 2 mEq/kg of body weight by slow push (1 mEq/min). This step may have to be repeated in a very difficult resuscitation.

7. When the baby appears pink, ventilation of the lungs should be stopped briefly to see if the baby will breathe spontaneously. If he does so and remains pink, he should be extubated and stimulated to cry. If he does not, ventilation should be continued, stopping at frequent intervals, and possibly some more bicarbonate should be given.

8. Any baby who requires prolonged intubation (more than 10 minutes) falls into a high-risk category and deserves close observation for 24 hours in the intensive care nursery.

9. Any further procedures (e.g., umbilical artery catheterization) should probably be carried out in the nursery rather than the delivery room, unless a suitably equipped treatment room is available in the delivery suite.

10. Naloxone (Narcan) may be used for narcotic depression in a dose of 0.1 mg/kg intravenously or intramuscularly and does not appear to have any obvious side effects. Use of this agent should probably be limited to the first 2 hours after birth.

11. The only other agents that may need to be used are 1:10,000 aqueous epinephrine (Adrenalin), which may be administered by endotracheal tube, and 10% glucose.

Although this procedure is not routinely performed, in cases in which fetal distress has occurred, it may be helpful to ask the obstetrician to double-clamp a portion of the umbilical cord. Blood from this segment can then be used to determine pH and blood gases, which may be helpful in deciding whether or not metabolic acidosis needs to be treated. If lactic acid levels are determined, they may have considerably more prognostic significance than do Apgar scores.

The consequences of asphyxia include persistent pulmonary hypertension, bleeding tendency, seizures, renal shutdown, disordered liver function, predisposition to infection, ineffective cardiac contractility, and tricuspid insufficiency.

PROBLEMS ASSOCIATED WITH INTRAPARTUM EVENTS

CESAREAN SECTION. Sometimes the reason for performing the cesarean section (e.g., placenta previa) may present problems for the neonate, but with all section deliveries, the possibility of aspiration of amniotic fluid or retention of lung fluid may cause respiratory difficulty. Aspiration may occur as the result of tactile stimulations' initiating gasping. Lung fluid may be retained because of lack of thoracic compression at delivery.

BREECH PRESENTATION. Not all breech presentations are delivered vaginally, so problems related to cesarean section may be encountered. One of the reasons for abdominal delivery of the premature infant in a breech presentation is that, after delivery of the body, the cervix may prevent delivery of the head because of insufficient dilatation. With a frank breech presentation (legs extended), the prevalence of congenital dislocation of the hip is increased. In addition, various other congenital malformations may be associated with breech presentation.

MECONIUM-STAINED AMNIOTIC FLUID. Meconium staining of amniotic fluid occurs in 10% or more of all term deliveries and is more common with postterm deliveries. It is uncommon before 38 weeks' gestation and rare before 34 weeks' gestation. Appropriate management in the delivery room remains controversial with debate centering on the need for intervention in the presence of thin, or light, meconium staining. In the presence of thick or particulate meconium staining (also called "pea soup" meconium), it is generally acknowledged that a combined obstetric-pediatric approach is needed to minimize the aspiration of such fluid into the baby's lungs. The obstetrician should suction the pharynx before the body is delivered, and the pediatrician should pass an endotracheal tube and suction the trachea after delivery.

Accompanying fetal heart rate abnormalities may reflect fetal asphyxia. Although meconium aspiration syndrome can be life threatening, this risk may be due more to persistent pulmonary hypertension than to aspiration of meconium itself (see also Chapter 9).

ANTEPARTUM HEMORRHAGE. Bleeding as the result of such conditions as placenta previa, abruptio placentae, and vasa praevia may initiate delivery by cesarean section. Whether or not delivery is by the abdominal or vaginal route, the risk of hypovolemia and shock in the infant is great.

PROLAPSED CORD. If a prolapsed umbilical cord is noted and treated appropriately, no problem may arise with the baby. However, if the prolapse is occult or management complicated, the risk of asphyxia is great.

MIDFORCEPS DELIVERY. Whenever midforceps are used, there is an increased risk of cephalhematoma, with a linear skull fracture underlying it.

VACUUM-EXTRACTOR DELIVERY. Inappropriate use of the vacuum extractor may result in laceration or abrasion of the fetal scalp.

FETAL SCALP ELECTRODE. Whenever an internal electrode has been placed on the scalp for fetal heart rate monitoring, the break in the skin should be cleansed with an antiseptic (povidone-iodine) because the risk of infection is increased.

BIBLIOGRAPHY

Events Occurring at Delivery

Nelson, N. M., Enkin, M. W., Saigal, S., et al.: A randomized clinical trial of the Leboyer approach to childbirth. *N. Engl. J. Med.* 1980, 302:655.

Resuscitation in the Delivery Room

Steiner, H., and Neligan, G.: Perinatal cardiac arrest: Quality of survivors. *Arch. Dis. Child.* 1975, 50:696.

Hey, E.: Resuscitation at birth. *Br. J. Anaesth.* 1977, 49:25.

Standards and guidelines for cardiopulmonary resuscitation and emergency cardiac care: Part V. Advanced cardiac life support for neonates. *J.A.M.A.* 1980, 244:495–500.

Editorial: The value of the Apgar score. *Lancet* 1982, i:1393–1394.

Lindemann, R.: Resuscitation of the newborn: Endotracheal administration of epinephrine. *Acta Paediatr. Scand.* 1984, 73:210–212.

Goldenberg, R. L., Huddleston, J. F., and Nelson, K. G.: Apgar scores and umbilical arterial pH in preterm newborn infants. *Am. J. Obstet. Gynecol.* 1984, 149:651–654.

Palme, C., Nystrom, B., and Tunell, R.: An evaluation of the efficiency of face masks in the resuscitation of newborn infants. *Lancet* 1985, i:207–210.

Levene, M. L., Kornberg, J., and Williams, T. H. C.: The incidence and severity of post-asphyxial encephalopathy in full-term infants. *Early Hum. Dev.* 1985, 11:21–26.

Winkler, C. L., Hauth, J. C., Tucker, J. M., et al.: Neonatal complications at term as related to the degree of umbilical artery acidemia. *Am. J. Obstet. Gynecol.* 1991, 164:637–641.

American Academy of Pediatrics Committee on Drugs: Naloxone dosage and route of administration for infants and children. *Pediatrics* 1990, 86:484–485.

Hird, M. F., Greenough, A., and Gamsu, H. R.: Inflating pressures for effective resuscitation of preterm infants. *Early Hum. Dev.* 1991, 26:69–72.

Jain, L., Ferre, C., Vidyasagar D., et al.: Cardiopulmonary resuscitation of apparently stillborn infants: Survival and long-term outcome. *J. Pediatr.* 1991, 118:778–782.

Upton, C. J., and Milner, A. D.: Endotracheal resuscitation of neonates using a rebreathing bag. *Arch. Dis. Child.* 1991, 66:39–42.

Problems Associated with Intrapartum Events

Brauer, F. H. T., Jones, K. L., and Smith, D. W.: Breech presentation as an indicator of fetal abnormality. *J. Pediatr.* 1975, 86:419.

Gresham, E. L.: Birth trauma. *Pediatr. Clin. North Am.* 1975, 22:317.

Faxelius, G., Raye, J., Gutberlet, R., et al.: Red cell volume measurements and acute blood loss in high-risk newborn infants. *J. Pediatr.* 1977, 90:273.

Davis, J. P., Moggio, M. V., Klein, D., et al.: Vertical transmission of group B streptococcus: Relation to intra-uterine fetal monitoring. *J.A.M.A.* 1979, 242:42.

Vyas, H., Milner, A. D., and Hopkin, I. E.: Intrathoracic pressure and volume changes during the spontaneous onset of respiration in babies born by cesarean section and by vaginal delivery. *J. Pediatr.* 1981, 99:787–791.

Editorial: Delivery of small breech babies. *Lancet* 1983, i:336–337.

Katz, V. L., and Bowes, W. A., Jr.: Meconium aspiration syndrome: Reflections on a murky subject. *Am. J. Obstet. Gynecol.* 1992, 166:171–183.

Ross, M. G.: Vacuum delivery by soft cup extraction. *Contemp. Obstet. Gynecol.* 1994, June:48–53.

3

THE NORMAL NEWBORN

NEONATAL HISTORY

It is a common misconception that the neonate does not have a history until the moment of birth. This is, of course, quite wrong because all the events occurring in utero from the time of implantation (and indeed many factors occurring before conception) may contribute to the well-being of the infant at delivery.

A typical neonatal history might read something like this: "Baby boy born to a 16-year-old primigravida, blood group O Rh-positive, hepatitis B surface antigen–negative, rubella-immune, at 38 weeks' gestation, after a pregnancy complicated by mild bleeding at the end of the first trimester and toxemia (manifested by hypertension and proteinuria) in the 3 weeks before delivery. Labor lasted 8 hours 40 minutes, with membranes rupturing spontaneously approximately 2 hours before delivery. Delivery was by low forceps, and the Apgar scores were 7 and 9 at 1 and 5 minutes, respectively. The baby weighed 6 pounds 2 ounces (2780 g), was active, and had a good color on arrival in the nursery."

The factors influencing the neonatal course can be thought of as preconceptional, prenatal, intranatal, and postnatal.

PRECONCEPTIONAL

Many problems occurring before conception may influence the health of the mother and hence the fetus. In the young mother in our example, the nutrition before pregnancy may well have been deficient in protein. This problem might have been further exacerbated if her prepregnancy weight was low (< 50 kg). Other problems include diabetes mellitus, cardiac disease, and chronic renal disease. Previous obstetric loss and/or previous premature baby or congenital abnormality may increase the chances of a similar occurrence in another pregnancy.

PRENATAL

Maternal-fetal blood group incompatibility may produce hemolytic disease of the newborn (see Chapter 10). Infections in the mother may produce either a pattern of malformations (e.g., rubella) or a small-for-gestational age baby (see Chapter 16) or result in prematurity. Hypertensive disorders (e.g., toxemia, essential hypertension, and renal disease) may result in a poorly perfused placenta and insufficient fetal growth. Polyhydramnios may indicate upper intestinal obstruction or inability of the fetus to swallow. Oligohydramnios may portend urinary tract abnormalities or a growth-retarded fetus.

INTRANATAL

With progression of labor, more acute events may affect the fetus. Prolonged (premature) rupture of the membranes may predispose to neonatal infection and so, too, may prolong labor (longer than 24 hours) or maternal infection (see sections on Sepsis and Meningitis in Chapter 15). Ability to adequately perfuse the placenta may be compromised as labor progresses, with uteroplacental insufficiency patterns (late deceleration) demonstrated on fetal monitoring. Accidents of the umbilical cord (e.g., prolapse) or brisk hemorrhage from placenta previa or abruptio placentae may result in fetal asphyxia and hence neonatal asphyxia. The method of delivery may adversely affect the fetus (e.g., the premature breech), and timing of clamping of the umbilical cord may profoundly affect the resulting neonatal course (i.e., allowing or preventing a placental transfusion).

POSTNATAL

The events occurring in the delivery room are the beginnings of extrauterine existence. The most common assessment of neonatal adjustment is the Apgar score, which assesses heart rate, respiratory rate, reflex irritability, tone, and color (see section on Resuscitation in The Delivery Room, Chapter 2). The score is usually assessed at 1 and 5 minutes, although some clinicians like to record it at 2 minutes; in depressed babies, further scores may be recorded at 10 and 15 minutes. The aim is to assess the situation in the first minute and correct any depressed (asphyxiated) infant by 5 minutes. Low Apgar scores have been correlated with poor neurologic performance at 1 year of age, but low cord pH is probably more predictive of poor outcome. The other problems likely to influence outcome are discussed in subsequent chapters.

INITIAL EXAMINATION

Having established the most important facts in a neonatal history, one may then approach the infant with a data base that allows the examination to be more purposeful. The major purposes are: (1) to establish whether or not any congenital abnormality exists, (2) to determine a birth weight–gestational age category (see Chapter 6), and (3) to detect any other abnormality that may affect the neonatal course. (Further interpretation of these observations can be found in Part II, pp. 281 to 362.)

The neonatal examination is not essentially different from the pediatric examination, but certain points require amplification. First, many abnormalities are readily apparent (see Chapter 8) and do not require careful attention to be noticed. Those aspects that are not obvious are stressed here. Second, although one does not need to gain the confidence of the newborn infant (unlike the older child) before proceeding to the physical examination, certain parts of the examination are better performed at the beginning.

In the approach to the newborn infant, the baby's weight and temperature should be noted, and the baby should be observed briefly before being disturbed (see Part II). Observations should be continued throughout the examination, and attention should be paid to color, posture, pattern of respiration, fullness of the abdomen, unusual movement of the limbs, alertness, and cry (later). A hand may be placed over the head to assess the size and tension of the anterior and posterior fontanel. The blankets should then be gently disturbed (if the baby is in a bassinet) before the examiner listens to the heart sounds and the lung fields anteriorly. This action usually disturbs the baby a little, so a brief withdrawal (which usually quiets the baby) should preface examination of the abdomen. Observation of the umbilical cord to determine the number of blood vessels should reveal a single vein and two arteries. It is usually easy to feel the baby's abdomen in the first 24 hours of life, including bimanual palpation of the kidneys. (An alternative technique for examining the kidneys is to use the thumb of one hand for palpation, with the fingers supporting the back. The other hand can be used to manipulate the legs.) The liver is almost invariably palpable, but the beginner frequently has difficulty locating it because it is somewhat soft, and the edges are rounded. Liver size may be estimated by percussion (i.e., span) rather than by relation to the costal margin.

By this time, the baby is usually aroused, and the examiner's ability to complete the remainder of the examination may depend on the level of arousal. To remember to examine all the essential areas, the examiner should start with the baby's head and progress toward the feet.

HEAD

Head size (occipitofrontal circumference) should be measured; normal is 33.0 to 37.0 cm. The shape should be noted: molding is frequent (accompanied by overriding bones at the suture lines), particularly if the labor has been prolonged. The heads of babies born by breech delivery or cesarean section usually have a more globular shape. Babies born by vertex vaginal delivery usually have a soft swelling over the occipital region (caput succedaneum). This swelling frequently crosses the suture lines and is thereby distinguished from cephalhematoma (Fig. 3–1), which results from subperiosteal bleeding and is therefore limited by the sutures.

A larger, more extensive, swelling over the head may be the result of bleeding under the scalp (sub-galeal hemorrhage). This phenomenon is more likely to occur after delivery by vacuum extraction. The anterior fontanel usually admits one or two fingertips but is variable in size and is likely to be smaller soon after birth than it is a few days later because of overriding bones. The

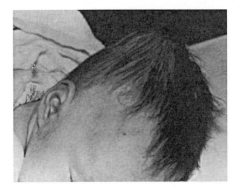

FIGURE 3–1. Head of a newborn infant exhibits a cephalhematoma over the right occipitoparietal region.

posterior fontanel usually is almost closed at birth in the term baby. Soft areas that pop in and out (like a Ping-Pong ball) are called craniotabes and may result from prolonged engagement of the fetal head.

EYES

The eyes are sometimes difficult to examine because of swelling of the eyelids that results from chemical conjunctivitis secondary to instillation of silver nitrate eyedrops (to prevent gonococcal ophthalmia), although this problem is now less common as a result of the use of erythromycin or tetracycline eyedrops or ointment.

The sclerae are usually slightly blue. Subconjunctival hemorrhage is common. The size and symmetry of the iris and pupil should be noted. (In dark-eyed babies, this is sometimes not as easy as it sounds.) The red reflex should then be checked by use of a small light source (pen flashlight), and in so doing, one may note a cloudy cornea or cataract. One maneuver to open the eyes (that sometimes works!) is to rock the baby from horizontal to vertical. The eyes usually open in the vertical position.

NOSE

Because newborn babies seem to be obligatory nose breathers, any obstruction is likely to cause respiratory difficulty, with mouth breathing or gasping movements. Passage of a soft catheter may be resisted by babies with all types of choanal atresia (tissue webs to bony bridges) (see also Chapter 24).

Deviation of the septum may also be present as a result of dislocation of the triangular cartilage. The nose may appear twisted. Diagnosis is made by compressing the tip of the nose or returning it to the midline, which shows the dislocated septum in either nasal aperture. This problem needs to be corrected by the third day to prevent deformity.

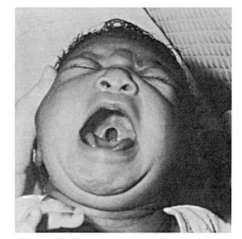

FIGURE 3–2. Posterior defect of the palate that may allow milk to enter the naso-pharynx.

MOUTH

Cleft lip is readily apparent, but cleft palate needs to be looked for carefully, including posterior palatal defects, which can give rise to feeding problems (Fig. 3–2). Pressing down on the chin with the thumb while holding the baby in a vertical position usually produces a good view of the palate, with or without crying. Occasionally, all attempts fail, and the fifth finger must be gently inserted into the mouth to palpate the palate. Retention cysts in one location or another are frequently seen and have fancy names (e.g., Epstein's pearls, Bohn's nodules) but are of little significance. Natal or neonatal teeth are occasionally seen and are more common in Native Americans (Fig. 3–3). The tongue appears to be

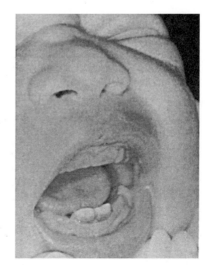

FIGURE 3–3. Newborn infant at 2 days of age demonstrating two teeth (natal teeth).

large in the neonate and may cause respiratory embarrassment if the jaw is very small and undershot (micrognathia). This phenomenon is known as glossoptosis. A truly large tongue is called macroglossia and may be associated with an omphalocele (see Chapter 28). During crying, the mouth may move asymmetrically because of facial palsy (see Chapter 30).

NECK

The muscles of the neck can be quickly palpated to look for a so-called sternomastoid tumor (Fig. 3–4), but major attention should be paid to the clavicles, particularly in the large baby (> 4 kg). The clavicle in the neonate describes a much more obvious S-shape than that in the older child or adult. Placing fingers over the lateral and medial ends and wiggling them usually elicits crepitus in the presence of a fractured clavicle, seen in 0.2 to 3.5% of newborns. (Failing to perform this test may result in embarrassment at 10 days to 2 weeks of age, when exuberant callus formation alarms the mother by producing a lump in the neck.) A short neck may indicate Klippel-Feil syndrome. Other anomalies include branchial and thyroglossal cysts. Neonatal goiter is occasionally encountered.

CHEST (See Chapters 25 and 26)

An increased anteroposterior diameter should suggest an aspiration syndrome. Hemangiomas and lymphangiomas (e.g., cystic hygroma) may involve the upper chest and extend into the neck. Accessory (supernumerary) nipples are occasionally noted in the nipple line in as many as 2.5% of live births. Infrequently at birth, but not uncommonly after several days, one may encounter breast hypertrophy with or without expression of milk ("witch's milk") (Fig. 3–5).

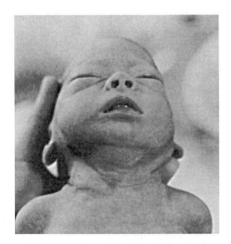

FIGURE 3–4. A swelling is present on the right side of the neck, resulting from a hematoma ("tumor") of the sternomastoid muscle.

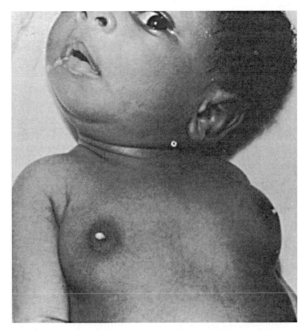

FIGURE 3–5. Breast hypertrophy with witch's milk in a female newborn infant at 3 days of age.

ARMS

The newborn infant carried to term usually adopts a flexed posture, and an arm lying in extension for more than brief periods raises the suspicion of brachial nerve palsy. Involvement of the upper cervical roots produces Erb's palsy, whereas lower root involvement produces Klumpke's paralysis. Reduction deformities of the upper extremity may be encountered, and the terms phocomelia, hemimelia, and amelia indicate varying degrees of abnormality (for terminology, see Warkany, J.: Congenital Malformations, Year Book Medical Publishers, Chicago, 1971 [reprinted 1981], pp. 939–957).

HANDS

The skin creases and folds on the hands and feet may provide a wealth of information to the initiated, but examining the newborn in this much detail is generally difficult. This subject is called dermatoglyphics. A single palmar crease (simian line) is seen unilaterally in 4% and bilaterally in 1% of the normal population, but it is associated with many syndromes (e.g., Down's syndrome).

ABDOMEN

See Chapter 28 for a complete discussion of the initial examination of the abdomen.

HIPS

Perhaps the most important examination in the well newborn infant is that of the hips, to detect congenital dislocation. Ability to make the diagnosis early may result in several weeks of simple treatment. Failure to do so may result in prolonged hospitalization, surgical procedures, and a lifetime of difficulties. Two basic maneuvers are used. The first is the Ortolani maneuver—with the baby's knees flexed, the physician's thumbs over the inner aspects of the thighs, and the physician's middle fingers pressing over the greater trochanters of the femurs, the hips are abducted. A dislocated hip returns to the acetabulum and gives a sensation of movement (generally referred to as a "clunk" rather than a "click", but the better term is a "jerk" because this indicates movement rather than sound). The second maneuver is the dislocation provocation maneuver (Barlow's)—as the baby's hips are now adducted, the physician's thumbs press backward and may displace the head of the femur from the acetabulum; Ortolani's maneuver should be repeated to test this. If the hip is dislocated or dislocatable, an orthopedic surgeon should be consulted. Crepitus under the fingers is usually the result of infolding of the ligamentum teres of the head of the femur.

The femoral pulses also require careful examination. Decreased pulses should initiate an evaluation of blood pressure in the upper and lower extremities (looking for coarctation of the aorta).

GENITALS

In the female infant, the labia should be spread to detect an imperforate hymen with hydrocolpos (or hydrometrocolpos). If not detected, diagnosis may be deferred until early puberty, when primary amenorrhea and a suprapubic mass may be presenting features. Some cases may resolve spontaneously. Occasionally, inclusion cysts arise from the wall of the vagina, and hymenal polyps are common and also resolve spontaneously (Fig. 3–6).

A more common finding is the presence of white mucoid discharge (which may be profuse), which is probably a result of the influence of estrogen being transmitted across the placenta. A related phenomenon, seen less frequently, is pseudomenses, or bleeding from the vagina, which is presumably a result of estrogen withdrawal.

The male infant may demonstrate abnormalities of the opening of the urethra. Hypospadias (Fig. 3–7), with or without a chordee (shortening of the ventral aspect of the penis), is seen much more commonly than is epispadias. If the testes are not present in the scrotum, they can occasionally be brought into normal position by pushing down gently over the inguinal canal (Fig. 3–8). The

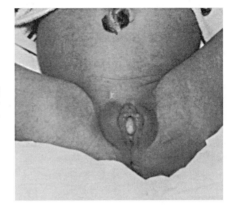

FIGURE 3–6. An example of a hymenal cyst (or vaginal cyst). In contrast to hydrocolpos, an opening is present posteriorly.

scrotum may be traumatized during breech delivery (Fig. 3–9). Swelling of the scrotum is usually the result of hydrocele, but inguinal hernia should be considered (see Chapter 33).

Great confusion generally arises when the genitalia are ambiguous (or indeterminate). Generally, it is unwise to hazard a guess, but if pressed, it is preferable to say that the baby is probably a girl (see Ambiguous Genitalia in Chapter 33).

LEGS

Flexion of the legs is the usual posture of the term neonate, but babies born by frank breech delivery may have the legs in extension. Similarly, limitation of

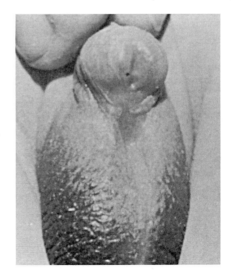

FIGURE 3–7. First-degree hypospadias with the urethral opening just below the mark. It should open in the crease above the mark.

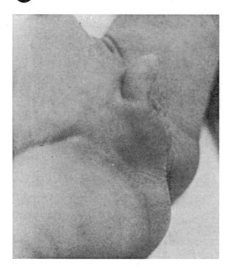

FIGURE 3–8. When the testes are not located in the scrotum, the condition is called cryptorchidism. By pressing down on the inguinal canal, the testes were palpable high in the scrotum in this baby.

the size of the uterine cavity, as in double uterus (uterus didelphys), may result in abnormal posture of the legs, the most dramatic being genu recurvatum (dislocation of the knee). Constriction deformities may involve any limb but are most striking in the leg (Figs. 3–10 and 3–11). Alternative names for this abnormality are amniotic bands and Streeter's dysplasia.

FEET

Abnormalities of the feet are frequently positional and may produce a transient, or false, clubfoot. The most common type of true clubfoot, which

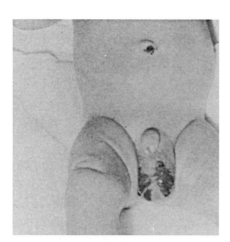

FIGURE 3–9. Scrotal hematoma, which might result from a frank breech presentation.

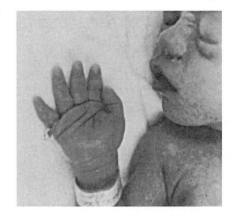

FIGURE 3–10. An amniotic fluid band is clearly seen encircling the base of the fifth finger, producing a constriction ring (sometimes called Streeter's dysplasia).

is distinguished by its being a fixed deformity, is talipes equinovarus (see Chapter 8).

NAILS

The nails of both the hands and feet require careful examination. They are usually obvious in the term neonate and may be excessively long and stained greenish-brown in the postterm (postmature) baby. Either absence of the nails or marked decrease in size is seen in the different forms of ectodermal dysplasia.

BACK

Before the baby is turned from supine to prone for an examination of the back, the anus should be observed for patency (Fig. 3–12). A finger should be

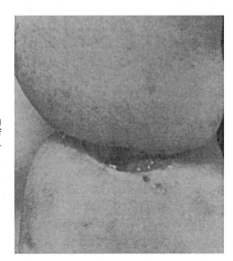

FIGURE 3–11. Close-up of a constriction ring deformity of the ankle (presumably of the same cause as that shown in Figure 3–10).

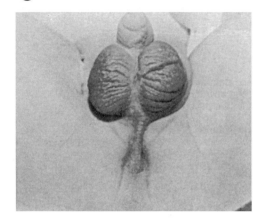

FIGURE 3–12. Male newborn infant with an imperforate anus.

run down the back to make sure that no obvious defects are present and that the sacrum is normal in size.

NEUROLOGIC EXAMINATION

A brief neurologic examination should be carried out. The tone may be determined while gestational age is assessed (see Dubowitz score, Chapter 6). In addition, a few reflexes may be elicited, such as the Moro, rooting, suck, grasp, and crossed extensor reflexes. The traditional neurologic examination has great limitations but if used appropriately can give valuable information. The Brazelton examination, which provides an assessment of the baby's responsiveness and ability to cope with his or her environment, seems to be more valuable than the traditional examination in predicting subsequent performance. Unfortunately, this examination takes much longer than the average physician can usually afford, but modifications may become available.

BIBLIOGRAPHY

Illingworth, R. S.: *The Development of the Infant and Young Child*, 8th ed. Churchill Livingstone, New York, 1983.
Kendig, J. W.: Care of the normal newborn. *Pediatr. Rev.* 1992, 13:262–268.

Neonatal History

Schmidt, R., Nitowsky, H. M., and Dar, H.: Cytogenetic studies in reproductive loss. *J.A.M.A.* 1976, 236:369.
Nadler, H. L.: Polyhydramnios, congenital malformations, and intrauterine detection. *Pediatrics* 1977, 59:785.
Berkowitz, R. L. (ed): High-risk pregnancy—1980. *Clin. Perinatol.* 1980, 7:225–445.

Initial Examination

Perlman, M., and Williams, J.: Detection of renal anomalies by abdominal palpation in newborn infants. *B.M.J.* 1976, 2:347.

Reiff, M. I., and Osborn, L. M.: Clinical estimation of liver size in newborn infants. *Pediatrics* 1983, 71:46–48.

Head

Zelson, C., Lee, S. J., and Pearl, M.: The incidence of skull fractures underlying cephalhematomas in newborn infants. *J. Pediatr.* 1974, 85:371.
Davies, D., Ansari, B. M., and Cooke, T. J. H.: Anterior fontanelle size in the neonate. *Arch. Dis. Child.* 1975, 50:81.
Graham, J. M., and Smith, D. W.: Parietal craniotabes in the neonate—Its origin and significance. *J. Pediatr.* 1979, 95:114.

Nose

Moss, M. L.: The veloepiglottic sphincter and obligate nose breathing in the neonate. *J. Pediatr.* 1965, 67:330.
Silverman, S. H., and Leibow, S. G.: Dislocation of the triangular cartilage of the nasal septum. *J. Pediatr.* 1975, 87:456–458.

Mouth

Gordon, R. C., and Langley, R. N.: Natal teeth in American Indian children. *J. Pediatr.* 1970, 76:613.
Sibert, J. R., and Porteous, J. R.: Erupted teeth in the newborn: Six members in a family. *Arch. Dis. Child.* 1974, 49:492.
Jorgensen, R. J., Shapiro, S. D., Salinas, C. F., and Levin, L. S.: Intra-oral findings and anomalies in neonates. *Pediatrics* 1982, 69:577–582.

Neck

Joseph, P. R. and Rosenfeld, W.: Clavicular fractures in neonates. *Am. J. Dis. Child.* 1990, 144:165–167.

Chest

Mimouni, F., Merlob, P., and Reisner, S. H.: Occurrence of supernumerary nipples in newborns. *Am. J. Dis. Child.* 1983, 137:952–953.
Sivan, Y., Merlob, P., and Reisner, S. H.: Sternum length, torso length, and inter-nipple distance in newborn infants. *Pediatrics* 1983, 72:523–525.

Arms

Molnar, G. E.: Brachial plexus injury in the newborn infant. *Pediatr. Rev.* 1984, 6:110–115.

Hands

Shisno, H., and Kadowaki, J.: Dermatoglyphics of congenital abnormalities without chromosomal aberrations: A review of the clinical applications. *Clin. Pediatr.* 1975, 14:1003.

Hips

Ritter, M. A.: Congenital dislocation of the hip in the newborn. *Am. J. Dis. Child.* 1973, 125:30.
Editorial: Detecting the dislocated hip. *Lancet* 1977, ii:909.
Ortolani, M.: Detecting the dislocated hip (Letter). *Lancet* 1978, i:506.

Genitals

Borglin, N. E., and Selander, P.: Hymenal polyps in newborn infants. *Acta Paediatr. Suppl.* 1962, 135:28.

Simpson, J. L.: Diagnosis and management of the infant with genital ambiguity. *Am. J. Obstet. Gynecol.* 1977, 128:137.

Merlob, P., Bahari, C., Liban, E., and Reisner, S. H.: Cysts of the female external genitalia in the newborn infant. *Am. J. Obstet. Gynecol.* 1978, 132:607.

Duckett, J. W.: Hypospadias. *Pediatr. Rev.* 1989, 11:37–42.

Neurologic Examination

Brazelton, T. B.: Neonatal Behavioral Assessment Scale. *Clinics in Developmental Medicine,* 2nd ed., No. 50. S.I.M.P., J. B. Lippincott, Philadelphia, 1984.

Volpe, J. J.: Value of the neonatal neurological examination. *Pediatrics* 1979, 64:547.

Bierman-van Eendenberg, M. E. C., Jurgens-van der Zee, A. D., Olinga, A. A., et al.: Predictive value of neonatal neurological examination: A follow-up study of 18 months. *Dev. Med. Child. Neurol.* 1981, 23:296–305.

4

ROUTINE PROCEDURES

Many procedures currently practiced in newborn nurseries are hardly noticed by those not directly involved with them. Others may forget the reasons for doing them. (For further information, consult *Guidelines for Perinatal Care*, 3rd edition, published jointly by the American Academy of Pediatrics and the American College of Obstetricians and Gynecologists, 1992.)

NURSERY TECHNIQUE

The fundamental principle of good nursery technique is good hand and arm washing both on arrival in the nursery and between patients.

Initial wash should be for 2 to 3 minutes with an iodinated or hexachlorophene-impregnated scrub sponge. Washing between babies can be limited to approximately 1 minute. Even a brief (15-second) wash between babies has been shown to be beneficial. All jewelry (including watches) except flat wedding bands should be removed before washing.

Babies in incubators with portholes may be examined by personnel not wearing a gown, but the personnel should wash before and after the examination. If a baby is examined out of an incubator in the intensive care nursery, and the examination involves holding the baby, a new gown must be worn for each examination.

In the well-baby nursery, as in the neonatal intensive care unit, the need to wear gowns has been questioned. This may be an unnecessary expense that does not increase infection control. If gowns are used, they should be short-sleeved (or the sleeves should be rolled up on long-sleeved gowns) so that arms can be washed between babies. Again, if the baby is held against the gown, a new gown must be worn for each examination.

Masks are not routinely required but should be worn by persons who have mild upper respiratory infections.

In the intensive care nursery, it is important for personnel to not lean on the incubators (and other pieces of equipment), particularly when making rounds, to prevent contaminating the arms and hands and consequently spreading the contamination to the next incubator. Equipment (e.g., stethoscope) should be cleaned between babies. IF IN DOUBT, WASH YOUR HANDS.

ISOLATION TECHNIQUE

Any baby with obvious or suspected infection should be placed in an incubator for isolation and observation. When isolation is ordered, the reason should be stated, and a note should be included about possible, probable, or definite infection.

Traditionally, babies born out of asepsis (e.g., in a taxi, an elevator, or a corridor) or those born to mothers with no prenatal care have been regarded as highly suspect for infection and have been observed for a minimum of 24 hours in an incubator. However, at least one study casts considerable doubt on the necessity for this practice.

Incubator isolation seems to be effective, even for infants with diarrhea and viral infections, provided adequate technique is used. The incubators holding such babies should be labeled appropriately, and a notice reading "WASH HANDS CAREFULLY" should be placed on the incubator to reinforce nursery technique. In addition, to further emphasize care in handling, separate gowns and gloves should be used for these babies.

Infants in isolation may not be taken out for feedings, but the mother may feed the baby in the incubator. A covered diaper pail should be used for the disposal of used diapers and other fomites.

Infants in open cribs should not be in the same area as sick, septic infants in incubators. Infants with respiratory infections (e.g., caused by respiratory syncytial virus) are best cared for in separate isolation rooms.

IDENTIFICATION

Because most hospitals deliver large numbers of babies, some method of identification should be used. The most usual method is some type of bracelet or band placed around the baby's wrist or ankle. This is sometimes difficult to maintain in very preterm babies, but there is less likelihood that such babies will be mixed up (except for multiple pregnancies).

One traditional method that gave the impression of reliability was footprinting. This method has proved to be of little value for identification purposes, particularly in term infants. For this reason, it should be abandoned.

VITAL SIGNS

Vital signs are generally considered the key to a baby's condition and include temperature, pulse rate, and respiratory rate. In the neonate, pulse rate is usually replaced by heart rate. Blood pressure is not usually measured routinely but is frequently considered a vital sign in sick infants. Vital signs are usually measured hourly for the first 4 hours and thereafter can be measured just before feeding.

It is usually recommended that the first temperature be taken rectally to detect imperforate anus. Subsequent temperatures should be axillary because (1) rectal perforation and bleeding have been associated with overzealous determinations of rectal temperature, and (2) axillary temperature may provide an earlier indication that a baby is being subjected to cold stress. More recently, tympanic membrane temperatures have been used. The neonate may attempt (and be able) to maintain core temperature in response to cold stress, which means that a normal rectal temperature could be misleading. Normal limits for axillary temperature are 36.5 to 37.0°C (97.6 to 98.6°F). When a baby is in an incubator, the incubator temperature should be recorded as well because hypothermia can be masked by a high environmental temperature (see Chapter 5).

Heart rate is usually detected by listening to the apex with a stethoscope. The usual rate is 120 to 160 beats/min, but some normal infants have rates of 100 or 110 beats/min. With newer monitoring techniques, it may be possible to look at the beat-to-beat variability (i.e., the rate calculated on the basis of the time interval between successive R waves).

As with the fetus, the newborn usually has a good deal of variability of heart rate. Loss of variability is more likely to be seen in sick neonates. (The significance of bradycardia and tachycardia is discussed in Chapter 26.)

Respiration rate and pattern (regular and irregular) are assessed by observation of the chest wall and movements of the abdomen (diaphragmatic movement). The normal rate is frequently stated to be 30 to 50 breaths/min, but others use a range of 40 to 60 breaths/min. Most term newborn infants breathe regularly during quiet sleep, but many have irregularities during rapid eye movement (REM) sleep and when awake.

Premature infants frequently have brief periods of apnea interspersed with bursts of good ventilation (periodic breathing). This phenomenon is generally considered to be the result of an immature respiratory center. Other respiratory problems (grunting, retractions, or flaring of the alae nasi) are looked for during routine observation (see Chapter 9).

WEIGHING

One of the first steps usually performed on admission of a newborn infant to the nursery is weighing of the baby. In association with gestational age assessment (see Chapter 6), this step provides a birth weight–gestational age category that may allow anticipation of certain problems.

Subsequently, weighing should be carried out daily (possibly more frequently in the sick neonate), with the weight taken as near as possible to the same time each day, preferably before feeding. Excessive weight gain or weight loss may indicate overhydration or underhydration. Newer devices may provide accurate weights for babies in incubators.

POSITIONING

Although which position a baby is placed for sleep might seem to be a simple decision, this has recently been reevaluated. Although positioning may not be crucial in the newborn nursery, there may be important implications regarding advice at the time of discharge to home. Traditionally, in the United States, babies have been placed in the prone position (on their abdomens). However, data from other countries suggested an increase in sudden infant death syndrome was associated with the prone position. In 1992, an American Academy of Pediatrics Task Force recommended placing babies supine (on their backs) or on their sides.

There is lack of unanimity on this subject because of differing rates of sudden infant death syndrome in different countries. It does seem advisable to avoid the use of sheepskins and other soft bedding materials because rebreathing may occur.

Specific situations (e.g., symptomatic gastroesophageal reflux, micrognathia with glossoptosis, or soft thoracic walls in preterm infants) may dictate the use of the prone position for sleeping. However, for most infants, the governments of the Netherlands, the United Kingdom, New Zealand, and Germany have recommended against the prone position. The American Academy of Pediatrics stand seems reasonable, but the last word on this subject is probably not in.

BLOOD GLUCOSE SCREENING

Blood glucose level can be screened using either Dextrostix or Chemstrip bG. These test strips incorporate glucose oxidase, and the color of the strip changes with increasing glucose levels. With Dextrostix, a drop of blood is placed on the strip and is washed off after exactly 1 minute. Semiquantitative blood glucose levels are provided with a gray-to-blue scale. No change in color indicates a level below 25 mg/dl (or test strips that are old and nonfunctioning because of exposure to air—a new bottle should be tried if necessary). More intense color may be produced, suggesting higher levels of glucose than are actually present, if exact timing is not used. Because discrepancies occasionally exist at both ends of the scale, infants with symptomatic hypoglycemia should probably have a blood glucose determination in addition to the test strip.

Infants of diabetic mothers and all low-birth-weight infants (< 2500 g), especially those who are small for their gestational age, should routinely have a test strip check of blood glucose level every hour for the first 4 hours, every 4 hours for the next 24 hours, and as ordered thereafter. This test should be performed whether or not the infants are receiving parenteral fluids.

Levels less than 25 mg/dl require confirmation by blood glucose determination and, if not already started, a 10% dextrose infusion.

In recent years, there has been a reevaluation of what constitutes a low glucose level, and it is possible that moderate hypoglycemic (< 45 mg/dl or < 2.6 mmol/L) in preterm infants may contribute to neurodevelopmental deficit. Many consider the test strips to be too unreliable for routine use, and more reliable, but simple, methods of measuring blood glucose level are being sought.

EYE PROPHYLAXIS

Gonorrheal conjunctivitis is a serious infection that can result in blindness. Because of this, most states have laws requiring antibacterial prophylaxis of the eyes. Silver nitrate seems to be extremely effective in eliminating gonococcal infection when used properly. Recent reports indicate that erythromycin and tetracycline eyedrops or ointment are equally efficacious (without the associated conjunctivitis), and both have been approved for prophylaxis. If silver nitrate is to be used, several points should be emphasized. Many babies have a chemical conjunctivitis secondary to instillation of silver nitrate. Because of this, most people rinse the eyes after its administration. Water is preferred over saline because saline may produce a precipitate of silver chloride. A controlled study indicated that rinsing did not decrease the prevalence of chemical conjunctivitis.

VITAMIN K PROPHYLAXIS

The prevention of hemorrhagic disease of the newborn is discussed else-where (see Chapter 20). Some controversy has recently been generated by a paper from the United Kingdom suggesting an association between intramuscu-lar vitamin K in the neonate and childhood cancer. After reviewing all the evidence, an ad hoc task force of the American Academy of Pediatrics published a strong recommendation that vitamin K should continue to be given to all newborns as a single intramuscular injection to prevent this bleeding disorder. The dose is 1 mg for most newborns, but 0.5 mg for infants weighing less than 1500 g.

BATHING

Although most babies are bathed early, this is one of the least important routines in our nurseries. It should always be deferred if temperature instability is present.

Reduction of staphylococcal colonization may be achieved by bathing the baby with hexachlorophene. However, this practice is no longer recommended on a routine basis, because toxicity to the central nervous system is a potential problem.

Recent evidence suggests that bathing to remove vernix caseosa and to clean the skin is as efficacious as washing thoroughly. Bathing also produces less heat loss and makes babies calmer, quieter, and more comfortable than washing.

UMBILICAL CORD CARE

At the time of delivery, occlusion of the cord close to the baby's body is performed with either a clamp (plastic or metal) or a rubber band technique. This procedure is performed primarily to prevent bleeding, which is more likely to be from the umbilical vein, because the arteries quickly go into spasm.

Subsequently, management is directed at preventing staphylococcal coloni-zation. Various preparations have been applied to the umbilical area, including bacitracin, triple dye, povidone-iodine preparation, and sodium sulfadiazine. All these measures seem to be effective.

IMMUNIZATION

Babies who remain in the hospital (usually in the neonatal intensive care unit) at the age of 2 months are eligible to receive immunization. A good response has been seen to the diphtheria-pertussis-tetanus vaccine in preterm infants, and half-doses should not be used. Oral polio vaccine should not be given until the time of discharge.

The response to *Haemophilus influenzae* type B vaccine is less reliable in preterm infants, but vaccine administration may also be initiated at 2 months of chronologic age.

It has been recommended by the Centers for Disease Control and Prevention that all neonates be immunized against the hepatitis B virus, regardless of maternal status. Until recently, hepatitis B vaccine was administered only to high-risk mothers, but universal vaccination was recommended in 1991 and has been adopted in many hospitals. Again, the response to the vaccine is lower in preterm infants.

FEEDING (See Chapter 11)

SCREENING TECHNIQUES

Until the 1970s, screening techniques were largely confined to screening for phenylketonuria. Many disorders lend themselves to screening, but from a practical standpoint, it is important to have effective treatment for such disorders. Some of these have now been added to screening programs; others may follow.

Population screening as a medical service is recommended if

1. The disease or disorder is clearly defined,
2. The tests used have few false-positive and false-negative results,
3. Proved treatment or prevention programs exist, or
4. Full medical services are available, including genetic counseling.

Disorders with a low frequency cannot be screened practically, unless the cost is affordable. At present, screening for congenital hypothyroidism is now widely practiced and accepted because the incidence is approximately 1 in 3000 to 1 in 5000, compared with approximately 1 in 10,000 for phenylketonuria. This contrasts with screening for maple syrup urine disease, which has a reported incidence of 1 in 224,000. Undoubtedly, some disorders are found more frequently in certain areas, which may make the cost/benefit ratio acceptable in one place and not in another. In addition to phenylketonuria and hypothyroidism, the same filter paper technique may also be used for galactosemia screening, which has a lower yield (about 1 in 62,000).

The test for phenylketonuria is called the Guthrie test and is based on the fact that elevated levels of serum phenylalanine will enhance the growth of bacteria *(Bacillus subtilis)*. It is therefore a waste of time and effort to obtain a sample from a baby who is receiving antibiotics. It is also preferable to allow a minimum of 48 hours of milk feeding before sending the sample. However, in

TABLE 4–1. TENTATIVE SCREENING RECOMMENDATIONS*

Disease or Condition	Group to Be Screened	Test Method	Intervention
Erythroblastosis fetalis	Pregnant women	Serologic test for Rh-negative blood	Administration of anti-Rh immunoglobulin after delivery or abortion
Down's syndrome and other chromosomal abnormalities	Pregnant women (> age 38)	Amniocentesis with cytogenetic study	Therapeutic abortion
Tay-Sachs disease	Pregnant women of Ashkenazi Jewish background	Leukocyte hexosaminidase activity	Test of father, test of fetus, therapeutic abortion
Sickle cell diseases and β-thalassemia	Pregnant women	Hemoglobin electrophoresis and RBC indices	Test of father, test of newborn, special management of affected neonate
Neural tube defects, abdominal wall defects	Pregnant women	Serum α-fetoprotein determination	Therapeutic abortion
	Pregnant women with family history of neural tube defects	Amniocentesis with α-fetoprotein determinations Ultrasonography	Notify pediatric surgeon
Gastrointestinal obstruction	Pregnant women and newborn infants	Observation for polyhydramnios Observation of feeding and bowel patterns	Special study of newborn and surgical correction
Urinary tract obstruction	Pregnant women and newborn infants	Observation for oligohydramnios Observation of voiding	Special study of newborn and surgical correction
Phenylketonuria	Newborn infants	Blood level	Diet
Galactosemia	Newborn infants	Blood level	Diet
Hypothyroidism	Newborn infants	Blood level	Thyroid medication
Biotinidase deficiency	Newborn infants	Blood level	Biotin administration

Table continued on following page

TABLE 4-1. TENTATIVE SCREENING RECOMMENDATIONS* *Continued*

Disease or Condition	Group to Be Screened	Test Method	Intervention
Risk of parenting disorders	Newborn infants and parturient mothers	Behavioral observations	Monitoring for child abuse, neglect
Congenital hip dysplasia	Newborns and 6-month-old infants	Ortolani's and Barlow's maneuvers	Positional splinting
Impaired vision	Infants from birth to age 3	Developmental screening	Various
Impaired hearing	Infants from birth to age 3	Developmental screening	Various
Anemia	Newborn infants	Hemoglobin and/or hematocrit level	Various
Congenital heart disease	Infants from birth to age 1	Auscultation, femoral pulses	Various

*Reproduced with modifications from: North, A. F., Jr.: *South. Med. J.* 1977, 70:1232.
RBC = red blood cell.

many cases, phenylalanine levels are elevated within hours of birth. Thus, it is always advisable to send a sample for screening before discharge from the hospital, even though early discharge (i.e., within 24 hours) is becoming more common. A follow-up sample is recommended under such circumstances. Not all babies who have hyperphenylalaninemia subsequently prove to have phenylketonuria.

Debate continues about the best test for hypothyroidism. In the United States and Canada, assessment of thyroxine level has been favored, but in Europe, thyrotropin (thyroid-stimulating hormone) level assessment has been used. Suspicious samples should initiate evaluation of both thyroxine and thyrotropin. In some preterm and sick infants, transient hypothyroidism has been observed, but more usually this is transient hypothyroxinemia without an increased thyrotropin.

Table 4-1 lists screening procedures that can be performed, although not all have been proved cost-effective. After extended evaluation of meconium testing for cystic fibrosis, the use of immunoreactive trypsin on dried blood spots seems likely to prove more valuable, although this latter technique may also give false-positive results that may cause unnecessary parental anxiety. A recent addition to screening tests is that for biotinidase deficiency.

There has recently been a suggestion that hearing screening should be performed on all neonates. However, with the duration of hospital stay in the United States now being so short, it is difficult to know how this screening could be effectively organized in a cost-efficient way. It should probably be reserved for high-risk populations.

CAR SEATS

Thanks in part to the American Academy of Pediatrics' promotion of *The First Ride: A Safe Ride* most nurseries provide information about infant restraints as part of their routine care. Many have set up programs to lease infant car seats to those who are less able to afford them. This type of preventive care may be as important as immunization in saving lives and should be endorsed enthusiastically. In preterm infants, special precautions may need to be taken because of their small size, to avoid oxygen desaturation while still affording protection (see American Academy of Pediatrics Committees on Injury and Poison Prevention and Fetus and Newborn, 1991).

BIBLIOGRAPHY

Nursery Technique

Sprunt, R., Redman, W., and Leidy, G.: Antibacterial effectiveness of routine hand washing. *Pediatrics* 1973, 52:264.
Davies, P. A.: Please wash your hands. *Arch. Dis. Child.* 1982, 57:647–648.
Cloney, D. L., and Donowitz, L. G.: Overgown use for infection control in nurseries and neonatal intensive care units. *Am. J. Dis. Child.* 1986, 140:680–683.

Isolation Technique

Sacks, L. M., McKitrick, J. C., and MacGregor, R. R.: Surface cultures and isolation procedures in infants born under unsterile conditions. *Am. J. Dis. Child.* 1983, 137:351–353.

Identification

Thompson, J. E., Clark, D. A., Salisbury, B., and Cahill, J.: Footprinting the newborn infant: Not cost-effective. *J. Pediatr.* 1981, 99:797–798.

Vital Signs

Frank, J. D., and Brown, S.: Thermometers and rectal perforations in the neonate. *Arch. Dis. Child.* 1978, 53:824.

Positioning

American Academy of Pediatrics Task Force on Infant Positioning and SIDS: Positioning and SIDS. *Pediatrics* 1992, 89:1120–1126.
News Commentary: Infant death in Europe. *B.M.J.* 1992, 305:139.
Orenstein, S. R., Mitchell, A. A., and Ward, S. D.: Concerning the American Academy of Pediatrics recommendation on sleep position for infants. *Pediatrics* 1993, 91:497–499.

Dextrostix and Chemstrip bG

Perelman, R. H., Gutcher, G. R., Engle, M. J., and MacDonald, M. J.: Comparative analysis of four methods for rapid glucose determination in neonates. *Am. J. Dis. Child.* 1982, 136:1051–1053.
Herrera, A. J., and Hsiang, Y. H.: Comparison of various methods of blood sugar screening in newborn infants. *J. Pediatr.* 1983, 102:769–772.
Lucas, A., Morley, R., and Cole, T. J.: Adverse neurodevelopmental outcome of moderate neonatal hypoglycemia. *B.M.J.* 1988, 297:1304–1308.

Cornblath, M., Schwartz, R., Aynsley-Green, A., and Lloyd, J. K.: Hypoglycemia in infancy: The need for a rational definition. *Pediatrics* 1990, 85:834–837.

Eye and Vitamin K Prophylaxis

Committees on Drugs, Fetus and Newborn, and Infectious Diseases, AAP: Prophylaxis and treatment of neonatal gonococcal infections. *Pediatrics* 1980, 65:1047–1048.
American Academy of Pediatrics Vitamin K Ad Hoc Task Force: Controversies concerning vitamin K and the newborn. *Pediatrics* 1993, 91:1001–1003.
Bell, T. A., Grayston, J. T., Krohn, M. A., et al.: Randomized trial of silver nitrate, erythromycin and no eye prophylaxis for the prevention of conjunctivitis among newborns not at risk for gonococcal ophthalmitis. *Pediatrics* 1993, 92:755–760.

Bathing

Henningson, A., Nystrom, B., and Tunnell, R.: Bathing or washing babies after birth. *Lancet* 1981, ii:1401–1403.

Umbilical Cord Care

Meberg, A., and Schoyen, R.: Bacterial colonization and neonatal infections: Effects of skin and umbilical disinfection in the nursery. *Acta Paediatr. Scand.* 1985, 74:366–371.

Immunization

Bernbaum, J., Daft, A., Samuelson, J., and Polin, R. A.: Half-dose immunization for diphtheria, tetanus, pertussis: Response of preterm infants. *Pediatrics* 1989, 83:471–476.
Centers for Disease Control: Hepatitis B virus: A comprehensive strategy for eliminating transmission in the United States through universal childhood vaccination. *Morb. Mortal. Wkly. Rep.* 1991, 40:1–24.
Lau, Y. L., Tam, A. Y. C., Ng, K. W., et al.: Response of preterm infants to hepatitis B vaccine. *J. Pediatr.* 1992, 121:962–965.
Washburn, L. K., O'Shea, T. M., Gillis, D. C., et al.: Response to *Haemophilus influenzae* type B conjugate vaccine in chronically ill premature infants. *J. Pediatr.* 1993, 123:791–794.
Mulligan, M. J., and Stiehm, E. R.: Neonatal hepatitis B infection: Clinical and immunologic considerations. *J. Perinatol.* 1994, 14:2–9.

Screening Techniques

Holtzman, N. A.: Newborn screening for inborn errors of metabolism. *Pediatr. Clin. North Am.* 1978, 25:411.
Levy, H. L., and Hammerson, G.: Newborn screening for galactosemia and other galactose metabolic defects. *J. Pediatr.* 1978, 92:871.
Naylor, E. W., and Guthrie, R.: Newborn screening for maple syrup urine disease (branched-chain ketoaciduria). *Pediatrics* 1978, 61:262.
Place, M., Parkin, D. M., and Fitton, J. M.: Effectiveness of neonatal screening for congenital dislocation of the hip. *Lancet* 1978, ii:249.
Hulse, J. A., Grant, D. B., Jackson, D., and Clayton, B. E.: Growth, development, and reassessment of hypothyroid infants diagnosed by screening. *B.M.J.* 1982, 284:1435–1437.
Mitchell, M. L., Bapat, V., Larsen, P. R., et al.: Pitfalls in screening for neonatal hypothyroidism. *Pediatrics* 1982, 70:16–20.
McCabe, E. R. B., McCabe, L., Mosher, G. A., et al.: Newborn screening for phenylketonuria: Predictive validity as a function of age. *Pediatrics* 1983, 72:390–398.
Schneider, A. J.: Newborn phenylalanine/tyrosine metabolism. Implications for screening for phenylketonuria. *Am. J. Dis. Child.* 1983, 137:427–432.
Stein, L., Ozdamar, O., Kraus, N., and Paton, J.: Follow-up of infants screened by auditory brainstem response in the neonatal intensive care unit. *J. Pediatr.* 1983, 103:447–453.
Holtzman, N. A.: Routine screening of newborns for cystic fibrosis: Not yet (Commentary). *Pediatrics.* 1984, 73:98–99.

Tada, K., Tateda, H., Arashima, S., et al.: Follow-up study of a nation-wide neonatal metabolic screening program in Japan. *Eur. J. Pediatr.* 1984, 142:204–207.

Grossman, L. K., Holtzman, N. A., Chasney, E., and Schwartz, D.: Neonatal screening and genetic couseling for sickle cell trait. *Am. J. Dis. Child.* 1985, 139:241–244.

Nyhan, W. L.: Neonatal screening for inherited disease. *N. Engl. J. Med.* 1985, 313:43–44.

Ranieri, E., Ryall, R. G., Morris, C. P., et al.: Neonatal screening strategy for cystic fibrosis using immunoreactive trypsinogen and direct gene analysis. *B.M.J.* 1991, 302:1237–1240.

Bess, F. H., and Paradise, J. L.: Universal screening for infant hearing impairment: Not simple, not risk-free, not necessarily beneficial and not presently justified. *Pediatrics* 1994, 93:330–334.

Car Seats

Colleti, R. B.: Hospital-based rental programs to increase car seat usage. *Pediatrics* 1983, 71:771–773.

American Academy of Pediatrics Committees on Injury and Poison Prevention and Fetus and Newborn: Safe transportation of premature infants. *Pediatrics* 1991, 87:120–122.

Bass, J. L., Mehta, K. A., and Camara, J.: Monitoring premature infants in car seats: Implementing the AAP policy in a community hospital. *Pediatrics* 1993, 91:1137–1141.

5

THERMOREGULATION

The regulation of body temperature is basically a matter of whether heat production can keep pace with heat loss. In the newborn infant, certain problems make it difficult for the baby to maintain its body temperature. Such problems are exaggerated if the baby is premature or small for gestational age. The current emphasis on maintaining body temperature of newborn infants was stimulated by the work of Dr. W. A. Silverman and his colleagues in the 1950s, who showed that even small changes in environmental temperature could significantly influence neonatal mortality (see Chapter 23).

The production of heat may be considered to be primarily the result of oxidative metabolism involving glucose and oxygen, and it therefore depends on the supply of both. The neonate can produce heat at a maximum rate of about 75 cal/kg/min, which compares with a basal heat production of 26 to 30 cal/kg/min. This maximum rate is only a little lower than that of adult man.

The major factor contributing to the difficulty in maintaining body temperature in the newborn infant is its capacity for heat loss. Heat loss occurs in four major ways: (1) radiation, (2) evaporation, (3) conduction, and (4) convection.

The first two ways are the most important in the newborn infant—evaporation, because the baby is wet at birth (and should be quickly dried), and radiation, because of the increased surface area to body weight ratio. A lack of subcutaneous tissue also plays a role, making the body of the newborn infant poorly insulated.

IMPORTANCE OF COOLING

In addition to the effect of hypothermia on neonatal mortality noted earlier, there may be long-term effects. An association between hypothermia shortly after birth and the risk of subsequent neurologic handicap in small preterm babies has been documented (Davies and Tizard). Initial cooling may have far-reaching effects, as can be seen in Figure 5–1.

SPECIAL DISADVANTAGES IN PREMATURE AND INTRAUTERINE GROWTH RETARDATION INFANTS

Both premature infants and those who have intrauterine growth retardation have poor stores of glycogen and fat. They tend to use available glucose quickly

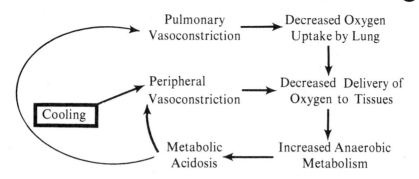

FIGURE 5–1. The effects of cooling on neonatal physiology.

and cannot replace it because of limitations of intake. In addition, the premature infant often has respiratory problems and is compromised as far as oxygen uptake is concerned. Heat loss is exaggerated because of minimal fat insulation. Because the head is relatively larger than the rest of the body, the increased surface area to body weight ratio is further accentuated.

RESPONSE TO COLD STRESS

Basal metabolic rate does not decrease with cooling in the newborn. On the contrary, the oxygen consumption increases with a decrease in environmental temperature. The range in which there is minimal oxygen consumption is the zone of minimum heat production; within this zone is a narrower thermoneutral zone. Body temperature can be maintained down to a certain environmental temperature (when summit metabolism is achieved), beyond which decreasing body temperature (hypothermia) occurs.

The decrease in environmental temperature stimulates heat production by increasing oxygen consumption initially utilized in the metabolism of glucose. However, the amount of glucose available is limited, and another substrate (brown fat) is brought into play. Brown fat is found in term babies in specific locations, principally between the scapulae, in the axillae, in the neck, around the mediastinum, and in the paravertebral region. Heat production from brown fat seems to be mediated by norepinephrine released by cold stress. Neonates appear to be incapable of shivering, and this mechanism using brown adipose tissue is referred to as nonshivering thermogenesis. This mechanism may release excessive amounts of free fatty acids that can potentially displace bilirubin from binding sites on albumin.

ENVIRONMENTAL TEMPERATURE

Thermal neutrality can be maintained by modifying the environmental temperature. The smaller (lighter) the baby, the higher the initial environmental temperature needs to be. Most term newborn babies can adapt to the average environmental temperatures (18 to 20°C) provided that they are clothed and wrapped in blankets. In comparison with the naked infant, such wrapping may lower the minimum temperature tolerated by 20°C. In other words, temperatures of 13 to 15°C can be tolerated in some babies. This finding contrasts with the recommendations for low-birth-weight infants in incubators, approximate values of which are shown in Table 5–1. In infants weighing less than 1000 g, even higher temperatures may be required. A complicating factor that is not always appreciated is that oxygen consumption increases when cold air is blown over the trigeminal region of the face, even though the general environmental temperature may be appropriate. This problem can be avoided by using heated nebulizers when oxygen is administered by head hood.

FEVER

Although cooling is the most important problem of thermoregulation, it is possible for some (term) babies not to be able to dissipate heat rapidly enough to avoid becoming febrile. In some cultures, it is considered very important to keep a baby well wrapped. If the environmental temperature is high (e.g., a hot summer day, with temperature over 90°F, or 32°C), bundling the baby can cause fever.

The environmental temperature of the fetus immediately before delivery is the same as the mother's temperature. Maternal fever can result in fever in the neonate immediately after birth. Epidural anesthesia can cause both maternal and neonatal fever, because heat dissipation in the mother is compromised.

INFANT SERVOCONTROL

Because of the need to prevent hypothermia (provoking a cold stress), many nurseries have used either incubators or radiant heat warmers (closed and open heating units), the heating units of which are switched on or off, depending on the baby's temperature. The temperature is determined with a skin thermistor,

TABLE 5–1. APPROPRIATE INCUBATOR (ENVIRONMENTAL) TEMPERATURES FOR BABIES OF DIFFERENT BIRTH WEIGHTS AT INTERVALS AFTER BIRTH*

Birth Weight (kg)	Environmental Temperature			
	35°C	*34°C*	*33°C*	*32°C*
>2.5	—	—	For 2 days	>2 days
2.0	—	For 2 days	>2 days	>3 weeks
1.5	—	For 10 days	>10 days	>4 weeks
1.0	For 10 days	>10 days	>3 weeks	>5 weeks

*Reproduced with modifications from: Hey, E.: Thermal neutrality. *Br. Med. Bull.* 1975, 31:69.

usually placed over the liver area or between the scapulae with the temperature set at 36.5°C. Such units are termed infant servocontrol devices. When treating a baby in a servocontrolled incubator, one should watch the fluctuations in incubator temperature rather than those of the baby. In other words, a rise in incubator temperature might reflect hypothermia in the baby. Some nurseries prefer to use the approximate temperatures listed in Table 5–1 and follow the fluctuations of the baby's temperature. Economic considerations play a role because servocontrol units are an additional cost. The use of infant servocontrol may cause greater fluctuations in temperature. In particular, shielding (insulating) the probe may cause increased skin-environmental temperature gradients.

CONSERVATION OF BODY TEMPERATURE

In addition to the measures already stated, babies at term are capable of two other methods of modifying body temperature. The first is by increased muscular activity, and the second is by adoption of a more flexed (fetal) position, which minimizes the surface area from which heat is lost. Premature babies are at a disadvantage in both respects because they usually conserve muscular activity for vital functions and lie in a more extended (open) position. If cooling occurs rapidly after birth, rapid rewarming seems to be the best management. Other methods of conserving heat include using bonnets to minimize heat loss from the head, providing intermediate surfaces (plastic heat shields or double-walled incubators) to decrease conductive heat loss, and avoiding drafts (convective loss).

COLD INJURY

If the baby is unable to keep pace with heat loss, neonatal cold injury may develop. This condition is manifested by redness of the face, hands, and feet in marked contrast to pallor of the rest of the body. The body is cold to the touch, and core temperature is markedly decreased. There may be edema of the hands and feet, and the baby is usually very lethargic. Treatment is by warming (usually relatively slowly, 0.5 to 1°C/hr, although rapid rewarming has recently been recommended) together with an intravenous infusion of glucose. Many cases of hypothermia are associated with sepsis, particularly in some countries, so that the possibility of infection should always be considered and antibiotics administered after appropriate cultures are taken. If cold injury is not recognized at an early stage, death may ensue, usually as a result of pulmonary hemorrhage (see also Chapter 24).

CONCLUSION

An understanding of the role that cooling may play in contributing to overall mortality, neurologic sequelae, metabolic acidosis, and other problems leads to the conclusion that prevention of cooling should be the cornerstone of neonatal management.

BIBLIOGRAPHY

Hull, D.: The structure and function of brown adipose tissue. *Br. Med. Bull.* 1966, 22:92.

Cummings, R., and Lykke, A. W. J.: Increased vascular permeability evoked by cold injury. *Pathology* 1973, 5:107.

Commentary: Comments on speed of rewarming after postnatal chilling. *J. Pediatr.* 1974, 85:551.

Hey, E.: Thermal neutrality. *Br. Med. Bull.* 1975, 31:69.

Davies, P. A., and Tizard, J. P. M.: Very low birth weight and subsequent neurological defect. Dev. Med. Child Neurol. 1975, 3:17.

Smales, O. R. C., and Kime, R.: Thermoregulation in babies immediately after birth. *Arch. Dis. Child.* 1978, 53:58.

Harpin, V. A., Chellappah, G., and Rutter, N.: Responses of the newborn infant to overheating. *Biol. Neonate* 1983, 44:65–75.

Sahib El-Radhi, A., Jawad, M., Mansor, N., et al.: Sepsis and hypothermia in the newborn infant: Value of gastric aspirate examination. *J. Pediatr.* 1983, 103:300–302.

Kaplan, M., and Eidelman, A. I.: Improved prognosis in severely hypothermic newborn infants treated by rapid rewarming. *J. Pediatr.* 1984, 105:470–474.

Sauer, P. J. J., and Visser, H. K. A.: Neutral temperature of very low-birth-weight infants. *Pediatrics* 1984, 74:288–289.

Baumgart, S.: Reduction of oxygen consumption, insensible water loss, and radiant heat demand with use of a plastic blanket for low-birth-weight infants under radiant warmers. *Pediatrics* 1984, 74:1022–1028.

Topper, W. H., and Stewart, T. P.: Thermal support for the very-low-birth-weight infant: Role of supplemental conductive heat. *J. Pediatr.* 1984, 105:810–814.

Ducker, D. A., Lyon, A. J., Russell, R. R., et al.: Incubator temperature control: Effects on the very low birthweight infant. *Arch. Dis. Child.* 1985, 60:902–907.

Fusi, L., Steer, P. J., Maresh, M. J. A., and Beard, R. W.: Maternal pyrexia associated with the use of epidural analgesia in labour. *Lancet* 1989, i:1250–1252.

LeBlanc, M. H.: Thermoregulation: Incubators, radiant warmers, artificial skin and body hoods. *Clin. Perinatol.* 1991, 18:403–422.

Hurgoiu, V.: Thermal regulation in preterm infants. *Early Hum. Dev.* 1992, 28:1–5.

Dollberg, S., Atherton, H. D., Sigda, M., et al.: Effect of insulated skin probes to increase skin-to-environmental temperature gradients of preterm infants cared for in convective incubators. *J. Pediatr.* 1994, 124:799–801.

6
ASSESSMENT OF GESTATIONAL AGE

Before 1970, the primary method of assessing gestational age after birth in North America was by examination of a handful of physical characteristics. These features were most helpful in the last 6 weeks of gestation (i.e., 34 to 40 weeks). In France, the examination of neurologic features was considered more reliable and seemed to be valuable over a broad range of gestational ages. In Britain, the range of physical characteristics was extended, and eventually, a scoring system was devised that used both neurologic and physical features. This is usually referred to as the Dubowitz score, and when performed carefully, it gives an estimate within 1 week of actual gestational age (Figs. 6–1 and 6–2 and Tables 6–1 and 6–2). This assessment may (1) confirm the stated gestation, (2) reveal 4-week discrepancies (e.g., a baby who scores at 35½ weeks when the stated gestational age is 32 weeks is probably 36 weeks' gestation), or (3) provide a reliable estimate when uncertainty exists. Even in different racial groups and in twins with similar birth weights, the scoring system has proved reliable. When twins have discordant birth weights, the lighter twin may score slightly less. Infants who are very sick or extremely premature (preterm) may require some modification that eliminates head lag and ventral suspension (Ballard et al., 1979, 1991).

Despite its usefulness, there are several pitfalls to be avoided. First, the baby who is depressed at birth as a result of asphyxia, anesthesia, or analgesia is likely to have a poor neurologic performance. Similarly, when the examination is performed later, the sick infant (e.g., with sepsis or respiratory distress syndrome) also scores less well on this portion of the assessment. Second, the infant who is small for gestational age (intrauterine growth retardation, small or light for dates), in the author's experience, frequently is underscored on physical features when the baby is close to term. This is the result of three features in particular, which are distorted in such babies. These features are softness of ear cartilage, lack of breast tissue, and decreased skin thickness (lack of subcutaneous tissue), despite other features indicating term maturity. Advanced neurologic maturation in association with these findings has been described. This finding may balance the score and give a reliable estimate.

It is best to look at both halves of the score, and if a discrepancy of more than five or six points exists, it is probably wise to rely more on physical

Text continued on page 54

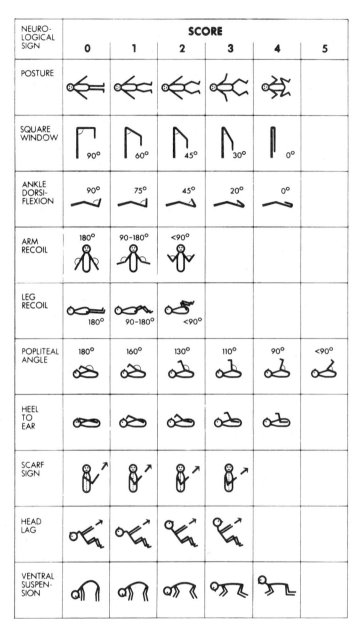

FIGURE 6–1. Neurologic criteria for evaluation of a Dubowitz score.

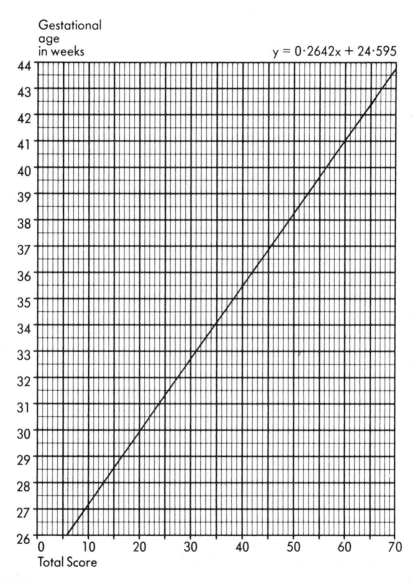

FIGURE 6–2. Graph used to estimate gestational age from the score of neurologic and external criteria (Dubowitz score).

TABLE 6-1. HOW TO PERFORM EVALUATION OF NEUROLOGIC CRITERIA FOR THE DUBOWITZ SCORE*

Posture: Observed with infant quiet and in supine position. Score 0: arms and legs extended; 1: beginning of flexion of hips and knees, arms extended; 2: stronger flexion of legs, arms extended; 3: arms slightly flexed, legs flexed and abducted; 4: full flexion of arms and legs.

Square Window: The hand is flexed on the forearm between the thumb and index finger of the examiner. Enough pressure is applied to get as full a flexion as possible, and the angle between the hypothenar eminence and the ventral aspect of the forearm is measured and graded according to diagram. (Care is taken not to rotate the infant's wrist while performing this maneuver.)

Ankle Dorsiflexion: The foot is dorsiflexed onto the anterior aspect of the leg, with the examiner's thumb on the sole of the foot and other fingers behind the leg. Enough pressure is applied to get as full flexion as possible, and the angle between the dorsum of the foot and the anterior aspect of the leg is measured.

Arm Recoil: With the infant in the supine position, the forearms are first flexed for 5 seconds, then fully extended by pulling on the hands, and then released. The sign is fully positive if the arms return briskly to full flexion (score 2). If the arms return to incomplete flexion or the response is sluggish, it is graded as score 1. If they remain extended or are only followed by random movements, the score is 0.

Leg Recoil: With the infant supine, the hips and knees are fully flexed for 5 seconds, then extended by traction on the feet and released. A maximal response is one of full flexion of the hips and knees (score 2). A partial flexion scores 1, and minimal or no movement scores 0.

Popliteal Angle: With the infant supine and the pelvis flat on the examining couch, the thigh is held in the knee-chest position by the examiner's left index finger and thumb supporting the knee. The leg is then extended by gentle pressure from the examiner's right index finger behind the ankle, and the popliteal angle is measured.

Heel-to-Ear Maneuver: With the baby supine, the baby's foot is drawn as near to the head as it will go without forcing it. The distance between the foot and the head, as well as the degree of extension at the knee, is observed. The score is graded, according to diagram (see Fig. 6–1). Note that the knee is left free and may draw down alongside the abdomen.

Scarf Sign: With the baby supine, the infant's hand is taken, and an attempt is made to put it around the neck and as far posteriorly as possible around the opposite shoulder. This maneuver is assisted by lifting the elbow across the body. The investigator sees how far the elbow will go across the grade according to illustrations (see Fig. 6–1). Score 0: elbow reaches opposite axillary line; 1: elbow is between midline and opposite axillary line; 2: elbow reaches midline; 3: elbow does not reach midline.

Head Lag: With the baby supine, the hands (or the arms if the infant is very small) are grasped, and the infant is pulled slowly toward the sitting position. The position of the head is observed in relation to the trunk, and the score is graded accordingly. In a small infant, the head may initially be supported by one hand. Score 0: complete lag; 1: partial head control; 2: able to maintain head in line with body; 3: brings head anterior to body.

Ventral Suspension: The infant is suspended in the prone position, with examiner's hand under the infant's chest (one hand in a small infant, two in a large infant). The degree of extension of the back and the amount of flexion of the arms and legs are observed. In addition, the relation of the head to the trunk is observed. The score is graded, according to the diagram (see Fig. 6–1).

If score differs on the two sides, the mean is taken.

---

*Reproduced from: Dubowitz, L., Dubowitz, V., Goldberg, C.: Clinical assessment of gestational age in the newborn infant. *J. Pediatr.* 1970, 77:1–10, with permission of the publisher.

TABLE 6-2. EXTERNAL CRITERIA FOR EVALUATION OF THE DUBOWITZ SCORE*

External Sign	Score				
	0	1	2	3	4
Edema	Obvious edema of hands and feet; pitting over tibia	No obvious edema of hands and feet; pitting over tibia	No edema		
Skin texture	Very thin, gelatinous	Thin and smooth	Smooth; medium thickness; rash or superficial peeling	Slight thickening; superficial cracking and peeling, especially hands and feet	Thick and parchment-like; superficial or deep cracking
Skin color (infant not crying)	Dark red	Uniformly pink	Pale pink; variable over body	Pale; only pink over ears, lips, palms, or soles	
Skin opacity (trunk)	Numerous veins and venules clearly seen, especially over abdomen	Veins and tributaries seen	A few large vessels clearly seen over abdomen	A few large vessels seen indistinctly over abdomen	No blood vessels seen
Lanugo (over back)	No lanugo	Abundant; long and thick over whole back	Hair thinning, especially over lower back	Small amount of lanugo and bald areas	At least half of back devoid of lanugo
Plantar creases	No skin creases	Faint red marks over anterior half of sole	Definite red marks over more than anterior half; indentations over less than anterior third	Indentations over more than anterior third	Definite deep indentations over more than anterior third
Nipple formation	Nipple barely visible; no areola	Nipple well defined; areola smooth and flat; diameter, <0.75 cm	Areola stippled; edge not raised; diameter <0.75 cm	Areola stippled; edge raised; diameter, >0.75 cm	
Breast size	No breast tissue palpable	Breast tissue on one or both sides; diameter, <0.5 cm	Breast tissue on both sides; one or both diameters, 0.5–1.0 cm	Breast tissue on both sides; one or both diameters, >1 cm	

Table continued on following page

TABLE 6-2. EXTERNAL CRITERIA FOR EVALUATION OF THE DUBOWITZ SCORE* *Continued*

External Sign	Score				
	0	1	2	3	4
Ear form	Pinna flat and shapeless; little or no incurving of edge	Incurving of part of edge of pinna	Partial incurving whole of upper pinna	Well-defined incurving whole of upper pinna	
Ear firmness	Pinna soft, easily folded; no recoil	Pinna soft, easily folded; slow recoil	Cartilage to edge of pinna, but soft in places; ready recoil	Pinna firm, cartilage to edge, instant recoil	
Genitalia					
Male	Neither testis in scrotum	At least one testis high in scrotum	At least one testis right down		
Female (with hips half abducted)	Labia majora widely separated; labia minora protruding	Labia majora almost covers labia minora	Labia majora completely covers labia minora		

*Reproduced with modification from: Farr, V., Mitchell, R. G., Neligan, G. A., Perkin, J. M.: The definition of some external characteristics used in the assessment of gestational age in the newborn infant. *Devel. Med. Child. Neurol.* 1966, 8:507.

characteristics (with the previously mentioned exception) and double that portion of the score to derive gestational age from the graph. The Ballard modification of the Dubowitz score has been further refined into the New Ballard score, which seems to be reliable down to 26 weeks' gestation and possibly lower if the examination is performed within 12 hours after delivery (Fig. 6–3). Further refinements can be made in the difficult case by assessing a number of reflexes (e.g., Moro, glabellar tap, crossed extensor), which appear at reasonably predictable gestational ages (Fig. 6–4). Another evaluative technique that may improve accuracy, especially in the extremely premature infant (in whom most difficulty arises), is examination of the eye. The anterior vascular capsule of the lens gradually disappears between the 27th and 34th weeks of gestation. Despite attempts to derive accurate estimates in the very immature baby (24 to 28 weeks' gestation), this remains an area for continued investigation. What seems clear is that eye opening is not an accurate indication of gestational age (i.e., the eyes may or may not be fused before or after 26 weeks' gestation) and does not accurately predict outcome (survival or death).

The student may, by now, be wondering why it is important to get an accurate assessment of gestational age. The major reason is to provide a birth weight–gestational age classification (Fig. 6–5), which is important for at least two reasons: first, to anticipate the problems a baby is likely to develop, and

Neuromuscular Maturity

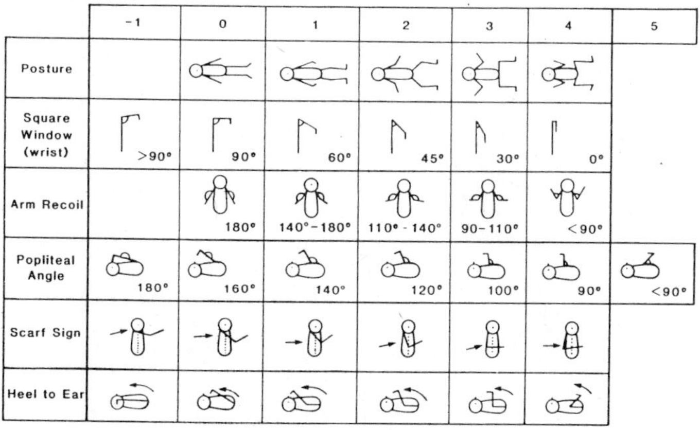

	−1	0	1	2	3	4	5
Posture							
Square Window (wrist)	>90°	90°	60°	45°	30°	0°	
Arm Recoil		180°	140°–180°	110°–140°	90–110°	<90°	
Popliteal Angle	180°	160°	140°	120°	100°	90°	<90°
Scarf Sign							
Heel to Ear							

Physical Maturity

Skin	sticky friable transparent	gelatinous red, translucent	smooth pink, visible veins	superficial peeling &/or rash. few veins	cracking pale areas rare veins	parchment deep cracking no vessels	leathery cracked wrinkled
Lanugo	none	sparse	abundant	thinning	bald areas	mostly bald	
Plantar Surface	heel–toe 40–50mm:−1 <40mm:−2	>50mm no crease	faint red marks	anterior transverse crease only	creases ant. 2/3	creases over entire sole	
Breast	imperceptible	barely perceptible	flat areola no bud	stippled areola 1–2mm bud	raised areola 3-4mm bud	full areola 5–10mm bud	
Eye/Ear	lids fused loosely:−1 tightly:−2	lids open pinna flat stays folded	sl. curved pinna; soft; slow recoil	well–curved pinna; soft but ready recoil	formed &firm instant recoil	thick cartilage ear stiff	
Genitals male	scrotum flat, smooth	scrotum empty faint rugae	testes in upper canal rare rugae	testes descending few rugae	testes down good rugae	testes pendulous deep rugae	
Genitals female	clitoris prominent labia flat	prominent clitoris small labia minora	prominent clitoris enlarging minora	majora & minora equally prominent	majora large minora small	majora cover clitoris & minora	

Maturity Rating

score	weeks
−10	20
−5	22
0	24
5	26
10	28
15	30
20	32
25	34
30	36
35	38
40	40
45	42
50	44

FIGURE 6–3. Expanded Ballard score, the New Ballard score, includes extremely premature infants and has been refined to improve accuracy in more mature infants. (From: Ballard, J. L., Khoury, J. C., Wedig, K., et al.: New Ballard score, expanded to include extremely premature infants. *J. Pediatr.* 1991, 119:417–423.)

FIGURE 6-4. A guide to the clinical estimation of gestational age.

PHYSICAL FINDINGS	EST GA	WEEKS GESTATION
		24 25 26 27 28 29 30 31 32 33 34 35 36 37 38 39 40 41 42 43 44
EXAMINATION FIRST HOURS		
VERNIX		APPEARS → COVERS BODY → DECREASE IN AMOUNT → NO VERNIX
BREAST TISSUE		
NIPPLES		BARELY VISIBLE / NONE → WELL DEFINED FLAT AREOLA 1–2 MM → 2, ANTERIOR 4 MM → WELL DEFINED, RAISED AREOLA 7 MM OR MORE
SOLE CREASES		NONE → 1, ANTERIOR TRANSVERSE → 2/3 SOLE → CREASES INVOLVING HEEL
EAR CARTILAGE		PINNA SOFT, STAYS FOLDED → RETURNS SLOWLY FROM FOLDING → THIN CARTILAGE, SPRINGS BACK → FIRM, REMAINS ERECT FROM HEAD
EAR FORM		FLAT, SHAPELESS → BEGINNING INCURVING OF PERIPHERY → PARTIAL INCURVING UPPER PINNA → WELL DEFINED INCURVING ALL OF UPPER PINNA
GENITALIA – TESTES & SCROTUM		UNDESCENDED → TESTES HIGH IN CANAL, FEW RUGAE → TESTES LOWER MORE RUGAE → TESTES DESCENDED, PENDULOUS SCROTUM, RUGAE COMPLETE
LABIA & CLITORIS		LABIA MAJORA WIDELY SEPARATED, PROMINENT CLITORIS → LABIA MAJORA NEARLY COVER LABIA MINORA → LABIA MINORA & CLITORIS COVERED
HAIR (APPEARS ON HEAD @ 20 WKS)		EYEBROWS & LASHES → FINE, WOOLLY HAIR → HAIR SILKY, SINGLE STRANDS
LANUGO (APPEARS @ 20 WKS)		LANUGO OVER ENTIRE BODY → VANISHES FROM FACE → SLIGHT LANUGO OVER SHOULDERS → NO LANUGO
SKIN TEXTURE		THIN → SMOOTH, MEDIUM THICKNESS → DESQUAMATION
SKIN COLOR & OPACITY		TRANSLUCENT, PLETHORIC, NUMEROUS VENULES (ABDOMEN) → PINK, FEW LARGE VESSELS OVERALL → PALE PINK, NO VESSELS SEEN
SKULL FIRMNESS		SOFT TO 1 INCH FROM ANTERIOR FONTANELLE → SPRINGY AT EDGES OF FONTANELLE CENTER FIRM → BONES HARD SUTURES EASILY DISPLACED → BONES HARD, CANNOT BE DISPLACED
POSTURE – RESTING		HYPOTONIA / LATERAL DECUBITUS → HYPOTONIA → SLIGHT INCREASE IN TONE, FROG-LIKE → TOTAL FLEXION
RECOIL		ABSENT → NONE UPPER EXTREMITIES GOOD LOWER EXTREMITIES → SLOW UPPER EXTREMITIES → GOOD UPPER EXTREMITIES
LATER EXAMINATION		
TONE – HEEL TO EAR		NO RESISTANCE → SLIGHT RESISTANCE → DIFFICULT ALMOST IMPOSSIBLE → IMPOSSIBLE
SCARF MANEUVER		NO RESISTANCE → MINIMAL RESISTANCE → FAIR RESISTANCE → DIFFICULT
NECK EXTENSORS		ABSENT → SLIGHT → FAIR → GOOD
NECK FLEXORS		ABSENT → MINIMAL → FAIR
MORO		BARELY APPARENT → COMPLETE, EXHAUSTIBLE → GOOD, COMPLETE → NO ADDUCTION → COMPLETE WITH ADDUCTION
REFLEXES – PUPILS TO LIGHT		REACT
GRASP		FEEBLE → FAIR → SOLID, INVOLVES ARMS → MAY PICK INFANT UP
ROOTING		MINIMAL & REINFORCEMENT → GOOD & REINFORCEMENT → GOOD
CROSSED EXTENSION		SLIGHT WITHDRAWAL → WITHDRAWAL → WITHDRAWAL & EXTENSION → WITHDRAWAL, EXTENSION, ADDUCTION
AUTOMATIC WALK		ABSENT → MINIMAL → GOOD, HEELS
TRUNK ELEVATION		ABSENT → SLIGHT → FAIR, TOES → GOOD
GLABELLAR TAP		ABSENT → APPEARS → PRESENT
HEAD TURNS TO LIGHT		ABSENT → APPEARS → PRESENT
CLINICAL ESTIMATE, GA		
CALCULATED GA		24 25 26 27 28 29 30 31 32 33 34 35 36 37 38 39 40 41 42 43 44 WEEKS GESTATION

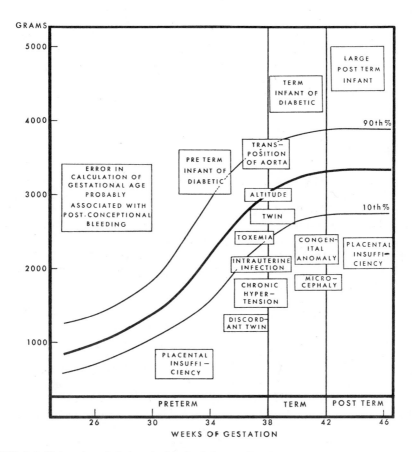

FIGURE 6-5. University of Colorado Medical Center Newborn and Premature Center: Problems associated with deviations of intrauterine growth.

second, to provide valid comparisons with respect to mortality and morbidity statistics. Two examples are given to explain these in more detail.

EXAMPLE 1

Two babies weighing 1800 g are delivered, one at 32 weeks', the other at 36 weeks' gestation. The former is an appropriate for gestational age baby, the latter is a small for gestational age baby. The appropriate for gestational age baby is very likely to develop respiratory distress syndrome (hyaline membrane disease); the small for gestational age baby is quite unlikely to develop respiratory distress syndrome. Any technique employed to prevent respiratory distress syndrome is likely to appear to be successful in the small for gestational age baby, largely because one is comparing similar but different things (e.g., apples and oranges).

EXAMPLE 2

A baby weighing 4500 g is admitted to the nursery, having been born to a mother who had little prenatal care but whose previous baby weighed 4200 g at an unknown gestational age. The natural inclination is to think of this baby as a term infant. Although the baby appears quite fat, the gestational age assessment is 36 weeks by Dubowitz score. This makes the baby markedly large for gestational age and preterm. Such a baby is likely to be an infant of a gestational diabetic and is more likely to have a variety of problems (see Chapter 16).

The importance of accurate birth weight–gestational age assessments becomes more apparent when one looks at the data for mortality risk (see Appendix 9). The appropriate for gestational age baby in example 1 has a higher mortality risk than an appropriate for gestational age baby at 36 weeks' gestation. Term is regarded as 38 to 42 weeks; birth after 42 weeks is postterm (or postmature) and before 38 weeks is preterm or premature. The former definition of prematurity (now obsolete) applied to any baby weighing less than 2500 g. Such babies are now referred to as babies of low birth weight, and gestational age categories are appended. Thus, a baby with a birth weight of 2150 g who is born at 39 weeks' gestation would be categorized as a low-birth-weight baby (< 2500 g) who is small for gestational age at term. (Other examples are shown in Figures 6–6 through 6–11.) Neonatal mortality and morbidity are closely linked to the low-birth-weight rate. Consequently, any reduction in low-birth-weight rate is likely to be reflected in lower neonatal (and infant) mortality (see Chapter 22).

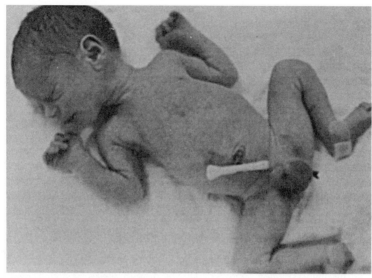

FIGURE 6–6. This small-for-gestational age baby weighed approximately 1700 g at term. The flexed posture is typical of the infant born close to term. This photograph also demonstrates mature ear formation, and the testes appear to be in the scrotum. The baby was pale pink.

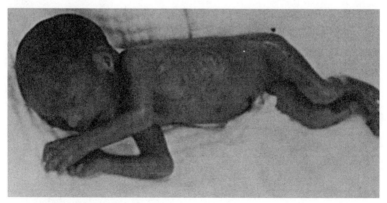

FIGURE 6–7. This baby weighed approximately 550 g at 25 weeks' gestation. The limbs are in extension, and the skin is dark red and appears thin and shiny. The ears are also poorly formed. (The baby died.)

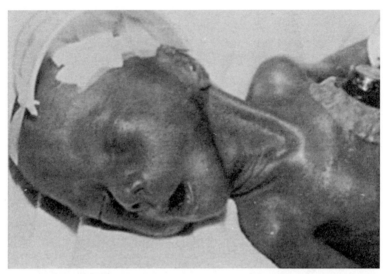

FIGURE 6–8. This baby weighed approximately 750 g at 26 weeks' gestation. By 1 week of age (when this photograph was taken), the right eye had opened, and the left eye remained fused. (The baby survived.)

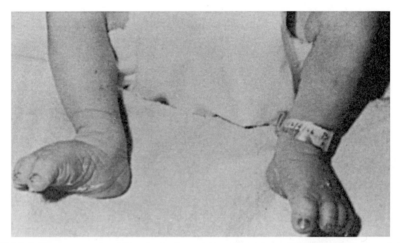

FIGURE 6–9. Postmature (postterm) newborn infant showing peeling of the skin of the soles of the feet. The nails were stained a green-brown color.

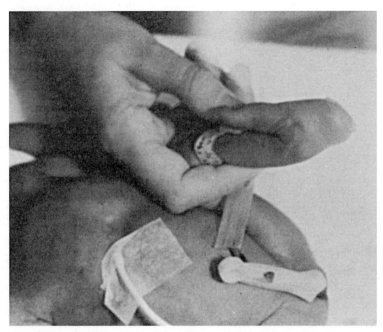

FIGURE 6–10. Demonstration of the ankle dorsiflexion maneuver in a term baby who was markedly small for gestational age. The angle is 0° (no force was used).

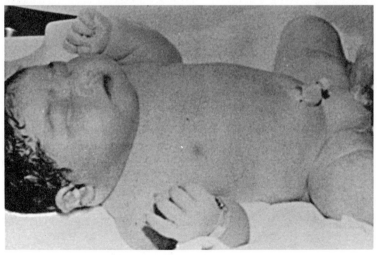

FIGURE 6–11. Typical example of an infant of a diabetic mother. This baby was markedly large for gestational age, weighing approximately 6 kg at 37 weeks' gestation.

BIBLIOGRAPHY

Dubowitz, L. M. S., and Dubowitz, V.: *Gestational Age of the Newborn.* Addison-Wesley Publishing Company, Menlo Park, CA, 1977.

Hittner, H. M., Hirsh, N. J., and Rudolph, A. J.: Assessment of gestational age by examination of the anterior vascular capsule of the lens. *J. Pediatr.* 1977, 91:455.

Woods, D. L., and Malan, A. F.: Assessment of gestational age in twins. *Arch. Dis. Child.* 1977, 52:735.

Ballard, J. L., Novak, K. K., and Driver, M.: A simplified score for assessment of fetal maturation of newly born infants. *J. Pediatr.* 1979, 95:769.

Amiel-Tison, C.: Possible acceleration of neurological maturation following high-risk pregnancy. *Am. J. Obstet. Gynecol.* 1980, 138:303–306.

Anderson, H. F., Johnson, T. R. B., Jr., Flora, J. D., Jr., and Barclay, M. L.: Gestational age assessment: II. Prediction from combined clinical observations. *Am. J. Obstet. Gynecol.* 1981, 140:770–774.

Philip, A. G. S., Little, G. A., Polivy, D. R., and Lucey, J. F.: Neonatal mortality risk for the eighties: The importance of birth weight/gestational age groups. *Pediatrics* 1981, 68:122–130.

Narayanan, I., Dua, K., Gujral, V. V., et al.: A simple method of assessment of gestational age in newborn infants. *Pediatrics* 1982, 69:27–32.

Forbes, J. F., and Smalls, M. J.: A comparative analysis of birthweight for gestational age standards. *Br. J. Obstet. Gynaecol.* 1983, 90:297–303.

Jimenez, J. M., Tyson, J. E., and Reisch, J. S.: Clinical measures of gestational age in normal pregnancies. *Obstet. Gynecol.* 1983, 61:438–443.

Rennie, J. M., and Cooke, R. W. I.: Do fused eyelids indicate inevitable neonatal death (Letter)? *Lancet* 1983, i:1157–1158.

Ballard, J. L., Khoury, J. C., Wedig, K., et al.: New Ballard Score, expanded to include extremely premature infants. *J. Pediatr.* 1991, 119:417–423.

Sanders, M., Allen, M., Alexander, G. R., et al.: Gestational age assessment in preterm neonates weighing less than 1500 grams. *Pediatrics* 1991, 88:542–546.

Alexander, G. R., DeCaunes, F., Hulsey, T. C., et al.: Validity of post-natal assessments of gestational age: A comparison of the method of Ballard et al. and early ultrasonography. *Am. J. Obstet. Gynecol.* 1992, 166:891–895.

1
REGIONALIZED CARE AND TRANSPORT OF THE SICK NEONATE

REGIONALIZATION

When the care of premature infants was largely a matter of waiting to see if the baby survived the first 2 days and then feeding it, there was little reason to transfer a baby from one hospital to another, except perhaps for cardiac evaluation or surgery. With the explosion of knowledge about the neonate, the university and large community hospital centers were able to demonstrate a significant reduction in neonatal and perinatal mortality as a result of the special care provided for the infant. With this demonstration, considerable sums of money were invested to equip hospitals with facilities that would match those of the centers. It soon became obvious that there was considerable duplication of equipment that was rarely used. What could not easily be duplicated were the nursing, respiratory therapy, radiology, and laboratory services so essential to modern-day management of the sick neonate. As the changes continued, a move to regionalize care emerged in North America. In many places, the medical center of the community started to assume responsibility for the care of neonates in the whole region rather than concentrating on only those babies born at the center. Results from many centers suggest that well-organized regionalization can have a significant impact on perinatal mortality and delivery of health care in community hospitals.

Several concepts are intrinsic to successful regionalization, including (1) an educational program for community nurses and physicians about stabilization techniques and recent developments in perinatal care, (2) a full range of antenatal (prenatal) diagnostic services at the medical center, (3) easy accessibility of consultation, (4) delivery in the community hospital if antenatal diagnostic services indicate low risk, (5) delivery at the medical center with careful intrapartum monitoring when the fetus is considered to be at high risk, (6) an intensive care nursery at the medical center that is capable of providing a full range of diagnostic and therapeutic services, (7) an effective and efficient system for transporting the sick infant from the community hospital to the center, (8) careful discharge planning to provide parental support when the baby goes home (social worker and nursing referral), and (9) follow-up of infants to assess outcome.

INTENSIVE CARE "BURNOUT"

Despite the clear benefits to be derived from a regionalized program, certain difficulties may be encountered that became apparent only after several years of experience with neonatal intensive care had elapsed. When this type of care was first started, there was a good deal of skepticism about the outcome for recipients of such care. This doubt led to a slow trickle of referrals from the community, which later became a steady stream and now seems to have become a flood, in some places. In recent years, this flow has included an increasingly large number of maternal-fetal referrals, as is discussed later.

The result of this change was that most intensive care nurseries no longer had peaks and troughs of activity but had to provide continual high-intensity care. Under such circumstances, many staff members are unable to function constantly at full efficiency; they may start out enthusiastically but end up apathetic and "burnt out." One of the tricks of running a regional center is to avoid such burnout in the staff. This task may be accomplished by a number of mechanisms, such as rotation of staff to less intensive areas, group therapy sessions to discuss chronically sick patients, attendance at educational programs, and social service rounds, not the least of which is the ability to retain a sense of humor.

TRANSPORT

"The best transport incubator is the uterus" is an oft-quoted aphorism. When this form of transport is available, it can be referred to as maternal-fetal transport. In other words, before delivery, the baby who is at high risk of developing neonatal problems may be transported in utero to the hospital where the intensive care nursery is located. With increasing recognition of the high-risk pregnancy, such referrals may be accomplished long before labor begins, whereas others may not occur until after the onset of labor. If preterm labor can be prevented or suppressed, referral back to the hospital of origin may be possible.

More frequently, the sick neonate is transferred after delivery, and this kind of transport usually requires the attendance of a skilled person (preferably two skilled people). Such transports have been classified as one way (community hospital to center) or two way (center to community hospital to center). Generally, the two-way transport is more reliable because personnel from the center who are familiar with the principles of neonatal transport accompany the baby. However, valuable time may be lost with this method, and if skilled personnel are available to travel with the baby, the one-way transport may be preferred (a good example would be an infant with diaphragmatic hernia; see Chapter 8).

For either method, it is desirable that a special incubator (a transport incubator) be used (Fig. 7–1). All incubators should provide (1) an unimpeded view of the infant, (2) ability to alter environmental temperature, (3) easy access to the baby, and (4) oxygen (the concentration of which can be regulated). In addition, the following items are important: (1) a heart rate monitor, (2) a constant infusion pump for intravenous or intraarterial fluids, (3) a bag and mask for ventilation, (4) emergency equipment (e.g., sodium bicarbonate, digoxin, endotracheal tubes, laryngoscope), (5) an oxygen analyzer, and (6) a portable respirator (if long distances or prolonged transport times are common). Many centers also include transcutaneous blood gas monitors or pulse oximeters in their transport equipment.

An additional advantage of the two-way transport is that members of the team who will be looking after the baby can make contact with the parents and provide first-hand information about the intensive care nursery. It is difficult to assess the importance of this personal contact, but it is frequently reassuring to parents to meet people who will be caring for the baby.

Infants who should be transported to a facility capable of providing intensive care nursing with 24-hour physician coverage are categorized as follows:

Almost Always Send
1. Infants weighing less than 1.5 kg (or less than 32 weeks' gestation)
2. Infants with obvious respiratory difficulty (including frequent apnea)
3. Infants with suspected sepsis, or meningitis, or both
4. Infants with convulsive disorder (or convulsive equivalents)
5. Infants requiring (or possibly requiring) neonatal surgery

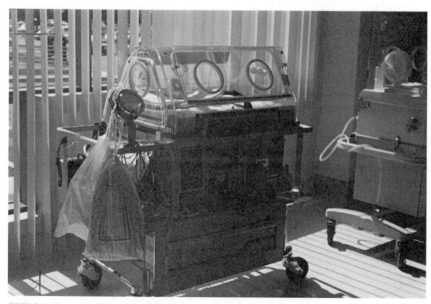

FIGURE 7–1. Example of equipment used to transport infants to a regional center. This incorporates a transport incubator, a gas-powered ventilator, physiologic monitoring equipment, and emergency equipment and medications.

6. Infants with central cyanosis (suspected congenital heart disease)

7. Infants with evidence of severe hemolytic disease of the newborn*

Consider Sending

1. Infants weighing less than 2 kg (or < 34 weeks' gestation)

2. Infants of insulin-dependent diabetic mothers (especially if the infants are macrosomic)*

3. Infants with obvious intrauterine growth retardation

4. Infants requiring prolonged resuscitation in the delivery room (> 10 to 15 minutes active resuscitation)

5. Infants with obvious pallor

6. Infants with evidence of meconium aspiration (via laryngoscopy or chest x-ray study)

7. Infants with severe congenital abnormalities (for evaluation)

STABILIZATION BEFORE TRANSPORT

Some of the principles outlined in other sections should be emphasized here. It is important to provide an adequate thermal environment (prevent cooling) and to provide oxygen to eliminate cyanosis. When the baby is pink, arterial or transcutaneous pO_2 levels should be determined, and if there is evidence of pallor or respiratory difficulty, pH and pCO_2 values will reveal whether or not metabolic or respiratory acidosis is present.

In any case in which significant respiratory difficulty exists (even though the baby may appear stable), it is preferable to insert an endotracheal tube before attempting to transport the baby. This is particularly true in cases of diaphragmatic hernia (see Chapter 8). It is much easier to assist ventilation in transit if an endotracheal tube is in place, and it is easier to insert the tube in the nursery than in the back of an ambulance.

Because most infants who require transfer are prone to hypoglycemia, it is also important to provide an adequate and reliable source of glucose. Umbilical artery catheters are the preferred route in infants with respiratory difficulty because blood gas analysis is required before and after transfer, and blood pressure measurements can be made directly. Alternative routes are peripheral venous or umbilical venous, using 10% dextrose at a rate of 4 ml/kg/hr (adjustments to daily intake can be made after arrival at the center).

When sepsis is strongly suspected, it is preferable to obtain blood and cerebrospinal fluid cultures and to start antibiotic therapy before the transfer is initiated because many cases of early onset sepsis have a rapid and fulminant course.

In an infant with suspected cyanotic congenital heart disease, keeping the ductus arteriosus patent with prostaglandin E (Prostin) is particularly important. Adminstration of this agent may be started at 10 to 25 ng/kg/min.

Many congenital abnormalities are now detected by ultrasonography prenatally, allowing earlier identification and maternal-fetal referral. Infants with ventral wall defects (omphalocele or gastroschisis) should preferably be referred

---

*Mothers should preferably be sent before delivery.

to a regional center with pediatric surgical capability for delivery. However, when these infants present unexpectedly, discussion with a surgeon is recommended. Wrapping the bowel may decrease fluid loss, and paying careful attention to maintaining a neutral thermal environment prevents cooling and its consequences (see Chapter 5).

Other circumstances that demand prompt attention are outlined in Chapter 24.

Whether or not there is a lower limit of weight below which aggressive intensive care is not justified is uncertain. Although it was suggested, from a center to which all admissions are referred, that assisted ventilation in an infant whose birth weight was smaller than 700 g may not be appropriate (because the outcome was so poor), other centers have shown a good outcome in babies born at their own center who survived with birth weights below this level, and results continue to improve. Gestational age and condition at birth may be more important than birth weight alone.

Considerable inconvenience to families may result from the transfer of babies. It is therefore important to consider sending the baby back to the referral hospital when intensive care is no longer needed. Such transfer should occur only after the wishes of the parents and the referring physician are considered. Many community hospitals have upgraded their capabilities by sending nursing staff to participate in on-site training in intensive care nurseries. This and similar activities are to be encouraged.

BIBLIOGRAPHY

Marshall, R. E., and Kasman, C.: Burnout in the neonatal intensive care unit. *Pediatrics* 1980, 65:1161–1165.

Harris, B. A., Wirtschafter, D. D., Huddleston, J. F., and Perlis, H. W.: In utero versus neonatal transportation of high-risk perinates: A comparison. *Obstet. Gynecol.* 1981, 57:496–499.

Sinclair, J. C., Torrance, G. W., Boyle, M. H., et al.: Evaluation of neonatal-intensive-care programs. *N. Engl. J. Med.* 1981, 305:489–494.

Harper, R. G., Little, G. A., and Sia, C. G.: The scope of nursing practice in level III neonatal intensive care units. *Pediatrics* 1982, 70:875–878.

Hirata, T., Epcar, J. T., Walsh, A., et al.: Survival and outcome of infants 501 to 750 mgs: A six-year experience. *J. Pediatr.* 1983, 102:741–748.

Lobb, M. O., Morgan, M. E. I., Bond, A. P., and Cooke, R. W. I.: Transfer before delivery on Merseyside: An analysis of the first 140 patients. *Br. J. Obstet. Gynaecol.* 1983, 90:338–341.

Clarke, T. A., Maniscalco, W., Taylor-Brown, S., et al.: Job satisfaction and stress among neonatologists. *Pediatrics* 1984, 74:52–57.

Campbell, A. N., Lightstone, A. D., Smith, J. M., et al.: Mechanical vibration and sound levels experienced in neonatal transport. *Am. J. Dis. Child.* 1984, 138:967–970.

McCormick, M. C., Shapiro, S., and Starfield, B. H.: The regionalization of perinatal services: Summary of the evaluation of a national demonstration program. *J.A.M.A.* 1985, 253:799–804.

Donn, S. M., Faix, R. G., and Gates, M. R.: Neonatal transport. *Curr. Prob. Pediatr.* 1985, 15:1–65.

Kellee, L. A. A., Brand, R., Schreuder, A. M., et al.: Five year outcome of preterm and very low birth weight infants: A comparison between maternal and neonatal transport. *Obstet. Gynecol.* 1992, 80:635–638.

8
COMMON CONGENITAL MALFORMATIONS

RECOGNIZABLE BY OBSERVATION

DOWN'S SYNDROME (MONGOLISM, OR TRISOMY 21)

Incidence

Down's syndrome is seen in approximately 1 in 800 live births. The risk is markedly increased in mothers over the age of 40 years. However, as a result of genetic amniocentesis (see Chapter 1), most babies with Down's syndrome are now born to mothers under the age of 35 years. The incidence is also increased in pregnant women with lower-than-normal levels of serum α-fetoprotein (see also triple testing under Maternal Screening for Fetal Disorders section in Chapter 1).

Etiology

Most cases of Down's syndrome are caused by the process of nondisjunction producing 47 chromosomes, with an extra chromosome in group G (21,22), which can now be identified as an extra chromosome 21, or trisomy 21. Sometimes, the extra chromosomal material is displaced onto another chromosome in the parent (who demonstrates 45 chromosomes) and is transmitted to the infant (who has 46 chromosomes). This process is called translocation (e.g., 15/21 translocation). This phenomenon is more likely to occur in younger mothers but nevertheless accounts for only 3 to 4% of all cases of Down's syndrome. In approximately 25% of cases, the genetic abnormality can be attributed to the father.

Diagnosis

The trained observer has little difficulty in spotting these babies (Figs. 8–1 through 8–4). This is as true in the Asian population as it is in the white population. The following are considered the most reliable features: generalized hypotonia; eyes slanting upward, from within outward; prominent epicanthic skin folds; flattened facies; flattened occiput; white speckled iris (Brushfield's

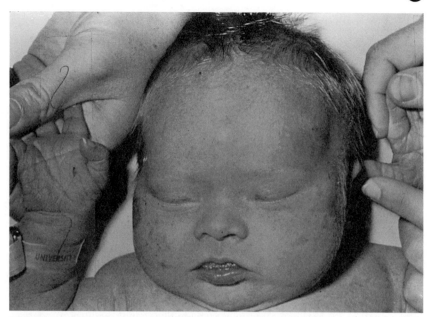

FIGURE 8–1. Baby with Down's syndrome (mongolism), showing the mongoloid slant of the eyes, the flattened facies, the protruding tongue, and the bilateral simian creases. The epicanthal folds are barely visible.

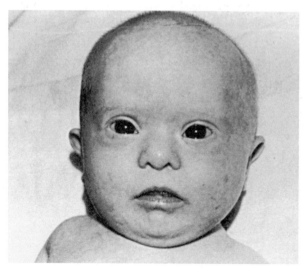

FIGURE 8–2. Another baby with Down's syndrome, showing flattened facies, prominent epicanthal skin folds, somewhat low-set ears, and slightly protruding tongue.

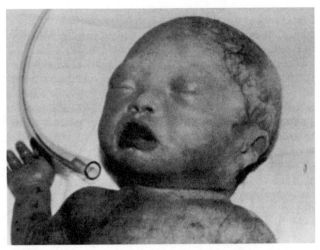

FIGURE 8–3. Premature infant with Down's syndrome, demonstrating flattened facies and protruding tongue. The left ear appears to be a little low set and abnormally shaped.

spots); small and misshapen ears; square (spade-like) hands, with short incurved fifth finger demonstrating the absence of one crease (and hypoplasia of middle phalanx on x-ray study); bilateral single palmar creases (simian crease, seen in only 50 to 60%); excessive skin over the back of the neck; and a characteristic pelvic x-ray study showing broadened ilial bones and narrow acetabular angle.

Infants with Down's syndrome are almost invariably below the 50th percentile for birth weight at a given gestational age. Frequently associated congenital anomalies are congenital heart disease (ventricular septal, atrial septal, and

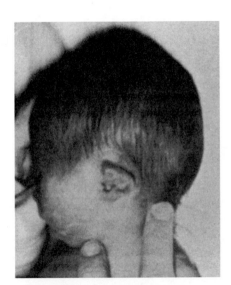

FIGURE 8–4. Same baby as in Figure 8–3, exhibiting a small, malformed left ear and flattening of the occiput.

endocardial cushion defects) and intestinal abnormalities (duodenal atresia being disporportionately represented). Examination of the skin creases (dermatoglyphics) also may be helpful.

Unusual laboratory findings may be a high hematocrit value ($> 60\%$) or a leukemoid response, with the total white blood cell count greater then $50.0 \times 10^9/L$. Rarely, true congenital leukemia is seen, or leukemia may develop at an older age.

Management

Because of the later association of Down's syndrome with variable degrees of mental retardation, there has been some debate about whether or not parents should care for these children. There is little doubt that the optimal potential for these children is achieved in a loving family environment rather than in an institution. The fact that these infants are usually easy to handle (nondestructive) and frequently progress through normal childhood development (but at a considerably reduced rate) makes discussion with these parents easier than discussion with parents of babies with some other abnormalities. It is best to discuss the situation fully with the parents soon after delivery (perhaps after the baby has been handled by the mother, to allow initial bonding). The decision about future care is theirs and may depend on whether or not other children's lives may be disrupted. A more positive attitude toward the baby may result from the use of nonthreatening words, such as avoidance of words like idiot and retarded. Occasionally, the child can be placed with foster parents if the parents feel that they would not be able to cope with a child who is likely to be mentally retarded.

In all cases, it is probably wise to perform chromosomal analysis on the baby. If the usual nondisjunction pattern is not observed, the parents should also have chromosomal analysis because translocation significantly increases the risk in subsequent pregnancies.

Summary

Down's syndrome is a fairly common chromosomal abnormality with easily recognizable features. It is more likely to occur in pregnancies with advanced maternal age or decreased maternal serum α-fetoprotein levels. Associated congenital abnormalities and mental retardation may make decisions about care difficult.

OTHER AUTOSOMAL TRISOMIES

Incidence

Trisomy 18 (trisomy E) occurs in about 1 in 3000 births, whereas trisomy 13 (trisomy D) occurs in approximately 1 in 5000 births.

Etiology

As with Down's syndrome, increased maternal age plays a role, but advanced paternal age also seems to be implicated. Most frequently, these disorders are the result of nondisjunction.

Diagnosis

Typical morphologic features are noted in trisomies 18 and 13, although some of these features overlap (Figs. 8–5 and 8–6). The presence of cleft lip and palate makes trisomy 13 the more likely diagnosis (Fig. 8–7). These babies are almost invariably small for gestational age and are born at term. A characteristic flexing of the fingers is seen in trisomy 18 (Fig. 8–8), as are rocker-bottom feet (Fig. 8–9), but similar features may be seen in trisomy 13.

Abnormally placed (low-set) and misshaped ears, simian creases, congenital heart defects, and mental retardation are also common to both disorders. The major findings of the three trisomies described are shown in Table 8–1. Firm diagnosis depends on chromosomal abnormalities, detected by karyotyping.

Management

Once the diagnosis is firmly established, aggressive management (e.g., cardiac massage and assisted ventilation) is contraindicated because of the severity of the psychomotor retardation. Most of these infants die within the first few months of life, frequently as a result of the associated cardiac abnormalities.

Summary

Small for gestational age babies with a constellation of abnormalities should be suspected of having trisomy 18 or 13. Chromosomal analysis confirms the diagnosis, but the outlook is uniformly poor.

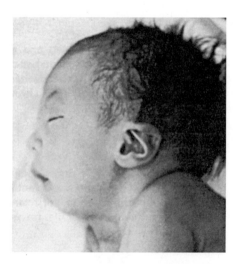

FIGURE 8–5. Newborn infant with trisomy 18 syndrome, showing the typical facies with mild micrognathia and a low-set misshapen ear.

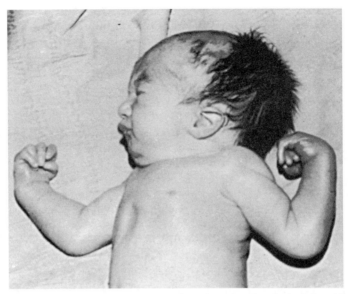

FIGURE 8–6. Another infant with trisomy 18 syndrome, showing limb deformities (fixed flexion) as well as the features seen in Figure 8–5.

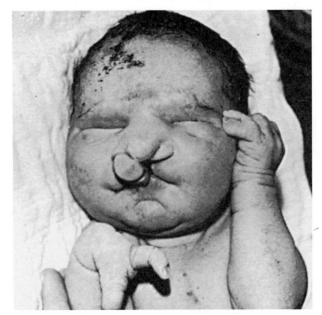

FIGURE 8–7. Baby with trisomy 13 syndrome, demonstrating the typical facies with flattened broad nose and bilateral cleft lip. Limb defects (hands) are also apparent.

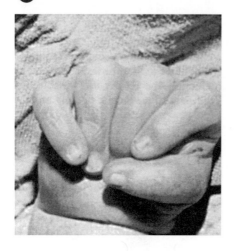

FIGURE 8–8. Close-up of the hand of the baby in Figure 8–6, showing the typical overriding position of the index and little fingers. There is also a fingerlike thumb.

OTHER AUTOSOMAL ABNORMALITIES

Many other potential problems with chromosomes exist. When a chromosome is missing (monosomy), the usual result is that the fetus is aborted in the first trimester. When a portion of a chromosome is missing (deletion), the results are variable. For instance, some cases of Prader-Willi syndrome have deletions of chromosome 15, and cri-du-chat syndrome is associated with a deletion of chromosome 5. In cases of balanced translocation, some chromosomal material is missing, but this lack does not seem to produce abnormality.

SEX CHROMOSOME ABNORMALITIES

Turner's syndrome (gonadal dysgenesis) is the most common sex chromosome abnormality and is characterized by an XO configuration, indicating that

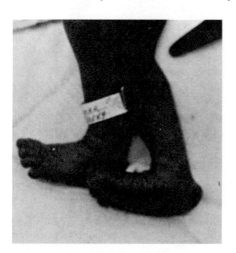

FIGURE 8–9. Rocker-bottom foot in trisomy 18 syndrome.

TABLE 8-1. MAJOR FINDINGS OF TRISOMIES AT BIRTH

Finding	Trisomy 21	Trisomy 18	Trisomy 13
Prevalence	1.5 in 1000	0.3 in 1000	0.2 in 1000
Gestation			
↓ Fetal activity	−	+ +	−
Pre, term, post	−	1/3, 1/3, 1/3	−
Polyhydramnios	−	+ +	−
Small placenta	−	+ +	−
Low birth weight	−	+ +	−
Single umbilical Artery	−	+ +	+ +
Neurologic			
Tone	Hypotonia + +	Hypertonia +	−
Seizure or apnea	−	−	+ +
Hearing	−	+ +	+ +
Craniofacial			
Facies	Flat + +	Narrow bifrontal +	Holoprosencephaly syndrome + +
Occiput	Flat + +	Prominent + +	−
Clefts	−	+	+ +
Ears	Small + +	Low + +	Shape + +
Eye fissure	Slanted + +	Short + +	−
Other eye problems	Brushfield's spots +	−	Microphthalmia +
Micrognathia	−	+ +	+
Skeletal			
Joint flexibility	Hyper + +	Hypo +	−
Pelvis	Hypoplasia + +	↓ Abduction + +	Hypoplasia + +
Radial aplasia	−	±	+
Rocker-bottom feet	−	+	−
Equinovarus	−	+	+
Hands			
Shape	Spade + +	Clenched + +	Clenched + +
Hypoplastic fifth	+ +	+ +	+
Simian crease	+ +	+	+ +
Hypoplastic nails	−	+ +	Toenails +
Dermatoglyphics	Ulnar loop +	Low arch + +	Low arch +
Cardiac defect	+	+ +	+ +
Abdominal defect	Duodenal atresia +	Omphalocele +	Omphalocele +
Genitals			
Cryptorchidism	−	+ +	+ +
Hypospadias	−	±	+
Hypoplastic labia	−	+	+
Prognosis (attrition)			
1 month	Congenital heart	30%*	45%
2 months	disease	50%	
6 months			70%
1 year		90%	85%
Adult	Variable	99.9%	99.9%

+ = minor; + + = major; − = uncommon; ↓ = decreased; ± = sometimes.
*% = death (i.e., attrition).

only one X chromosome is present with 44 autosomes. Phenotypically (physically), such individuals are female. The newborn may demonstrate webbing of the neck, there may be coarctation of the aorta, and edema of the hands and feet is often present. The neck webbing and edema may have a similar cause, with disordered lymphatic drainage being a common link. Lymphangioma (cystic hygroma) of the neck may be present in utero, and the peripheral edema seems to be much more prominent at birth than later.

The next most common sex chromosomal abnormality is Klinefelter's syndrome, in which an X chromosome is added, giving an XXY configuration. It is difficult to recognize this diagnosis in the neonate, although cryptorchidism (testes absent from the scrotum) is common.

CLEFT LIP AND PALATE

Introduction

The embryologic development of the face provides a good explanation of the different types of abnormalities encountered. Simply put, the two maxillary processes developing horizontally should fuse with the frontal process developing vertically. If fusion fails on one or both sides, then a unilateral or bilateral cleft results. A central single cleft lip indicates failure of the frontal process to develop normally and may reflect failure of forebrain development. This is obviously of more serious prognostic significance. The incidence is about 1 in 1000 live births.

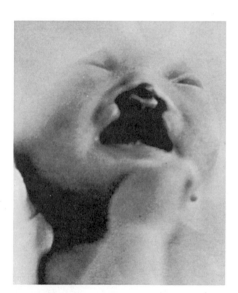

FIGURE 8–10. Bilateral cleft lip and palate, demonstrating the presence of the frontal process, which should fuse with the maxillary processes.

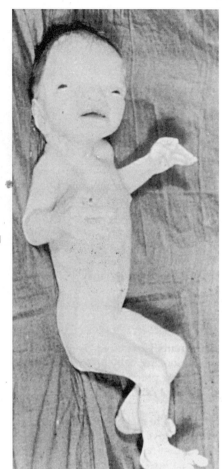

FIGURE 8–11. This baby exhibits marked hypertelorism.

Etiology

There is a definite genetic component, with the chance of siblings and offspring of affected individuals having cleft lip (Fig. 8–10), or cleft palate, or both, being 40 times that seen in the general population. Certain ethnic groups (e.g., Japanese) have a higher prevalence.

As indicated earlier, this disorder may occur in association with other abnormalities (e.g., trisomy D), and a search for other congenital defects should be made. It may be part of the first arch syndrome, which also includes micrognathia (with cleft palate, the Pierre Robin syndrome), hypertelorism (Fig. 8–11), and mandibulofacial dysostosis (Fig. 8–12). These disorders may result from maldevelopment or suppression of the stapedial artery (McKenzie, 1958).

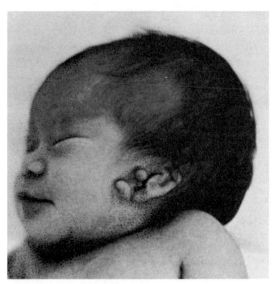

FIGURE 8–12. Several preauricular skin tags and a malformed ear make deafness a definite possibility in this baby.

Diagnosis

Cleft lip provides little difficulty, but palatal defects may be observed only by careful examination. Feeding difficulty may be the first indicator of a posterior palatal defect (see Fig. 3–2).

Management

Sympathetic interaction with the parents is required. Early repair of the cleft lip provides a more normal-looking baby and may facilitate parent-infant interaction. A generally good prognosis can be predicted for those with lateral defects in the lip, but a central cleft lip necessitates a more guarded outlook.

Various techniques have been employed to make feeding easier, with some workers using a palatal prosthesis to give the baby something firm to suck against (some babies can even breast-feed with such a prosthesis). Cleft palate repair is usually undertaken after 18 months of age. Speech therapy and orthodontics may also be necessary.

Summary

These easily recognized defects occur alone or in association with other abnormalities and are considered part of the first arch syndrome. Early management is directed at closure of the cleft lip and facilitation of feeding.

CLUBFOOT

Introduction

Although several different abnormalities of position of the foot exist (e.g., calcaneovalgus deformity and metatarsus varus deformity), the most common abnormality is talipes equinovarus. If a foot in this position can be brought to a normal position, it is probably a result of mechanical forces acting in utero and may be called a transient, or false, clubfoot. A fixed deformity, or one that cannot be completely corrected by manipulation of the foot, is a true clubfoot.

Etiology

Denis Browne considered all clubfeet to be mechanical in origin, but undoubtedly genetic factors are also involved. Talipes equinovarus is also seen in association with other abnormalities in which muscle activity has been compromised (e.g., meningomyelocele and arthrogryposis multiplex congenita).

Diagnosis

In addition to the distinctions made earlier regarding clubfoot, there is frequently a deep crease in the sole of the foot and another below the medial malleolus (Figs. 8–13 and 8–14). Radiographic evidence may confirm the diagnosis.

Management

At least three different kinds of correction of this deformity have been tried: taping, plaster casts, and shoe splints. Each has its advocates, but attention to the hind foot seems most important, and a heel cord–lengthening procedure

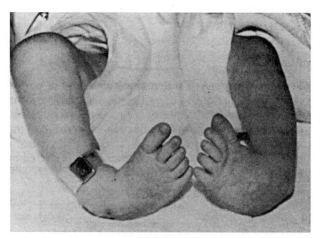

FIGURE 8–13. Bilateral talipes equinovarus (clubfeet).

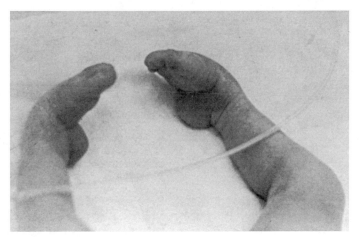

FIGURE 8–14. Another example of bilateral talipes equinovarus, with the obvious deep plantar creases commonly seen with true clubfoot.

may also be required to achieve a satisfactory position. These issues require a consultation from an orthopedic surgeon.

Summary

The classic form of clubfoot is talipes equinovarus, in which the foot cannot be manipulated into normal position. Both genetic and mechanical factors are implicated in the cause, and immediate and long-term orthopedic management is required.

POLYDACTYLY

The presence of extra fingers and toes may occur alone or in combination with other abnormalities (Fig. 8–15). It is more common in the black population. If there is a very narrow pedicle between the fingers and the hand, simple ligation may be effective treatment, but frequently, operative intervention is required.

SYNDACTYLY

Minor degrees of syndactyly (fusion of fingers or toes) are seen in a significant proportion of the general population, especially between the second and third toes. More obvious syndactyly (Fig. 8–16) may be transmitted within families or may be seen as part of numerous syndromes (e.g., Apert's syndrome, or acrocephaly-syndactyly). Amniotic bands have also been implicated in the production of syndactyly.

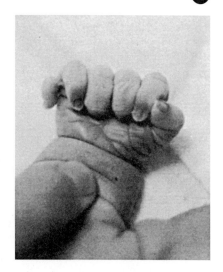

FIGURE 8–15. Polydactyly, with the super-numerary digit attached by a narrow pedicle.

NEURAL TUBE DEFECTS (MENINGOMYELOCELE AND ANENCEPHALY)

Introduction

Several different types of developmental failure of the neural tube exist. When the cerebral hemispheres fail to develop, the problem is called anenceph-aly. When the spinal column is involved, the defects are usually classified together as meningomyelocele (or spina bifida cystica). The location of the defect, together with certain associated features, may have considerable bearing on the outcome. After an era of immediate surgical closure in all cases, a more

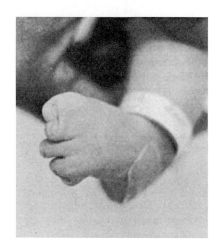

FIGURE 8–16. Syndactyly, showing fusion of the first and second and the fourth and fifth toes.

balanced approach is currently being adopted. Obviously, no treatment exists for anencephaly.

Etiology

One of the more intriguing aspects of the epidemiology of congenital abnormalities is that related to meningomyelocele and the related disorder of anencephaly. A particularly high incidence of these disorders is found in Ireland, with a decreasing incidence found in the United Kingdom as one moves from the northern and western regions toward the southeast corner. An association with potato blight is debatable, and the role of goitrogens is also controversial. Hyperthermia is another factor implicated, and the adequacy of intake of periconceptional vitamins has recently been cited. Initial, uncontrolled studies of multivitamin supplementation suggested that recurrences may be prevented. More recently, by use of a randomized double-blind approach, folic acid supplementation was shown to be substantially protective when used around the time of conception, but other vitamins were not. Folic acid supplementation following a previously affected pregnancy had a 72% protective effect. Under usual circumstances, the chance of either meningomyelocele or anencephaly recurring in

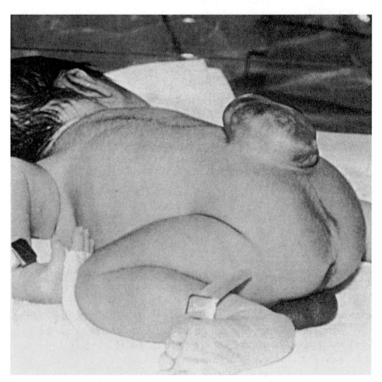

FIGURE 8–17. Lumbosacral meningomyelocele, showing the lower extremities in good position. Chances for successful surgical correction are good.

a subsequent pregnancy is considerably higher than that in the general population. However, another factor to be considered is the steady decline in the incidence of myelomeningocele in the northeastern region of the United States and elsewhere.

Embryologic development of the spinal cord provides a logical explanation of the different types of disorders. Arrest at the neural-plate stage results in a myelocele, partial invagination results in a true meningomyelocele, and almost complete invagination may leave a meningocele (Figs. 8–17 and 8–18). When a defect in the vertebral column only is present, the condition is called spina bifida occulta.

Diagnosis

There is usually little difficulty in making this diagnosis if one observes the baby carefully. Frequently, only a thin membrane covers the defect, although occasionally a thin layer of skin provides protection (usually a meningocele). Frequently, there is leakage of spinal fluid and predisposition to infection.

The most striking diagnostic advance in recent years has been the ability to detect neural tube defects prenatally with the use of amniotic fluid α-fetoprotein levels. Elevated levels may be detected when an open lesion is present (i.e., not covered by skin) at a stage (16 weeks' gestation) when the pregnancy may be safely terminated if so desired. α-Fetoprotein levels have also been determined

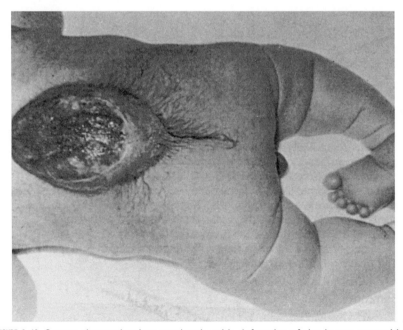

FIGURE 8–18. Severe thoracolumbar myelocele with deformity of the lower extremities. Chances for successful surgical correction are poor.

on maternal sera and have been used as a screening test for these disorders (see Chapter 1). At present, α-fetoprotein levels have been most helpful when a previous pregnancy has resulted in a neural tube defect (either anencephaly [Fig. 8–19] or meningomyelocele). Another useful prenatal test is diagnostic ultrasound. These techniques are probably more valuable in reassuring the mother of a normal fetus and allowing a pregnancy to continue than in deciding when pregnancy should be terminated. When doubt exists, it may be possible to perform ultrasonographically guided fetoscopy.

Management of Meningomyelocele

Rarely in neonatology is a team approach more desirable than in the treatment of a child with meningomyelocele. Although the pediatrician provides the focus for the family, the neurologist, neurosurgeon, orthopedic surgeon, urologist, and radiologist are all involved in the treatment of these children. Perhaps the most important team member of all is a sympathetic social worker.

After advocating early closure in the early 1960s, the Sheffield group in England moved to a more selective approach in the early 1970s. Findings more likely to be associated with a poor prognosis (and hence a delay in surgery) are associated hydrocephalus, a thoracolumbar defect, loss of motor function below L-2, and loss of sensation below 1-3. The finding of a lacunar skull (Lükenschä-del) without apparent hydrocephalus may also indicate a poor prognosis. Debate continues regarding the best time to operate; recent evidence supports careful evaluation and discussion during the first week after delivery.

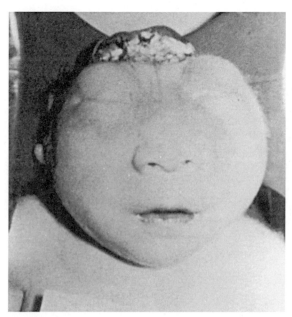

FIGURE 8–19. Anencephalus, showing small amounts of the cerebral hemispheres protruding where the skull should be.

Long-term management frequently revolves around orthopedic care and treatment of kidney infections.

Summary

Neural tube defects occur in several different forms, and geographic differences in incidence exist. Prenatal detection by α-fetoprotein level assessment and diagnostic ultrasonographic examination may be possible. Early surgical closure of meningomyelocele should be selective, and management is multidisciplinary. Prevention of recurrence may be possible.

HYDROCEPHALUS

Introduction

Although most frequently encountered as a complication of meningomyelocele, either preoperatively or postoperatively, dilation and excessive pressure within the ventricular system of the brain may be seen as an isolated congenital abnormality or may be an acquired problem in infants who have meningitis or intracranial hemorrhage (see p. 236).

Etiology

Blockage at some point in the circulation of cerebrospinal fluid is implicated in practically all cases, the most common obstruction being at the aqueduct of Sylvius (usually noncommunicating). Destruction as a result of viral infection has been documented in experimental animals and can produce hydrocephalus or, more likely, hydranencephalus.

Diagnosis

The more obvious cases of hydrocephalus can be easily spotted prenatally with diagnostic ultrasonographic study. Even less obvious cases may be detected by use of ventricle to cerebral hemisphere ratio. However, associated anomalies make prenatal intervention of limited value. Problems may occur at the time of delivery, particularly if the diagnosis has not been made prenatally. The infant with hydrocephalus and a large head (Fig. 8–20) has to be differentiated from the infant with hydranencephaly (fluid-filled skull but no cerebral hemispheres) and macrocephaly (excessive amount of brain substance). Hydranencephaly is easily recognized by transillumination (Figs. 8–21 and 8–22). Pneumoencephalography has now been replaced by either computed tomography or cerebral ultrasonography (see Chapter 34).

In the absence of a computed tomographic scanner or diagnostic ultrasonographic equipment, careful measurements of head circumference (occipitofrontal) are most likely to detect hydrocephalus early in those cases that are not obvious at birth. Even a normal rate of head growth may be an ominous sign

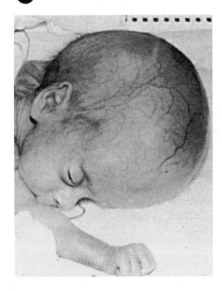

FIGURE 8–20. Baby with hydrocephalus, showing both the disproportionately large calvarium when compared with the face and the prominence of the scalp veins.

in the sick infant (i.e., if there is minimal increase in weight, the head growth may be disproportionate).

Management

Early diagnosis (using computed tomographic or ultrasonographic study), is likely to give the most satisfactory results. In cases of posthemorrhagic hydrocephalus, some infants can be treated with sequential lumbar punctures and others with ventriculostomy drainage to remove cerebrospinal fluid so that operative intervention is not required. If unsuccessful, or in patients with congenital hydrocephalus, a ventriculoperitoneal shunt is usually inserted. Compressive head wrapping was used in selected cases, but this now seems to have been abandoned. Complications with the shunt are blockage and infection, and it is difficult to predict which infants will develop such problems.

Many infants who were formerly considered to have posthemorrhagic hydrocephalus have proved to have ventriculomegaly that either resolved spontaneously or did not progress.

Summary

Hydrocephalus is the result of increased intraventricular pressure caused by blockage in the circulation of cerebrospinal fluid. It may be congenital or acquired but often requires surgical management. Early recognition seems to offer the most hope for a good prognosis.

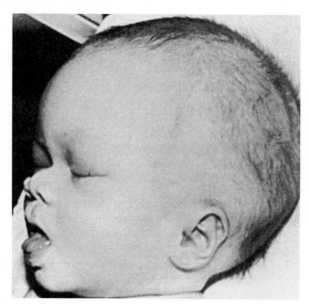

FIGURE 8–21. Baby with a large head that proved to be hydranencephaly. The head became much larger later.

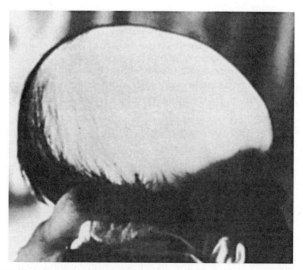

FIGURE 8–22. Transillumination of the skull of a baby with hydranencephaly. The same dramatic picture was seen in the baby in Figure 8–21, showing fluid replacing the cerebral hemispheres.

ABDOMINAL WALL DEFECTS (see pp. 314 to 317)

It is important to distinguish omphalocele (in which the intestines remain in the body stalk or umbilical cord) from gastroschisis (a defect to the right of the insertion of the umbilical cord) because omphalocele may have associated abnormalities, whereas gastroschisis usually does not.

IMPERFORATE ANUS

Introduction

This easily recognized abnormality (see Fig. 3–12) is important because it is part of an association between different types of congenital malformation. This link has been described as the VATER association, the acronym for *v*ertebral and *v*ascular, *a*nal, *t*racheo*e*sophageal, and *r*enal and *r*adial abnormalities. More recently, the acronym has been designated VACTERL, with C for cardiovascular and L for limb, instead of radial, abnormalities.

Etiology

Imperforate anus results from breakdown of the anorectal membrane and may be associated with a defective urorectal membrane, which may result in rectovaginal fistula in the female or rectovesical fistula in the male.

Diagnosis

This disorder is frequently encountered by the nurse who takes the first temperature on the baby (and for this reason, initial temperature is often taken rectally). Apart from a search for associated anomalies, diagnosis centers around radiologic assessment of the distance of the rectum from the anus and whether or not a fistulous communication is present. If air has entered the large bowel, an x-ray study of the abdomen with the baby in an inverted position and a marker over the anus should provide an adequate assessment of the distance between the rectum and the anus (Fig. 8–23). It may also outline a fistulous connection.

Management

The surgeon's task is made easier by the diagnostic technique just mentioned. A short segment defect (anal membrane) can be corrected in one stage. When a longer segment is involved, a colostomy is usually performed first, and a more definitive repair is undertaken at a later date. The timing of such decisions is inevitably related to any associated malformation. A urine examination should be followed by an intravenous pyelogram and voiding cystourethrogram, but these tests may be supplemented or preceded by ultrasonography of the kidney (nephrosonography).

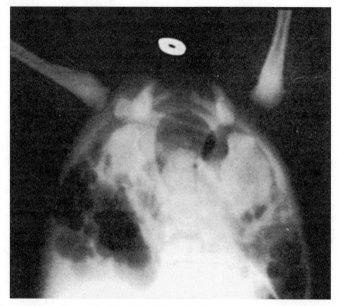

FIGURE 8–23. An inverted (upside-down) radiograph showing a considerable gap between a marker placed over an imperforate anus and the lower end of the bowel.

Summary

Imperforate anus is frequently associated with other anomalies in the VATER association and frequently has an associated fistula. Definitive surgical correction can sometimes be achieved early, but, more frequently, it is delayed.

RECOGNIZABLE BY EXAMINATION AND INVESTIGATION

TRACHEOESOPHAGEAL FISTULA

Introduction

The association of tracheoesophageal fistula with abnormalities such as imperforate anus (VATER association), mentioned earlier, provides a natural link with the previous section. Although tracheoesophageal fistula is an infrequently encountered problem (incidence, approximately 1 in 2500 births), it is important that it be recognized as early as possible so that appropriate surgical intervention can be undertaken.

Etiology

When one remembers that the lungs develop from the foregut, it is a little easier to understand why this kind of anomaly occurs. Although several different types of defect exist, by far the most common is esophageal atresia with a communication (fistula) between the trachea and the lower part of the esophagus. This type is discussed further. Exogenous progestogens and estrogens have been implicated in the production of all the anomalies in the VATER association.

Diagnosis

High intestinal atresia may be anticipated prenatally when polyhydramnios is present. An excessive amount of mucus in a baby (the so-called mucusy or juicy baby) within the first few hours should always suggest esophageal atresia, with or without a fistula. If the defect is not recognized before the first feeding, the baby may vomit and aspirate whatever is being fed, possibly resulting in respiratory difficulty. It is also possible, when a fistula exists, that gastric secretions will be transmitted to the tracheobronchial tree. Passage of a soft rubber or plastic catheter into the esophagus frequently defines the level of esophageal atresia. Occasionally, the catheter curls up on itself in a dilated esophageal segment, so that one gains the impression that it may have entered the stomach. The pH of the aspirate should be tested and should be definitely acidic if from the stomach, although the pH of gastric secretions is less acidic in the immediate newborn period.

Radiographs of the upper chest show a dilated upper esophageal segment with air contrast in most cases. Only occasionally is injection of contrast material necessary. Abdominal x-ray study usually shows air in the bowel but does not if no true fistulous communication exists. A less common type, which can cause confusion because it is difficult to outline, is the H-type fistula. This may produce a classic triad of choking during feeding, abdominal distension, and pneumonitis, with persistent chest x-ray findings. It may be diagnosed by measurement of intragastric oxygen concentration while varying the oxygen concentration administered through an endotracheal tube.

Management

Early recognition of the baby at risk should initiate a search for an obstructive lesion before the first feeding. Surgical intervention is required and depends on the size of the infant, the type of defect, and the distance between the two portions of the esophagus. The outlook for infants with a single problem is quite good but becomes much worse when associated abnormalities are present. Despite repair, lower esophageal sphincter incompetence may be present that results in recurrent pneumonia.

Summary

Tracheoesophageal fistula usually accompanies esophageal atresia and may be part of the VATER association. Early recognition allows the best hope for successful surgical intervention.

DIAPHRAGMATIC HERNIA

Introduction

Several types of diaphragmatic hernia exist, most of which are not life threatening. The only type causing a major problem is herniation through a posterolateral defect in the diaphragm, which is approximately in the location of the foramen of Bochdalek. The incidence is about 1 in 2000 births.

Etiology

The failure in closure of the diaphragm occurs at approximately 8 weeks' gestation. The defect is encountered more frequently on the left, although this may be an erroneous impression because the liver may protect a defect on the right. As the intestines return to the abdominal cavity from the body stalk, they are able to pass through the defect into the thoracic cavity, where they inhibit the growth of the lung. If the defect is very large and other abdominal viscera herniate with the intestines, so much displacement may be present that the contralateral lung is also affected.

More recently, another possible cause of diaphragmatic hernia has been described. It is not clear whether this is an acquired disorder or whether a congenital lesion is revealed by respiratory difficulty, but several (26 in a 1989 review) babies with pneumonia caused by group B streptococci have demonstrated right-sided diaphragmatic hernias, which became apparent several days after birth (see Bibliography).

Diagnosis

Occasionally, the defect is so large and lung hypoplasia so great that it is impossible to resuscitate the baby in the delivery room. More frequently, the baby has relatively minor difficulty initially but begins to have increasing difficulty within the first few hours after delivery. Most babies have a somewhat scaphoid abdomen at delivery, but the infant with diaphragmatic hernia continues to have a scaphoid abdomen in most instances. In addition, a classic triad of symptoms has been described, namely (1) cyanosis, (2) dyspnea, and (3) "dextrocardia." This apparent dextrocardia is the result of displacement of the mediastinum, which tends to become progressively more pronounced as air fills the intestines within the thoracic cavity. Heart sounds are therefore more easily heard on the right side. Together with the hypoplasia of the lungs, mediastinal shift also produces respiratory distress and contributes to an inability to maintain adequate oxygenation.

The differential diagnosis includes a left tension pneumothorax (but this is usually much more acute in onset) and true dextrocardia with an intrinsic congenital heart defect. Chest x-ray study usually allows the diagnosis to be made rapidly (Fig. 8–24), although the appearance may be almost completely opaque until air enters the bowel. Because it produces a unilateral bubbly appearance, cystic adenomatoid malformation may also cause confusion.

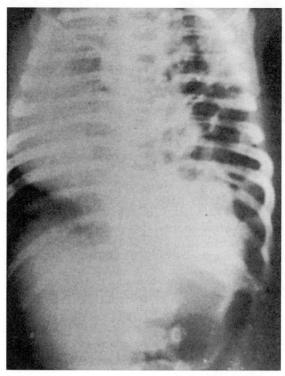

FIGURE 8–24. Diaphragmatic hernia, with displacement of the mediastinum to the right side and the air-filled intestine in the left thoracic cavity.

Management

Early diagnosis provides the best chance for early surgical correction, which is critical in the infant with hypoplastic lungs. Infants who survive for several days before a diagnosis is made have less severely affected lungs and are likely to do well.

Two important maneuvers should be initiated in any baby who needs to be transported to a center for neonatal surgery. The first should be performed in all cases (whether transported or not) and involves the passage of an orogastric tube to decompress the stomach and minimize air distention of the intestines. The second is the insertion of an endotracheal tube, so that if resuscitation is required during transfer, the air will pass directly to the lungs (bag-and-mask ventilation frequently produces gastric distension). A chest tube is usually left in place postoperatively to facilitate the reexpansion of the hypoplastic lung (Fig. 8–25). Postoperative management may also be complicated by a tendency toward persistent pulmonary hypertension (persistent fetal circulation). When persistent pulmonary hypertension is severe, it may be necessary to use extra corporeal membrane oxygenation or other adjunctive therapy (see Chapter 9). Despite the use of extracorporeal membrane oxygenation (sometimes before

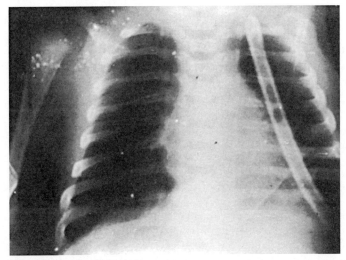

FIGURE 8–25. Same baby as in Figure 8–24, after surgery, with return of the mediastinum and reexpansion of the lungs (a chest tube is in the left thoracic cavity).

surgery), infants with diaphragmatic hernia with clinical manifestations at birth have a poor prognosis (approximately 50% survival).

Summary

This infrequently encountered problem is so life threatening that the essentials of diagnosis should be memorized by everybody caring for newborn infants. Prompt recognition allows the best chance for early surgical intervention, but hypoplastic lungs and persistent pulmonary hypertension may complicate recovery.

DIAPHRAGMATIC EVENTRATION OR PARALYSIS

Significant respiratory difficulty may be encountered with either eventration (incomplete development) or paralysis of the diaphragm (resulting from phrenic nerve palsy). Neither of these problems is as acutely life threatening as diaphragmatic hernia. The diaphragm usually appears higher on one side than on the other.

HIRSCHSPRUNG'S DISEASE (CONGENITAL MEGACOLON; AGANGLIONOSIS OF COLON)

Incidence

Hirschsprung's disease is relatively uncommon (approximately 1 in 3000 to 1 in 10,000 live births) but may be one of the more common causes of intestinal obstruction in the newborn. On the other hand, it is frequently overlooked in the first weeks (and even months) of life.

Pathophysiology

The absence (or paucity) of ganglion cells in the wall of the distal colon and/or rectum leads to persistent spasm of this portion of intestine. As a result of this obstruction, the proximal bowel becomes increasingly dilated, resulting in abdominal distension.

Diagnosis

Most babies with Hirschsprung's disease are born at term. There may be delay in the passage of the first meconium stool (see p. 312), or there may be evidence of the meconium plug syndrome with apparent improvement after passage of a plug of meconium. The abdominal x-ray study may show the nonspecific finding of dilated loops of bowel. The classic picture of megacolon above a narrowed segment may not develop for several weeks. Diagnosis can frequently be made by barium enema studies. The narrowed segment of rectosigmoid may not be seen, but the presence of barium on a follow-up film (taken 24 hours after insertion of the barium) is strongly suggestive of Hirschsprung's disease. In addition, anorectal manometry may be helpful in making a diagnosis, although not all authorities agree.

Management

On the basis of the suspicions mentioned earlier, the baby should be seen by a pediatric surgeon. Some surgeons may elect to perform a full-thickness rectal biopsy with the patient under anesthesia and then perform a colostomy if no ganglion cells are seen on frozen section. Others prefer to perform a biopsy of the mucosa and submucosa with a biopsy capsule kit. The advantage of performing a rectal biopsy at the bedside (or in the treatment room) is that anesthesia is not required, and the specimen can be evaluated more leisurely before a decision about the need for colostomy is made. Definitive treatment is carried out toward the end of the first year of life. Numerous surgical procedures have been used, the Duhamel procedure (or variations) being the most popular.

Summary

This relatively uncommon condition is one of the more common causes of intestinal obstruction and is the result of congenital absence of ganglion cells in the rectum and/or colon. Delay in passing meconium (with abdominal distension) initiates a barium enema study. Colostomy is performed in the neonatal period and definitive surgery deferred.

CONGENITAL DISLOCATION OF THE HIP

Incidence

This disorder occurs in approximately 1 in 800 deliveries. It is one of the few neonatal disorders with a significantly greater frequency in females (male to female = 1:8).

Etiology

Frank breech presentation and certain neuromuscular disorders (e.g., meningomyelocele) contribute to the occurrence of congenital dislocation of the hip. Several years ago, the estrogenic hormone relaxin was implicated as the predominant causative factor, but, in addition to mechanical factors, congenital hip dislocation seems to be a hereditary disorder. Development of a shallow acetabulum and generalized joint laxity seem to be the most important causal factors.

Diagnosis

Every newborn infant should be examined by use of the technique described in the section on physical examination (see p. 26). Early recognition may prevent months of misery. However, despite careful neonatal evaluation, some cases may not become apparent until later on in the first year. Late diagnosis may be related to a relatively short gestational period and a low mean birth weight as well as physician's failure to perform the examination correctly (if at all). There are three different phenomena that can occur with the use of Ortolani's and the dislocation provocation (Barlow's) maneuvers. The hips may be subluxable (slight movement), dislocatable (obvious movement), or dislocated (may be difficult to replace in the acetabulum). When the hip is dislocated, backward movement of the thigh (with one hand) is not transmitted to the pelvis (fixed with the other) and produces a sensation of floating free, or "telescoping." Asymmetry of the skin folds posteriorly is an unreliable sign in the neonate.

Although radiologic investigation has been traditionally used to confirm the diagnosis, considerable difficulty is encountered because of the lack of ossification of the head of the femur and the acetabular margins in the neonate. Introduction of ultrasonographic evaluation promises to alleviate this difficulty because cartilage can be demonstrated quite readily with this medium.

Management

Subluxable hips may be treated with the triple-diaper technique, but some form of splint technique is usually required to keep dislocatable and dislocated hips in abduction. Perhaps the best of these is the Malmo splint (Von Rosen splint), which is a malleable metal splint covered by washable rubber that grips the baby's shoulders, sides, and thighs. Because it is washable, it requires infrequent manipulation. However, orthopedic consultation is always indicated when hips are dislocatable or dislocated. Because some splints have maintained an overcorrection and have resulted in avascular necrosis of the femoral head, the Pavlik harness has gained favor. This harness positions the femur in flexion but allows motion within a restricted range and allows the hip to self-reduce.

Summary

Careful examination of the hips is one of the most important aspects of the routine neonatal examination. Hereditary, mechanical, and hormonal factors have been implicated in the etiology. Early treatment is relatively short, simple, and painless. Delay in diagnosis for several months may result in prolonged and complicated surgical management.

CONGENITAL HEART DISEASE

Introduction

Many forms of congenital heart disease may present in the neonatal period. It is impossible to give a detailed account of all types that may be encountered, but there are certain broad categories that may allow one to make an intelligent guess before seeking consultation from a cardiologist. Another important fact to remember is that heart murmurs heard on the first day of life are unlikely to be associated with intrinsic congenital heart disease; such murmurs probably result from changes in flow through the ductus arteriosus.

Etiology

Most cardiac defects can be timed between 6 and 8 weeks' gestation. There is undoubtedly a genetic predisposition, and the chance of a subsequent infant having congenital heart disease rises to 1 in 50 (from 1 in 250) after one affected infant. The more complicated defects are likely to arise earliest in gestation. It is therefore not surprising that congenital heart disease is frequently associated with other defects or syndromes. Numerous viral agents (particularly coxsackie-viruses) have been implicated in the production of congenital heart disease.

Diagnosis

Most infants with congenital heart disease are of appropriate weight for gestational age, although infants with transposition of the great vessels are frequently larger than average. However, for other forms of congenital heart disease, there is a slight preponderance for low birth weight (12% versus 7 to 8%). The most commonly encountered cardiac defect with present-day pulmonary management is patent ductus arteriosus, the main features of which are a systolic murmur at the second or third left interspace, which may radiate down the left sternal edge. Only rarely is the classic "machinery murmur" heard early in the neonatal period, although the diastolic component tends to become more obvious with age. Bounding peripheral pulses (dorsalis pedis and posterior tibial) or a wide pulse pressure are almost invariably found when shunting through the ductus is significant. In some babies, echocardiography reveals significant ductal shunting, without evidence of a murmur.

Signs of congestive cardiac failure also may be present. These are (roughly in decreasing order of frequency) (1) enlarging liver, (2) large heart on chest x-ray study, (3) slight fullness of the anterior fontanel, (4) peripheral edema, and (5) moist rales (crepitations) in the lungs. Tachypnea is also an early finding, but it may be present for many reasons.

Patent ductus arteriosus is included in the category of potentially cyanotic congenital heart disease. This category also includes ventricular septal defect, atrial septal defect, endocardial cushion defects, and tetralogy of Fallot. With ventricular septal defect, a murmur may not be apparent for 2 weeks or more and consequently may not be detected until the first follow-up visit after discharge from the nursery. In addition, tachypnea, poor weight gain, and plethoric lung fields on x-ray study are usually found. Pure atrial septal defect does not usually present in the neonatal period. Tetralogy of Fallot is frequently overlooked in the neonatal period, but the component of pulmonary stenosis may produce a soft systolic murmur, which does not necessitate further investigation unless cyanosis is present.

A hyperoxia test frequently fails to relieve cyanosis (see p. 376). The most commonly encountered types of congenital heart disease in this category are (1) transposition of the great vessels, (2) complicated truncus arteriosus, (3) tricuspid atresia, (4) total anomalous pulmonary venous return, (5) hypoplastic left heart syndrome, and (6) hypoplastic right heart syndrome.

Helpful indicators for each of these are (1) normal or heavy birth weight, (2) no splitting of the second heart sound, (3) pulsatile liver, (4) confusion with pulmonary disease, (5) poor peripheral pulses, and (6) prominent left-sided forces on the electrocardiograph (compared with the prominent right-sided forces usually seen in the neonate).

An estimated 75% of congenital heart disease remains undetected in the neonatal period or does not have signs or symptoms significant enough to warrant complete investigation. Attention is given to disorders that produce cyanosis or distress in the early neonatal period. Enough shunting may occur through a patent ductus arteriosus (soon after birth) to keep the baby pink. However, when the ductus starts to close, increasing difficulty may be seen. In the first or second day of life, changes in heart size may not have occurred, which confuses the picture further. Most classifications (that have a functional basis) divide cyanotic heart disease into three major categories associated with (1) decreased pulmonary blood flow, (2) increased pulmonary blood flow, or (3) pulmonary venous congestion, but the last two are usually combined when the chest x-ray study is considered to have increased pulmonary vascular markings. Combinations of these or complex lesions may also exist.

Table 8–2 is a simplification that may allow a tentative diagnosis to be made when cyanosis is prominent. However, the opinion of a pediatric cardiologist should be obtained as soon as possible because cyanotic congenital heart disease is usually a medical emergency, and most forms and cases of congenital heart disease are amenable to surgery.

Heart disease that does not produce cyanosis may still result in significant distress in the neonatal period, although this is unlikely to occur in the first few

TABLE 8–2. DIFFERENTIATION OF CYANOTIC CONGENITAL HEART DISEASE

Pulmonary Vascular Markings (X-ray Study)	Heart Size (X-ray Study)	ECG	Systolic Murmur	Diagnosis
Decreased	Small	LVH	No	Tricuspid atresia
	Small	RVH	±	Pulmonary atresia or stenosis (with VSD)
	Small	RVH	Yes	Tetralogy of Fallot
			No	TGA (early)
	Large	LVH	±	Ebstein's anomaly (tricuspid valve)
	Large	RVH	No	Pulmonary atresia
			Yes	Severe pulmonary stenosis
Increased	Small or large	LVH	No	Tricuspid atresia and TGA
	Small or large	RVH	±	Hypoplastic left heart
		RVH	No	TGA
		RVH	Yes (soft)	TAPVR
		RVH	±	TGA and VSD
	Large	BVH	Yes	Single ventricle Truncus arteriosus Double outlet RV

BVH = biventricular hypertrophy; ECG = electrocardiogram; LVH = left ventricular hypertrophy; RVH = right ventricular hypertrophy; TGA = transposition of great arteries; TAPVR = total anomalous pulmonary venous return; VSD = ventricular septal defect; ± = sometimes.

days of life. The major diagnoses are provided in Table 8–3. Most of these conditions give rise to congestive heart failure with tachypnea and poor feeding, and poor weight gain is almost invariable.

Management

There are several principles of management to be followed:

1. Murmurs in the first 24 hours are usually benign and should be reevaluated.

2. Differentiation from pulmonary disease is sometimes difficult but may be helped by the hyperoxia test (see Chapter 34).

3. Recognition of probable (or even possible) congenital heart disease is the goal.

4. Definitive diagnosis usually requires the opinion and investigations of a cardiologist.

Blood pressure should always be measured, most reliably with an intraarterial catheter and a pressure transducer; however, newer noninvasive methods using oscillometry can provide reliable and continuous measurements. Doppler

TABLE 8-3. ACYANOTIC CONGENITAL HEART DISEASE

Pulmonary Vascular Markings (x-ray Study)	Heart Size (x-ray Study)	ECG	Systolic Murmur	Diagnosis
Normal	Normal or large	RVH	Yes	Pulmonary stenosis
	Normal or large	RVH	No	Mitral stenosis
	Normal or large	LVH	Yes	Coarctation of the aorta
	Normal or large	LVH	Yes	Aortic stenosis
	Normal or large	LVH	?	Mitral regurgitation
	Large	LVH	No	Endocardial fibroelastosis
	Large	LVH	No	Glycogen storage disease Type II (Pompe's disease)
	Large	LVH	No	Myocarditis
Increased	Normal or large	RVH	No	ASD
		RVH	?	L→R shunts with pulmonary HT
	Normal or large	LVH	Yes	PDA
		LVH	Yes	VSD
		LVH	?	Arteriovenous fistula

ASD = atrial septal defect; ECG = electrocardiogram; HT = hypertension; PDA = patent ductus arteriosus; VSD = ventricular septal defect.

ultrasonographic devices can also provide good systolic pressures. Less reliable techniques may still demonstrate differences between upper and lower extremities or reveal very low pressures. Thus, if more sophisticated methods are not available, either flush blood pressure or detection of return of flow by manual palpation of the radial artery as cuff pressure is lowered can be used. Whenever coarctation of the aorta is suspected, blood pressure in the upper and lower limbs should be measured.

The hematocrit should always be measured when cyanotic congenital heart disease is suspected. This initially may be estimated by a hematocrit level obtained by warm heel stick. If this value is over 70%, the venous hematocrit should be measured. If this is greater than 65%, hyperviscosity is almost certainly present and should be corrected by phlebotomy and infusion of a plasma expander or by partial exchange transfusion. In some centers, a large number of cases of high hematocrit syndrome are included among babies referred for cyanotic heart disease (see pp. 242 to 243).

Experience with echocardiography suggests that many diagnoses can be made with this technique without resorting to cardiac catheterization. Such decisions are in the hands of the cardiologist. The protective effect of a patent ductus arteriosus in some babies with cyanotic congenital heart disease has been a stimulus to maintain the patency of the ductus arteriosus by administration of prostaglandin E. On the other hand, patent ductus arteriosus has been treated in many cases by administration of a prostaglandin synthetase inhibitor, such as indomethacin.

Congestive failure should be managed with digoxin (0.03 to 0.05 mg/kg digitalizing dose in divided doses) and diuretics (furosemide or ethacrynic acid, 1 mg/kg). An alternative to digitalization (which seems to be safer) is administration of the maintenance dosage of digoxin daily for 1 week, after which a steady state level will be reached. A dose of 0.016 mg/kg has been suggested.

Summary

This brief review of congenital heart disease is a mere introduction to the subject, and other texts should be consulted for specific diagnoses. In addition to cyanosis, the findings of tachypnea, poor feeding, and failure to gain weight should all suggest congenital heart disease. The hyperoxia test may help to differentiate pulmonary disease, and hematocrit determination may eliminate the diagnosis of hyperviscosity. Further investigation is usually carried out under the guidance of a cardiologist.

GENETIC COUNSELING

INTRODUCTION

Whenever a child is born with a congenital abnormality that causes concern (i.e., more than a minor abnormality, e.g., low-set ears), it is important to determine the cause of the abnormality. When this information is available, an intelligent discussion can be held with the parents about the possibility of a similar occurrence in a subsequent pregnancy. With drug-related abnormalities, the chance of recurrence is negligible unless administration of the drug is continued, such as with anticonvulsants. With virally induced abnormalities, recurrence is unlikely; with genetic disease, the recurrence risk can be estimated; and with chromosomal abnormalities, it may be necessary to perform chromosomal analysis on the parents (especially with evidence of translocation).

Many obstetric techniques are available that can help predict whether or not a fetus has a congenital abnormality. These may either allow a decision to be made about termination of pregnancy before 20 weeks gestation or provide reassurance that the fetus is normal. These techniques become particularly valuable when a previous pregnancy has resulted in a baby with a congenital abnormality. These techniques include the following:

AMNIOCENTESIS FOR CELL CULTURE. This assessment is used for chromosomal analysis and enzyme defects (inborn errors of metabolism).

α-FETOPROTEIN. Serum levels are obtained for screening, and amniotic fluid levels are obtained for diagnosis. Elevated levels indicate open neural tube defects, omphalocele, congenital nephrosis, and other abnormalities. Normal levels do not exclude closed neural tube defects. Decreased levels may be associated with chromosomal abnormality, especially when other serum markers are abnormal.

ULTRASONOGRAPHY. Current techniques provide delineation of most external abnormalities and many internal (renal and cardiac) anomalies. This information may be particularly helpful in conjunction with abnormal amniotic fluid α-fetoprotein levels.

FETOSCOPY. The fetus may be directly visualized by use of a small fiberoptic telescope. It is also possible to obtain fetal blood with some accuracy when fetoscopy is combined with ultrasonographic visualization.

CHORIONIC VILLUS SAMPLING. This assessment yields information similar to that found with amniocentesis but can be performed earlier in pregnancy, which may offer psychological as well as technical advantages if termination of pregnancy is the decision (see Chapter 1).

TYPES OF INHERITANCE (FOR SINGLE-GENE DISORDERS)

AUTOSOMAL-DOMINANT. In this type of inheritance, one parent has the same disorder or a new mutation; examples are achondroplasia and polydactyly.

AUTOSOMAL-RECESSIVE. In this type, both parents appear normal, but both carry a defective gene; examples are cystic fibrosis, galactosemia, phenylketonuria, and Tay-Sachs disease (accumulation of sphingolipid).

X-LINKED (SEX-LINKED) RECESSIVE. In this type, the mother carries the defective gene, and only male offspring are affected; examples are hemophilia, color blindness, and Duchenne's muscular dystrophy.

X-LINKED DOMINANT. In this type, heterozygous females are affected as well as males but usually less severely; example is vitamin D–resistant rickets.

In recent years, the picture regarding patterns of inheritance has become more complicated. Formerly, it was assumed that both the father and mother each contributed one of a pair of chromosomes. It is now known that both chromosomes of a pair may come from only one parent. This situation is called uniparental disomy. Under certain circumstances, the parent of origin may have an important influence on the clinical picture produced.

The best-known examples demonstrating these differences are the Prader-Willi and Angelman (happy puppet) syndromes. Prader-Willi syndrome (see Chapter 33) occurs when a critical region of chromosome 15 inherited from the father is missing or when both chromosomes 15 come from the mother. If both copies of chromosome 15 come from the father or there is missing chromosomal material on the maternal chromosome 15, Angelman's syndrome occurs.

The phenotypic differences resulting from inheritance from the father rather than the mother seem to be the result of "genomic imprinting." This is a situation in which differences in structure or function (i.e., the phenotype) reflect which parent was the source of the genetic material (Hall, 1992).

Prader-Willi syndrome is also an example of a "contiguous gene syndrome," where two genes come into close proximity with one another (because chromosome material is deleted) and result in a recognizable clinical

TABLE 8-4. RECURRENCE RISKS FOR CHROMOSOMAL AND SINGLE-GENE ABNORMALITIES

Inheritance Pattern	Parent Affected	Recurrence Risk
Chromosomal		
All spontaneous chromosomal abnormalities (e.g., aneuploidy)		1–2%
Parental carrier (includes translocation, certain inversions, and mosaicism)	Father	5–10%
	Mother	10–20%
Single gene		
Autosomal-dominant	Mother affected	50%
	Father affected	50%
Autosomal-recessive	Both parents carriers	25%
X-linked recessive (likelihood of having an affected male)	Mother carrier	50%
	Father affected	mutation rate
X-linked recessive (likelihood of having a carrier female)	Mother carrier	50%
	Father affected	100%

syndrome. (Other examples are DiGeorge's syndrome and Beckwith-Wiedemann syndrome.) The inheritance pattern is generally sporadic.

When multiple genetic and environmental factors appear to interact, the inheritance is called polygenic or multifactorial.

In counseling for X-linked traits, the Lyon hypothesis has important implications, as stated clearly by Dr. Michael Kaback (1978):

> . . . this hypothesis states that in any one cell, only one X chromosome is active. Thus, in a normal male (46 XY), the one X is always active, whereas in a normal female (46 XX) or in a Klinefelter's male (47 XXY), in each cell only one X chromosome is active, the other being inactivated. The nuclear chromatin mass (Barr body) represents the inactivated X chromosome, and is always found to be one less in number than the number of X chromosomes (e.g., XXX = two chromatin bodies). The decision as to which X chromosome is inactivated in each cell is made early in embryonic life. All the daughter cells of each of these primordial cells have the same X chromosome inactivated. In carrier females, half of the cells on the average would have the mutant X active, and in the other half the normal X would be active. The proportion of mutant to normal X chromosomes inactivated, however, follows a normal distribution.
>
> Thus, in some cases, in almost all of the cells the mutant X is active; at the other end of the spectrum in almost all the cells the mutant X is inactive . . .
>
> . . . one cannot completely rule out the carrier state, as an apparently normal female might, by chance, have the abnormal X inactivated in most of her cells, and thus be phenotypically normal.

The recurrence risks for chromosomal and single-gene abnormalities are

TABLE 8–5. RECURRENCE RISKS FOR COMMON CONGENITAL MALFORMATIONS (POLYGENIC)

Abnormality	Sex Ratio (M:F)	Population Frequency (per 1000)	% Risk for Sibling* After 1 Affected Sibling (Parents Normal)
Anencephaly	1:2 to 1:7	0.2 to 5.0	4
Spina bifida	1:1.3 to 1:1.5	0.2 to 4.0	6
Congenital hydrocephalus	M > F	0.6 to 1.8	4 to 5
Cleft lip with or without cleft palate	1.6:1 to 2:1	1.0	4 to 5
Cleft palate alone	1:1.4	0.4	2 to 6
Congenital dislocation of the hip	1:3 to 1:8	1.2 to 4.0	4 to 14 (male, 0.5; female, 6.3)
Clubfoot (TEV)	2:1	1.2	2 to 8
Hirschsprung's disease	3.7:1	0.2	3 to 5
Imperforate anus	M > F	0.4	4 to 5
TE fistula	1:1	0.3	4 to 5
Diaphragmatic hernia	2:1	0.5	4 to 5
Pyloric stenosis	5:1	1.0 to 3.0	3 (male, 4; female, 2.4)
Congenital heart disease	Variable	5.8 to 8.0	VSD, 5 PDA, 3.5 ASD, 3.2† Tetralogy of Fallot, 3.2 Transposition, 2.2 Truncus arteriosus, 0.7

ASD = atrial septal defect; PDA = patent ductus arteriosus; TE = tracheoesophageal; TEV = talipes equinovirus; VSD = ventricular septal defect.

*Risk is similar in first child of affected parent. Risk may be higher with some disorders in which siblings are less frequently born (e.g., tracheoesophageal fistula), but all figures are approximations. With two offspring affected, the risk for siblings is two to three times greater than for one (i.e., 10 to 15%).

†Recent figures suggest substantially higher risk.

given in Table 8–4, and the recurrence risks for those common congenital malformations that have polygenic inheritance are given in Table 8–5.

BIBLIOGRAPHY

Kalter, H., and Warkany, J.: Congenital malformations: Etiologic factors and their role in prevention (parts I and II). *N. Engl. J. Med.* 1983, 308:424–431, 491–497.

Chromosomal Abnormalities

Smith, D. W.: Autosomal abnormalities. *Am. J. Obstet. Gynecol.* 1964, 90:1055.
Smith, D. W., and Wilson, A. A.: *The Child with Down's Syndrome (Mongolism).* W. B. Saunders, Philadelphia, 1973.

Ledbetter, D. H., Riccardi, V. M., Airhart, S. D., et al.: Deletions of chromosome 15 as a cause of the Prader-Willi syndrome. *N. Engl. J. Med.* 1981, 304:325–329.

Rex, A. P., and Preus, M.: A diagnostic index for Down syndrome. *J. Pediatr.* 1982, 100:903–906.

Chervenak, F. A., Isaacson, G., Blakemore, K. J., et al.: Fetal cystic hygroma: Cause and natural history. *N. Engl. J. Med.* 1983, 309:822–825.

Nyhan, W. L.: Cytogenetic disease. *Ciba Clin. Symp.* 1983, 35:1–32.

Seibel, N. L., Sommer, A., and Miser, J.: Transient neonatal leukemoid reactions in mosaic trisomy 21. *J. Pediatr.* 1984, 104:251–254.

Gaedicke, G., Kleihauer, E., and Terinde, R.: Acute non-lymphocytic leukaemia versus transient leukaemoid reaction in fetuses with Down syndrome (Letter). *Lancet* 1990, 335:857.

Haddow, J. E., Palomaki, G. E., Knight, G. J., et al.: Prenatal screening for Down's syndrome with use of maternal serum markers. *N. Engl. J. Med.* 1992, 327:588–593.

Cleft Lip and Palate

McKenzie, J.: The first arch syndrome. *Arch. Dis. Child.* 1958, 33:477.

Stewart, R. E.: Craniofacial malformations: Clinical and genetic considerations. *Pediatr. Clin. North Am.* 1978, 25:485.

Suslak, L. and Desposito, F.: Infants with cleft lip/cleft palate. *Pediatr. Rev.* 1988, 9:331–334.

Clubfoot

Dunn, P. M.: Congenital postural deformities. *Br. Med. Bull.* 1976, 32:71.

Swann, M.: The early management of the clubfoot. *Proc. R. Soc. Med.* 1977, 70:256.

Polydactyly and Syndactyly

Ornoy, A., Sekeles, E., and Sadovsky, E.: Amniogenic bands as a cause of syndactyly in a young human fetus. *Teratology* 1974, 9:129.

Neural Tube Defects and Hydrocephalus

Campbell, S., Pryse-Davies, J., Coltart, T. M., et al.: Ultrasound in diagnosis of spina bifida. *Lancet* 1975, i:1065.

Golden, G. S.: Neural tube defects. *Pediatr. Rev.* 1979, 1:187–190.

Lorber, J., and Salfield, S. A. W.: Results of selective treatment of spina bifida cystica. *Arch Dis. Child.* 1981, 56:822–830.

Palmer, D.: Neural tube defects in siblings of children with other malformations (Letter). *Lancet* 1982, ii:764.

Gross, R. H., Cox, A., Tatyrek, R., et al.: Early management and decision making for the treatment of myelomeningocele. *Pediatrics* 1983, 72:450–458.

Allan, W. C., Dransfield, D. A., and Tito, A. M.: Ventricular dilation following periventricular-intraventricular hemorrhage: Outcome at one year. *Pediatrics* 1984, 73:158–162.

Charney, E. B., Weller, S. C., Sutton, L. N., et al.: Management of the newborn with myelomeningocele; time for a decision-making process. *Pediatrics* 1985, 75:58–64.

Wald, N., Sneddon, J., Densem, J., et al.: Prevention of neural tube defects: Results of the Medical Research Council vitamin study. *Lancet* 1991, 338:131–137.

Milunsky, A., Ulcickas, M., Rothman, K. J., et al.: Maternal heat exposure and neural tube defects. *J.A.M.A.* 1992, 268:882–885.

Yen, I. H., Khoury, M. J., Erickson, J. D., et al.: The changing epidemiology of neural tube defects: United States, 1968–1989. *Am. J. Dis. Child.* 1992, 146:857–861.

Fernell, E., Hagberg, G., and Hagberg, B.: Infantile hydrocephalus in preterm, low-birth-weight infants—A nationwide Swedish cohort study 1979–88. *Acta Paediatr. Int. J. Paediatr.* 1993, 82:45–48.

The VATER Association

Apold, J., Dahl, E., and Aarskog, D.: The VATER association: Malformations of the male external genitalia. *Acta Paediatr.* 1976, 65:150.

Korones, S. B., and Evans, L. J.: Measurement of intragastric oxygen concentration for the diagnosis of H-type tracheoesophageal fistula. *Pediatrics* 1977, 60:450.

Boles, E. T.: Imperforate anus. *Clin. Perinatol.* 1978, 5:149.

Nora, J. J., Nora, A. H., Blu, J., et al.: Exogenous progestogen and estrogen implicated in birth defects. *J.A.M.A.* 1978, 240:837.

Schuster, S. R., and Teele, R. L.: An analysis of ultrasound scanning as a guide in determination of "high" or "low" imperforate anus. *J. Pediatr. Surg.* 1979, 14:798–800.

Kelsch, R. C., and Oliver, W. J.: Use of nephrosonography in evaluation of renal disease in infants. *Pediatr. Rev.* 1980, 2:25–29.

Touloukian, R. J.: Long-term results following repair of esophageal atresia by end-to-end anastomosis and ligation of the tracheoesophageal fistula. *J. Pediatr. Surg.* 1981, 16:983–988.

Khoury, M. J., Cordero, J. F., Greenberg, F., et al.: A population study of the VACTERL association: Evidence for its etiologic heterogeneity. *Pediatrics* 1983, 71:815–820.

Diaphragmatic Problems

Otherson, H. B., and Lorenzo, R. L.: Diaphragmatic paralysis and eventration: Newer approaches to diagnosis and operative correlation. *J. Pediatr. Surg.* 1977, 12:309.

Dibbins, A. W.: Congenital diaphragmatic hernia: Hypoplastic lung and pulmonary vasoconstriction. *Clin. Perinatol.* 1978, 5:93.

Gencik, A., Moser, H., Gencikova, A., and Kehrer, B.: Familial occurrence of congenital diaphragmatic defects in three families. *Helv. Paediatr. Acta* 1982, 37:289–293.

Rescorla, F. J., Yoder, M. C., West, K. W., and Grosfeld, J. L.: Delayed presentation of a right-sided diaphragmatic hernia and group B streptococcal sepsis: Two case reports and a review of the literature. *Arch. Surg.* 1989, 124:1083–1086.

Breaux, C. W., Jr., Rouse, T. M., Cain, W. S., and Georgeson, K. E.: Congenital diaphragmatic hernia in an era of delayed repair after medical and/or extra-corporeal membrane oxygenation stabilization: A prognostic and management classification. *J. Pediatr. Surg.* 1992, 27:1192–1196.

Hirschsprung's Disease

Boley, S. J., Dinari, G., and Cohen, M. I.: Hirschsprung's disease in the newborn. *Clin. Perinatol.* 1978, 5:45.

Foster, P., Cowan, G., and Wrenn, E. L., Jr.: Twenty-five years' experience with Hirschsprung's disease. *J. Pediatr. Surg.* 1990, 25:531–534.

Verder, H., Petersen, W., and Mauritzen, K.: Anal tonometry in the neonatal period for the diagnosis of Hirschsprung's disease. *Acta Paediatr.* 1991, 80:45–50.

Congenital Dislocation of the Hip

Cyvin, K. B.: Congenital dislocation of the hip joint. Clinical studies with special reference to the pathogenesis. *Acta Paediatr.* 1977, 66(Suppl):263.

Mubarak, S., Garfin, S., Vance, R., et al.: Pitfalls in the use of the Pavlik harness for treatment of congenital dysplasia, subluxation, and dislocation of the hip. *J. Bone Joint Surg.* 1981, 63A:1239–1248.

Catterall, A.: What is congenital dislocation of the hip? *J. Bone Joint Surg.* 1984, 66B:469–470.

Clarke, N. M. P., Harcke, H. T., McHugh, P., et al.: Real-time ultrasound in the diagnosis of congenital dislocation and dysplasia of the hip. *J. Bone Joint Surg.* 1985, 67B:406–412.

MacEwen, G. D., and Millet, C.: Congenital dislocation of the hip. *Pediatr. Rev.* 1990, 11:249–252.

Editorial: Screening for congenital hip dysplasia. *Lancet* 1991, 337:947–948.

Langkamer, V. G., Clarke, N. M. P., and Witherow, P.: Complications of splintage in congenital dislocation of the hip. *Arch. Dis. Child.* 1991, 66:1322–1325.

Walter, R. S., Donaldson, J. S., Davis, C. L., et al.: Ultrasound screening of high-risk infants: A method to increase early detection of congenital dysplasia of the hip. *Am. J. Dis. Child.* 1992, 146:230–234.

Congenital Heart Disease

Nora, J. J., and Nora, A. H.: Recurrence risks in children having one parent with a congenital heart disease. *Circulation* 1976, 53:701.
Friedman, W. F., Sahn, D. J., and Hirschklau, M. J.: A review: Newer, noninvasive cardiac diagnostic methods. *Pediatr. Res.* 1977, 11:190.
Lewis, A. B., Takahasi, M., and Lurie, P. R.: Administration of prostaglandin E in neonates with critical congenital cardiac defects. *J. Pediatr.* 1978, 93:481.
Noonan, J. A.: Association of congenital heart disease with syndromes or other defects. *Pediatr. Clin. North Am.* 1978, 25:797.
Lovorgna, L.: Neonatal cardiology. *Pediatr. Ann.* 1979, 8/2:12.
Report of the New England Regional Infant Cardiac Program. *Pediatrics* 1980, 65 (Suppl):377.
Nadas, A. S.: Indomethacin and the patent ductus arteriosus. *N. Engl. J. Med.* 1981, 305:97–98.
Bove, E. L., Bull, C., Stark, J., et al.: Congenital heart disease in the neonate: Results of surgical treatment. *Arch. Dis. Child.* 1983, 58:137–141.
Ward, K. E., Pryor, R. W., Matson, J. R., et al.: Delayed detection of coarctation in infancy: Implications for timing of newborn follow-up. *Pediatrics* 1990, 86:972–976.
Groves, A. M. M., Fagg, N. L. K., Cook, A. C., and Allan, L. D.: Cardiac tumours in intrauterine life. *Arch. Dis. Child.* 1992, 67:1189–1192.

Genetic Counseling

Kaback, M. M.: Medical genetics: An overview. *Pediatr. Clin. North Am.* 1978, 25:395.
Nadler, H. L.: Role of the general pediatrician in genetics. *Pediatr. Rev.* 1981, 3:4–12.
Gerald, P. S.: Cytogenetics in the practice of pediatrics. *Pediatr. Rev.* 1982, 3:333–340.
Kronick, J. B., Scriver, C. R., Goodyer, P. R., and Kaplan, P. B.: A perimortem protocol for suspected genetic disease. *Pediatrics* 1983, 71:960–963.
Leonard, C. O.: Counseling parents of a child with meningomyelocele. *Pediatr. Rev.* 1983, 4:317–321.
Rose, V., Gold, R. J. M., Lindsay, G., and Allen, M.: A possible increase in the incidence of congenital heart defects among the offspring of affected parents. *J. Am. Coll. Cardiol.* 1985, 6:376–382.
Schmickel, R. D.: Contiguous gene syndromes: A component of recognizable syndromes. *J. Pediatr.* 1986, 109:231–241.
Hall, J. G.: Genomic imprinting and its clinical implications. *N. Engl. J. Med.* 1992, 326: 827–829.

RESPIRATORY PROBLEMS

9

The importance of respiratory disorders in the neonatal period is evidenced by even a cursory examination of the number of infants with respiratory problems who are admitted to special care nurseries. A good working knowledge of the major disorders in this category is therefore essential.

RESPIRATORY DISTRESS SYNDROME (HYALINE MEMBRANE DISEASE)

INTRODUCTION AND INCIDENCE

Respiratory distress syndrome (RDS) has dominated neonatal mortality statistics until very recently, and although recent advances in management have resulted in improvement in outcome, many deaths are still attributed to this disorder. The disorder seems to occur worldwide, and the role of prematurity is dominant. The incidence is roughly 20% of all infants with birth weights between 1000 and 1500 g. The term progressive atelectasis of prematurity describes the disorder succinctly.

ETIOLOGY AND PATHOPHYSIOLOGY

Numerous predisposing factors have been associated with production or increased severity of RDS: (1) prematurity, (2) birth by cesarean section (especially without labor), (3) diabetic mother, (4) antepartum hemorrhage (acute), (5) second of twins, and (6) asphyxia at birth.

The disorder occurs approximately twice as frequently in males as in females. A previous low-birth-weight infant who had RDS makes the chances extremely high that any subsequent low-birth-weight infants will have RDS. Conversely, the factors making RDS unlikely are (1) term birth, (2) intrauterine growth retardation, (3) prolonged rupture of membranes, and (4) other fetal stress (including chronic retroplacental bleeding). The common thread may be cord serum cortisol levels, which are decreased in RDS.

There appear to be two major contributing factors in the pathophysiology of the disorder: (1) pulmonary hypoperfusion (or pulmonary ischemia), and (2) lack of surfactant (the lining substance of alveoli produced by type 2 pneumo-

107

cytes), particularly the phosphatidylglycerol component. One of the clearest statements has been made by Gluck.

> The infant making his respiratory adjustment at birth, even when not stressed, needs to synthesize surface-active lecithin at a phenomenal rate. . . . The premature infant who develops respiratory distress syndrome does so because he lacks the ability to synthesize lecithin at the required rapid rate. Consequently, he is unable to maintain alveolar stability on expiration, and the progressive atelectasis and the secondary changes that characterize respiratory distress syndrome develop. Thus, inability to meet the demands of postnatal respiratory adjustment by sufficiently rapid synthesis of surface-active pulmonary lecithin, and not the absence of surfactant per se, proves to be the limiting factor causing respiratory distress syndrome.

Figure 9–1 diagrams the causal factors in the development of RDS.

DIAGNOSIS

If one attempts to define RDS, the major features in diagnosis are stated. It may be defined as a developmental disorder starting at or soon after birth; occurring almost exclusively in infants with immature lungs; consisting of increasing respiratory difficulty in the first 3 to 6 hours manifest by rapid respirations, grunting, intercostal and sternal retractions, and flaring of the alae nasi, which is associated with hypoxemia; and radiographic picture revealing a reticu-

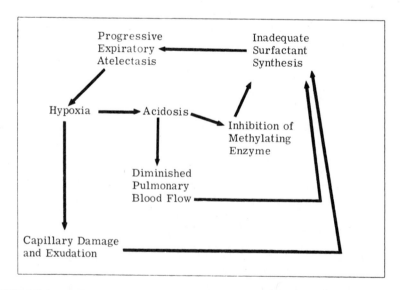

FIGURE 9–1. Schema showing the causal factors in the development of respiratory distress syndrome.

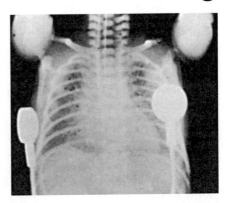

FIGURE 9–2. Radiograph of the chest of a baby with moderately severe respiratory distress syndrome. A reticulogranular appearance is present throughout both lung fields, and an air bronchogram is evident at both bases. The endotracheal tube is situated close to the carina. (Note the presence of an artifact over the apex of both lungs.)

logranular appearance, with or without an air bronchogram (Figs. 9–2 and 9–3). In severe cases that do not receive treatment, infants either progress to death or significantly improve within 48 to 72 hours. The improvement in uncomplicated or complicated RDS is almost invariably preceded by a diuresis.

Perhaps the simplest concept to describe RDS is that of progressive atelectasis, which helps explain many of the features. Unfortunately, the chest x-ray findings of RDS can also be seen with pneumonia caused by group B β-hemolytic streptococci and other organisms (pathologically, this type of pneumonia may show hyaline membranes with engulfed organisms). Help in differentiating between the two may be provided by a foam stability test of the gastric

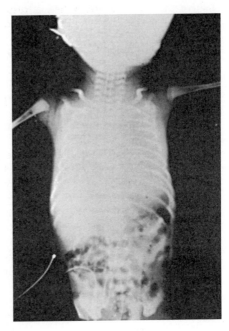

FIGURE 9–3. Radiograph of a baby with severe respiratory distress syndrome with virtual white-out of the chest (the air bronchograms can just be distinguished). The endotracheal tube is in good position, but the tip of the umbilical artery catheter is at L-2 and was withdrawn to L-4 shortly after this film was taken.

aspirate or pharyngeal secretions. A positive test result usually excludes RDS. Thymus size (which is large in RDS) and diagnostic tests for infection may also be helpful (see Chapter 15).

MANAGEMENT

With better understanding of the pathophysiology of RDS, its treatment has become more rational. Treatment in the early 1960s was primarily confined to the use of supplemental oxygen and intravenous dextrose, with or without bicarbonate. In the late 1960s, many babies who had profound hypoxemia or severe apnea were treated with different forms of mechanical ventilatory support (intermittent positive or negative pressure respirators). Thermoregulation was given increasing importance, and together these advances resulted in many survivors. Unfortunately, many babies went on to develop chronic lung disease (bronchopulmonary dysplasia), with a significant proportion eventually dying of cor pulmonale.

The 1970s heralded the age of continuous distending pressure, the principle of which is to provide a constant pressure across the lungs, which prevents collapse of alveoli at the end of expiration and thereby prevents atelectasis. This procedure may be performed by applying either (1) continuous positive airway pressure via an endotracheal tube, head box, face mask, or nasal cannulae (prongs or tubes) or (2) continuous negative pressure via a negative pressure respirator or a more portable device placed inside a regular incubator. By convention, when a baby is breathing completely alone and spontaneously on continuous distending pressure, the baby is considered to have continuous positive airway pressure. When a respirator is used with either control or intermittent mandatory ventilation modes, the term positive end-expiratory pressure is used.

There has been a general tendency in the past few years to use earlier continuous positive airway pressure, or positive end-expiratory pressure, with intermittent mandatory ventilation. Although this early use undoubtedly has reduced the number of babies that require mechanical ventilation and the duration of endotracheal intubation, no clear evidence shows that such use has had a direct effect on neonatal mortality resulting from RDS. Persistent patency of the ductus arteriosus also occurs in many infants with RDS. As a result of the observation that diuresis usually precedes clinical improvement and that delay in such diuresis may predispose to bronchopulmonary dysplasia, attempts have been made to induce a diuresis. However, it is not clear that this method has contributed to improved survival. Nevertheless, modern neonatal intensive care has resulted in a dramatic improvement in the survival rate of infants with RDS.

The 1980s saw the emergence of large trials to evaluate the efficacy of exogenous surfactants, and now, in the 1990s, these surfactants have assumed a primary role in the prevention and rescue of babies with RDS. Initial studies using single doses of exogenous surfactant showed rapid improvement in oxygenation and the ability to lower ventilator settings but did not influence mortality or later morbidity. Later studies with multiple doses of surfactant clearly demonstrated increased survival and lowered morbidity. In particular, air leaks (pneumothorax and pulmonary interstitial emphysema) were markedly decreased. In the United States, natural surfactants derived from calf lung extract (e.g., Survanta) and a synthetic surfactant (Exosurf) have been used. Natural surfactants seem to act more rapidly and to have a more dramatic effect. In Europe and Scandinavia, a porcine-derived surfactant (Curosurf) has been used extensively.

High-frequency ventilation has not proved to be superior to conventional ventilation for most babies with RDS, although it may offer advantages in tiny babies who develop pulmonary interstitial emphysema.

For a baby admitted to a special care nursery with a presumptive diagnosis of RDS, the following orders (with explanatory notes) might be required:

1. Give nothing by mouth.
2. Give oxygen to relieve cyanosis, or state concentration (use head box if high concentration is required).
3. Start intravenous line or insert umbilical artery catheter.
4. Give 10% dextrose in water at 100 ml/kg for the first 2 days; more fluid may be needed if baby is treated under an open radiant heat bed. Electrolyte solution should be used after 2 days (or earlier).
5. Check arterialized or arterial blood gases (preferably the latter).
6. Depending on the base deficit derived from pH and pCO_2 assessments, add sodium bicarbonate to the infusion fluid, using the following formula:

$$\text{mEq of bicarbonate} = \text{weight in kg} \times 0.3 \times \text{base deficit}$$

7. Obtain a complete blood count (especially hematocrit).
8. Get a chest x-ray study and/or an x-ray study of the abdomen for placement of umbilical artery catheter.
9. Keep humidity at 50 to 60% (do not obscure view of baby with high humidity).
10. Place the baby on heart rate monitor and oxygen saturation monitor (and transcutaneous oxygen and carbon dioxide monitor [$tcpO_2$/$tcpCO_2$], if available). Keep oxygen saturation at 93 to 97%.
11. Maintain the baby's body temperature via either a neutral thermal environment or infant servocontrol.
12. Adjust the inspired oxygen concentration to maintain arterial pO_2 at 50 to 70 mm Hg (35 to 50 mm Hg on capillary samples). Use $tcpO_2$ or an intraarterial device to measure continuously, if available. Arterial pO_2 as low as 40 mm Hg is acceptable if high oxygen concentration is required, if metabolic acidosis is not present.
13. Conduct other investigations as deemed appropriate, such as total protein, serum electrolytes, serum calcium, blood glucose level determinations.
14. Keep record of amount of blood removed for sampling and consider transfusion when 10% of blood volume has been removed (i.e., 8 ml in a 1-kg infant, 16 ml in a 2-kg infant).
15. Record blood pressure on admission and frequently while respiratory difficulty persists. If the pressure is low, the baby may need blood, and more frequent readings should be made (possibly continuously using a pressure

transducer attached to the arterial line or a noninvasive ultrasonographic or oscillometric technique).

16. If more than 40% oxygen is required to maintain an adequate paO_2 the baby should be treated with continuous positive airway pressure by nasal prongs starting at 4 cm H_2O pressure (up to 10 cm H_2O). Prepare to give assisted ventilation (using a ventilator) and exogenous surfactant.

A discussion of the management of RDS cannot be complete without a word about possible prevention. Undoubtedly, the most important single factor that would decrease overall mortality in this disorder is the prevention of premature delivery. Currently, such a goal seems unattainable. An acceptable compromise in the very immature baby (< 32 weeks' gestation and possibly < 34 weeks gestation) is to attempt to enhance pulmonary maturity in utero. This may be achieved, if premature labor can be suppressed and delivery deferred for 24 to 48 hours, by the use of corticosteroids administered to the mother. (The corticosteroid is most frequently in the form of betamethasone but dexamethasone is also successful.) Another preventive measure, which has yet to achieve universal acclaim, is to allow a placental transfusion to occur at the time of delivery and hence avoid relative hypovolemia.

In infants born at gestational ages of less than 29 weeks (especially < 27 weeks), many neonatologists use prophylactic exogenous surfactant in the delivery room (administered via an endotracheal tube). Independent effects of prenatal corticosteroids and exogenous surfactant seem to occur. A potential complication of surfactant therapy is persistent (patent) ductus arteriosus; closure with either indomethacin or surgery may be needed.

SUMMARY

This commonly encountered disorder is primarily seen in the premature infant and is the result of a deficiency of surfactant, which normally lowers surface tension in the alveoli. In its absence, progressive atelectasis occurs. Treatment is directed at improving pulmonary maturation prenatally (by administering betamethasone) or preventing atelectasis neonatally (by administering continuous distending pressure). Other supportive measures (e.g., nutrition and thermoregulation) are also important, and it may be possible to replace the deficiency of endogenous surfactant with an exogenous form.

INTRAUTERINE (CONGENITAL) PNEUMONIA

INTRODUCTION

Intrauterine pneumonia may be confused with RDS because it is seen more frequently in premature infants, and the manifestations may be quite similar.

PATHOPHYSIOLOGY

Prolonged labor (longer than 24 hours), prolonged rupture of membranes (longer than 24 hours), maternal fever, foul-smelling amniotic fluid, and other evidence of amnionitis have all been associated with intrauterine pneumonia. However, these findings are not prerequisite. The infecting organism can frequently be recovered from the maternal genital tract as well as the baby. Infection is either (1) bloodborne via the placenta or (2) ascending, in which the amniotic fluid becomes infected. Labor, via contractions, seems to predispose to ascending infection. Although many microorganisms have been implicated, the most commonly associated organism at the present time is group B β-hemolytic streptococcus (see Chapter 15). Hyaline membranes with embedded organisms have been observed pathologically in the lungs of babies who die.

DIAGNOSIS

Difficulty may be encountered in the delivery room, with infants demonstrating poor Apgar scores and a need for resuscitation, or it may be delayed for several hours. Rapid respirations, grunting, and retractions may be noted. Apnea and shock (poor peripheral perfusion) are more likely to be seen in the first 24 hours in intrauterine pneumonia than in RDS. Hypothermia also may be noted. In a term infant who first develops grunting and retractions after the first 12 hours, there are few other diagnoses to be considered. White blood count and differential may reveal neutropenia or an abnormally high band to total neutrophil ratio. The level of C-reactive protein may not be increased early with group B streptococcal infection but rises later. Chest x-ray is frequently diagnostic (Fig. 9–4), although this disorder may be confused with RDS in some premature infants.

MANAGEMENT

In cases in which infection may be suspected (e.g., prolonged rupture of membranes or maternal fever), it may be valuable to perform a smear of the gastric aspirate. Many pus cells (polymorphonuclear leukocytes) in the depressed (low-Apgar) premature infant suggest infection. In group B streptococcal infection, many cocci are usually seen in the gastric aspirate smear. The gastric aspirate can also be evaluated with the foam stability (shake) test. If the result is positive, pneumonia is more likely (and RDS very unlikely). A negative result may not distinguish between RDS and pneumonia. Evaluation of tracheal aspirate may be helpful. These findings, with or without an abnormal white blood count and differential, should initiate a sepsis evaluation, which includes blood, urine, and cerebrospinal fluid cultures. Treatment with broad-spectrum antibiotics is usually begun until the results of cultures and sensitivities are known. Treatment should consist of a penicillin and an aminoglycoside (we currently start therapy with ampicillin and gentamicin). Duration of therapy is usually 1 week, if C-reactive protein levels rapidly return to normal.

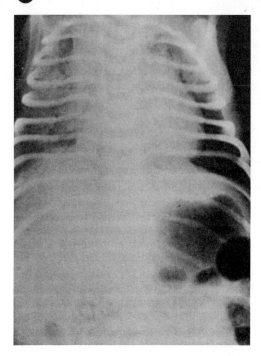

FIGURE 9–4. Radiograph of the chest in a baby with congenital (intrauterine) pneumonia involving most of the right lung and the left upper lobe.

SUMMARY

This disorder most frequently follows ascending infection of the maternal genital tract. Particularly with group B streptococcal infection, the clinical manifestations may resemble those of RDS. Apnea, shock, and hypothermia may occur. Chest x-ray study frequently provides the diagnosis, and broad-spectrum antibiotic therapy is used.

NEONATAL PNEUMONIA

Pneumonia that occurs after the first few days of life can no longer be considered congenital, or intrauterine. Many organisms have been associated with neonatal pneumonia, the most common being *Escherichia coli*, enterococci, staphylococci, and streptococci. However, particularly when assisted ventilation is used, the premature infant may succumb to organisms such as *Klebsiella* and *Pseudomonas* sp.

Another form of pneumonia is that caused by *Chlamydia trachomatis*, which may produce a chest x-ray picture of hyperinflation with diffuse interstitial or patchy infiltrates. It is usually seen later in (or beyond) the neonatal period. It is unclear whether the pneumonia is caused by direct infection or is a hypersensitivity reaction to the organism. The fact that eosinophilia is often prominent may support the latter concept.

Pneumonia caused by *Staphylococcus aureus* is not commonly seen at birth but may occur toward the end of the first month. The baby often appears much worse clinically than the chest x-ray study would suggest, but later the chest x-ray study may show pneumatoceles. Other organisms (*Klebsiella pneumoniae* and *E. coli*) have also been associated with pneumatocele formation in the newborn.

Antibiotic treatment is directed toward eradicating the specific organism. Erythromycin seems to be useful in the treatment of chlamydial pneumonia.

ASPIRATION SYNDROMES

Any foreign substance entering the tracheobronchial tree may give rise to aspiration syndrome. Amniotic fluid does not normally penetrate deeply into the fetal tracheobronchial tree (see Retained Lung Fluid Syndromes section further in this chapter), but under conditions that produce asphyxia, a sphincteric mechanism at the vocal cords may relax, and gasping may occur. This phenomenon usually produces a generalized picture of involvement on chest x-ray study. Milk aspiration may occur at any time in the neonatal course and is more likely to produce involvement of the right upper lobe (because the right mainstem bronchus comes off the trachea at a less acute angle than the left and predisposes to flow to that side). The most important aspiration syndrome is that caused by meconium-stained amniotic fluid, but blood-stained amniotic fluid may also be aspirated and produce a very similar picture.

MECONIUM ASPIRATION SYNDROME

Incidence

Eight to 10% of all pregnancies are complicated by the presence of some meconium staining of the amniotic fluid. This is presumptive evidence that at some time in the preceding few days, the fetus had been sufficiently stressed (asphyxiated) to pass meconium. A sizable proportion of these infants are depressed at birth, but others are not. Fetal heart rate monitoring and fetal scalp blood sampling may alter obstetric management when meconium-stained amniotic fluid is encountered.

Pathophysiology

Meconium aspiration syndrome may be most easily remembered as being the result of a relaxation and a stimulation "at both ends." Asphyxia tends to relax the anal sphincter and stimulate peristalsis, resulting in passage of meconium into amniotic fluid. The passage of meconium may occur in response to a substance called motilin, released during fetal distress. As stated earlier, asphyxia also produces relaxation of a sphincteric mechanism at the glottis and stimulates gasping. The result is aspiration of meconium. If this material is not cleared shortly after birth, it will migrate peripherally as continued respiration is established. Complete or partial obstruction may result, and atelectasis or ball-valve effects (with hyperinflation) may occur. Lastly, this irritating foreign material may produce a chemical pneumonitis.

One other problem may play a significant role in the morbidity and mortality of this condition: namely, persistent pulmonary hypertension (persistent fetal circulation, p. 122). The underlying asphyxia, which may be a reflection of more chronic hypoxia, predisposes to a morphologic change in the arterioles of the lung. The circular muscle, which is usually very sparse in the distal arterioles, is exaggerated and prolonged toward the capillaries. After delivery, the normally smooth transition may be difficult.

Diagnosis

One may anticipate problems in any labor in which evidence of placental insufficiency exists (e.g., via fetal heart rate monitoring). Presence of meconium-stained amniotic fluid should initiate appropriate prophylactic therapy (see the following discussion), and the child should be observed carefully thereafter. The baby is frequently depressed (flaccid) at birth and may be covered in meconium. The condition is more likely to be seen in infants who are postmature or small for gestational age at (or close to) term. Preterm babies may lack motilin. Rapid respirations, with cyanosis, soon develop, and an increase in the anteroposterior diameter of the chest is often seen (the result of air trapping). An increasing oxygen dependency occurs, with labored breathing. Sudden deterioration may be indicative of pneumothorax and pneumomediastinum. Testing the first specimen of urine for the presence of high levels of a specific pigment may provide a useful diagnostic test in cases in which it is doubtful whether or not meconium has been aspirated. Some infants have great difficulty with oxygenation, and the hyperoxia test (p. 376) may suggest the presence of persistent pulmonary hypertension, although cyanotic heart disease also has to be considered. Extreme lability of oxygenation (with rapid drops of paO_2 or $tcpO_2$ with crying or agitation) is also suggestive of persistent pulmonary hypertension.

Radiologic features are coarse bilateral pulmonary infiltrates, usually with some increase in the anteroposterior diameter of the chest, and frequently hyperinflation at the bases with flattening of the diaphragm. A small pneumomediastinum may be visible only on the lateral radiograph.

Management

Although some cases of meconium aspiration syndrome may occur many hours before delivery (and subsequently may result in death), an active intervention policy in the delivery room is to be strongly encouraged in the presence of thick or particulate meconium-stained amniotic fluid. The obstetrician may provide valuable assistance by suctioning the pharynx with a DeLee suction catheter (rather than a bulb syringe) while the head is on the perineum (see also Recusci-tation Technique section, Chapter 2.) Whenever a baby is depressed and flaccid, laryngoscopy and endotracheal suction should be performed before attempts are made to ventilate the baby. This may require high-pressure suction to remove thick, inspissated meconium. Bronchial lavage has been advocated but may do more harm than good. After respiration has been established, the stomach contents should be aspirated to remove any possible subsequent exposure to meconium (which might be vomited).

When definite evidence of meconium aspiration syndrome exists (either on chest x-ray study or when respiratory symptoms follow demonstrable meconium below the vocal cords), it is advisable to evaluate the baby for possible infection and to consider starting antibiotic administration (ampicillin and gentamicin). Suspecting infection is based on the following:

1. In the absence of a satisfactory etiology for asphyxia, infection may be the stress leading to meconium passage.

2. Meconium in amniotic fluid seems to be a good culture medium for *E. coli*, in contrast to most normal amniotic fluids.

3. At autopsy, the lungs of babies who die of meconium aspiration syndrome frequently show evidence of aspiration and infection.

The use of steroids has been suggested in the past but was shown to have no beneficial effect in a controlled study. On the other hand, continuous positive airway pressure has been shown to be of some value, despite the fact that unequal aeration exists, which may predispose to pneumothorax or pneumomediastinum (see p. 119). The worst cases may require high inspired oxygen concentration with ventilatory assistance. Chest physiotherapy is also extremely valuable but may need to be deferred in a "sensitive" baby (one who has lability of oxygenation with crying or agitation). The management of persistent pulmonary hypertension can be difficult. Attempts to hyperventilate are hindered by the other components of the syndrome, and tolazoline (Priscoline) is frequently ineffective. Consequently, despite all these measures, it may be impossible to adequately oxygenate these babies, and death may ensue. In recent years, survival of the sickest babies has improved in response to extracorporeal membrane oxygenation.

Summary

Meconium-stained amniotic fluid usually results from fetal stress (asphyxia or infection) at some time before delivery. Gasping may result in aspiration of this material, which may be recovered to a considerable extent by vigorous resuscitative efforts, including laryngoscopy and tracheal suctioning, in the delivery room. Inspissated meconium may produce air leaks (e.g., pneumothorax) or hyperinflation of the chest as a result of a ball-valve effect, and persistent pulmonary hypertension may be an additional complicating factor. Supportive measures, including administration of oxygen, antibiotics, chest physiotherapy, ventilatory assistance and extracorporeal membrane oxygenation, may be necessary, but death may still occur.

RETAINED LUNG FLUID SYNDROMES

INTRODUCTION

Circumstances that limit removal of lung fluid after birth may produce at least two distinct pictures. These diagnoses are frequently made only in retrospect (i.e., by exclusion).

PATHOPHYSIOLOGY

Although some doubt remains about the contribution of amniotic fluid to the fluid in the tracheobronchial tree, the major contribution is undoubtedly lung fluid. This fluid is probably a filtrate of blood, with selective reabsorption or secretion by the lung. With vaginal delivery, some of this fluid is usually expelled by thoracic compression. With cesarean section, the forces acting to expel lung fluid are not as great. Consequently, the tendency to retain lung fluid is greater. The removal of lung fluid, after air breathing is established, seems to be primarily via the lymphatics. When there is an excessive amount of fluid or a delay in removal of the fluid, respiratory symptoms may be seen.

DIAGNOSIS

Two distinct clinical pictures have been observed and described, although the radiologic features may be the same. The first was labeled transient tachypnea of the newborn, and the second was called respiratory distress syndrome, type II (RDS type II). In transient tachypnea of the newborn, the picture is quite simply one of a baby who appears to have no respiratory distress but who is breathing very fast (frequently at a rate of over 100/min). This phenomenon may last for up to 3 or 4 days. In RDS type II, the features of RDS (retractions, grunting, and flaring of the alae nasi) are seen. Biochemical derangement is usually not remarkable, and the course is usually transient (approximately 24 hours) and benign. The chest radiograph is most helpful, although the radiographic signs are not always distinguishable from those seen with other disorders (e.g., a similar picture may be seen in group B streptococcal pneumonia). A diffuse haziness in both lung fields is usually present with some clearing toward the periphery, and fluid is frequently seen in the interlobar fissures.

MANAGEMENT

Diagnosis is usually not conclusive early, although it may be suspected. A brief search for other disorders is probably warranted. Erythrocythemia (high hematocrit syndrome) may produce a similar radiographic picture. Tachypnea may warrant investigation of metabolic acidosis (via pH and blood gases) or congenital heart disease. Supportive management, with oxygen, temperature regulation, and intravenous fluids and calories, is usually all that is required.

SUMMARY

Retained lung fluid syndrome includes at least two benign disorders: (1) transient tachypnea of the newborn and (2) RDS type II. The cause seems to be a transient failure of the lymphatics to remove lung fluid. Although radiographs may suggest the diagnosis, it is frequently made by exclusion. Management is supportive.

PNEUMOTHORAX AND PNEUMOMEDIASTINUM

INTRODUCTION AND INCIDENCE

Although other kinds of air leaks have been described (pneumopericardium and pneumoperitoneum), the association between pneumothorax and pneumomediastinum is strong, and they may be considered together. Pulmonary interstitial emphysema (PIE) may also be included in this association but is discussed later (p. 122).

The incidence of spontaneous pneumothorax and pneumomediastinum has been documented as 0.5 to 1% in routine term newborn infants. Under special circumstances, the incidence is much higher. Spontaneous pneumothorax occurs in approximately 4% of cases of RDS. When continuous positive airway pressure is added to the management, the incidence may rise to 15%, and with intermittent mandatory (mechanical) ventilation, it may be as high as 20 to 25%. Since the advent of exogenous surfactant to treat RDS, the incidence has returned to baseline (3 to 6%), even with assisted ventilation. Infants with meconium aspiration syndrome have associated pneumothorax and/or pneumomediastinum in approximately 6% of cases.

ETIOLOGY AND PATHOPHYSIOLOGY

The pressures normally exerted to produce initial inflation of the lung may be very high (70 to 80 cm). If portions of the lung are expanded, the pressure needed to ventilate them is considerably lower (rapidly falls to 25 to 30 cm and later to 15 to 20 cm). When some areas are collapsed and others expanded, an inappropriate pressure may be applied to some areas of the lung, which may produce rupture and an air leak. This phenomenon can occur shortly after delivery, as the lung is adjusting to extrauterine life. This same situation tends to persist for several days in babies with RDS. It has been suggested that babies who are spontaneously breathing out of phase with the ventilator are more predisposed to air leak. Some evidence supports the use of paralysis (with pancuronium) to prevent air leak, but this has been disputed.

An alternative mechanism, which has been described earlier under meconium aspiration syndrome, is based on air trapping due to a ball-valve effect. If the rupture is on the outer aspect of the lung, pneumothorax will occur. If the rupture is on the inner aspect, air may track along the sheaths of blood vessels to the mediastinum, producing a pneumomediastinum. The air leak may be limited to the interstitial spaces of the lung (PIE), but pneumothorax and pneumomediastinum should be anticipated. In spontaneous pneumothorax and pneumomediastinum, particularly in the male, one should consider the possibility of an associated urinary tract anomaly. Although this relationship is not completely clear, it probably relates to pulmonary hypoplasia (see p. 124).

DIAGNOSIS AND MANAGEMENT

Pneumothorax (particularly tension pneumothorax) is suggested in any baby whose condition shows sudden deterioration, either with or without assisted ventilation. If the signs are conclusive (shift of the mediastinum—via position of maximal cardiac impulse or sound on auscultation—with marked decrease in air entry or hypotension, and baby's condition is poor), emergency treatment should be implemented. The use of transillumination to the chest wall (see Figs. 35–11 and 35–12) may provide rapid confirmation without having to wait for chest x-ray study. It may also be possible to detect pneumothorax by the use of transthoracic impedance; another mode of presentation is the onset of hypotension (see Pulmonary Interstitial Emphysema section, p. 122).

When doubt still exists or the condition is not critical, confirmation via chest x-ray study should be obtained as soon as possible. If a tension pneumothorax exists (Fig. 9–5), emergency treatment is to be instituted. If no tension is present, conservative management may be indicated (careful observation in increased oxygen concentration).

Emergency treatment consists of insertion of an Intracath-type needle attached to a three-way stopcock and large (30-ml) syringe. The needle should be inserted through the second or third intercostal space just outside the nipple line. After the chest has been entered, the catheter portion may be advanced somewhat while the needle portion is removed. Air is removed via the syringe and may be expelled via the stopcock (without removal of the syringe) after each filling.

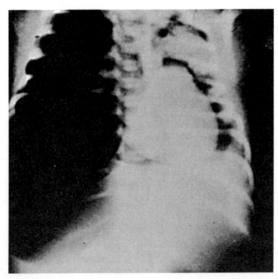

FIGURE 9–5. Radiograph of the chest of a baby, showing a huge right-sided tension pneumothorax. The "sail" on the left is the thymus, which is elevated by a pneumomediastinum.

Permanent placement of a chest tube to underwater seal drainage or to a suction device (e.g., the Pleur-Evac) is usually necessary.

Pneumomediastinum should be anticipated (along with pneumothorax) in all cases of meconium aspiration syndrome. There is usually an increased antero-posterior diameter of the chest, and the heart sounds may be heard indistinctly. A pneumomediastinum may produce a sail or spinnaker sign on chest x-ray study by elevating and outlining the thymus (Figs. 9–5 and 9–6).

Rapid resolution of the problem is frequently achieved by placing the infant in high oxygen concentration (80 to 100%) for 12 to 24 hours. The oxygen displaces nitrogen, and the oxygen is more easily absorbed. This condition usually occurs in term babies, and the management does not usually constitute a problem with respect to oxygen toxicity. In the premature infant, paO_2 levels should be monitored closely, and exposure to high oxygen concentration should be minimized as much as possible.

SUMMARY

Pneumothorax, pneumomediastinum, and other air leaks should be antici-pated with aspiration syndromes, RDS, or assisted ventilation. Abnormal forces or a ball-valve effect is implicated. Detection has been greatly helped by transil-lumination of the chest wall. Needle aspiration or chest tubes may be needed for tension pneumothorax.

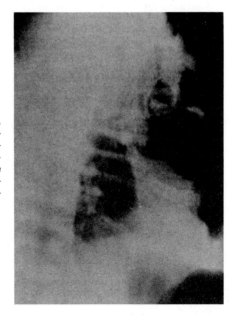

FIGURE 9–6. Another example of an air leak, showing the usefulness of a lateral ra-diograph in demonstrating a pneu-momediastinum as well as a pneumo-thorax. The pneumomediastinum is the radiolucent area just beneath the ster-num that has produced a sail, or spin-naker, sign.

PULMONARY INTERSTITIAL EMPHYSEMA

Another type of air leak, which may be more difficult to interpret, is PIE. In severe cases of RDS, the chest x-ray study may show apparently improved results on the second or third day because of a decrease in radiopacity. However, on closer inspection many microcystic areas are noted throughout one or both lungs. The lungs may be hyperinflated, with flattened diaphragms. Progression to pneumothorax and/or pneumomediastinum may occur, but considerable physiologic derangement may occur as a result of PIE alone (principally hypotension).

If PIE is unilateral and persists, selective intubation of the mainstem bronchus supplying the other lung may yield dramatic improvement. When PIE persists in both lungs, the prognosis for survival is poor, although high-frequency ventilation techniques have proved to be very beneficial in many cases. If the infant does survive, the chance of its developing chronic lung disease of prematurity (bronchopulmonary dysplasia) is very high. An intriguing possible therapy for bilateral PIE when high-frequency ventilation is not available, on the basis of improvement seen with spontaneous pneumothorax, is to create an artificial pneumothorax.

PERSISTENT PULMONARY HYPERTENSION
(PERSISTENT FETAL [TRANSITIONAL] CIRCULATION)

INTRODUCTION

It is unclear whether persistent pulmonary hypertension is increasing in frequency or whether it is being recognized more effectively. The diagnosis now seems to be made more often, pathologically as well as clinically.

ETIOLOGY

In fetal life, the pressure in the pulmonary artery is somewhat higher than that in the aorta, largely because the lungs are filled with fluid and are not being used as an organ of respiration. Consequently, the pulmonary vascular resistance is considerably higher than it will be subsequently. As a result, there is right-to-left flow of blood through the ductus arteriosus. When this arrangement continues after delivery, the term persistent fetal circulation has been used, but because the placenta is no longer in the circulation, it is more correctly termed persistent transitional circulation. The outstanding feature is that the pressure in the pulmonary artery remains high, and thus the term favored by some authors is persistent pulmonary hypertension. However, pulmonary artery pressure may be much more labile than previously thought, hence it may not be so much *persistence* as *reversion*. The most frequent predisposing factor to this persistent fetal state is asphyxia, which occurs either prenatally or at the time of delivery but may also be the result of intrinsic pulmonary disease that develops after delivery. Pathologically, the arterioles remain thick walled (rather than undergoing the normal developmental process), with persistence of an increased pulmonary vascular resistance.

Recent evidence suggests that a major stimulus to pulmonary vasoconstriction is the presence of leukotrienes (primarily C_4). The release of leukotrienes may be triggered by asphyxia, group B streptococcus, and so on.

DIAGNOSIS

The most striking clinical feature is persistent cyanosis, which is not relieved by increasing concentrations of oxygen. There may be associated respiratory difficulty, and it is frequently difficult to distinguish this condition from cyanotic congenital heart disease or severe pulmonary disease. A baby who was asphyxiated at birth and who has a normal chest x-ray study but remains cyanotic should be suspected of having persistent pulmonary hypertension. When the chest x-ray study shows pulmonary infiltrates, it may be difficult to be sure whether cyanosis is purely a result of the pulmonary disease or whether persistent pulmonary hypertension is complicating the picture (particularly with group B streptococcal pneumonia).

MANAGEMENT

One method of trying to differentiate between pulmonary disease and either congenital heart disease or persistent pulmonary hypertension is to use the hyperoxia test, which may be augmented with continuous positive airway pressure. With pulmonary disease there should be a significant increase in the paO_2 or $tcpO_2$. With cyanotic congenital heart disease or persistent fetal circulation, it is unlikely that a significant elevation in pO_2 will occur, although there may be enough improvement to eliminate cyanosis. If cyanosis persists, the first approach to treatment is assisted ventilation, which is accomplished using an endotracheal tube, with either a pressure- or volume-limited respirator. In many cases, satisfactory ventilation of the lungs is enough to decrease pulmonary vascular resistance and allow the usual transition with effective blood flow. It may be necessary to maintain pCO_2 around 25 mm Hg to produce a respiratory alkalosis. The improvement in pO_2 that may ensue is primarily the result of an increase in pH rather than a decrease in pCO_2.

Other methods of increasing the blood pH may be needed to decrease pulmonary vasoconstriction. Initially, sodium bicarbonate can be tried, but, if serum sodium levels are high, tris hydroxymethyl amino-methane (THAM) may be an alternative. It is usually necessary to raise the pH above 7.55 to achieve a satisfactory response.

Another approach is to increase systemic blood pressure, to eliminate right-to-left shunting at the atrial or ductal level caused by suprasystemic pressure in the pulmonary circuit. This may be accomplished by using boluses of fluid (crystalloid or colloid, preferably the latter) or vasopressor agents, such as dopamine.

Yet another approach is to use a pharmacologic agent that will have a preferential effect in vasodilating the pulmonary arteries. In the past, tolazoline was used for this purpose, but it tends to vasodilate the systemic arteries too and may produce a marked hypotension. It should be administered only after initiating a vasopressor agent. Leukotriene inhibitors have been successful in animal models, but the most exciting new therapy is the use of inhaled nitric oxide. Because it acts directly on pulmonary blood vessels but is rapidly converted, inhaled nitric oxide does not produce systemic hypotension. At this writing, this treatment is still experimental.

Finally, in many cases of persistent pulmonary hypertension that are unresponsive to these measures, it may be necessary to use extracorporeal membrane oxygenation.

SUMMARY

Persistent pulmonary hypertension seems to be the result of an asphyxial insult that produces persistence of the thickening of the arteriolar wall of pulmonary vessels. It may also be triggered by the release of leukotrienes. This condition may be difficult to distinguish from cyanotic congenital heart disease or severe pulmonary parenchymal disease. Resolution of the problem is frequently accomplished by the use of assisted ventilation, alkalinization, and pressor support, but extracorporeal membrane oxygenation may be required in some cases.

PULMONARY HYPOPLASIA

INTRODUCTION

Many clinical situations may be encountered in neonatology in which hypoplasia of the lungs may contribute to morbidity and mortality. Clearly, the degree of hypoplasia or the presence of other problems determines whether survival or death is the outcome.

PATHOGENESIS

Understanding of the possible pathogenesis of this disorder has been greatly enhanced by recent studies. Certain situations have been clear for some time; for example, compression and limitation of lung growth are seen in cases of diaphragmatic hernia. It has also been observed that chronic leakage of amniotic fluid and renal disorders that produce oligohydramnios (e.g., bilateral renal agenesis or posterior urethral valves) may be associated with pulmonary hypoplasia, possibly because of compression of the fetal thorax.

These last findings have been further explained by observations and experiments in which fetal breathing movements were obliterated. Absence of fetal breathing movements (which may be limited by thoracic compression) seems to result in pulmonary hypoplasia (Wigglesworth, 1982).

DIAGNOSIS

The conditions noted in the discussion of pathogenesis should strongly suggest pulmonary hypoplasia. The most usual presentation is significant respiratory distress. Considerably higher pressures than are usually needed to ventilate the lungs may be required. In addition, the chest x-ray study usually suggests a decreased thoracic volume, and the clinical picture of persistent pulmonary hypertension is frequently encountered.

MANAGEMENT

No obvious method of prevention is available. Supportive management with assisted ventilation and other treatment directed toward persistent pulmonary hypertension seems to be all that can be offered. It may be possible to maintain the conditions of some babies until continued lung growth allows their lungs to function adequately.

SUMMARY

Several circumstances are associated with pulmonary hypoplasia, including diaphragmatic hernia, congenital renal abnormalities, prolonged leakage of amniotic fluid, and disorders that prevent fetal breathing movements. Management is difficult and is complicated by persistent pulmonary hypertension.

CHRONIC LUNG DISEASE OF THE NEONATE

INTRODUCTION

The choice of this term is an attempt to avoid separating the two commonly employed terms of bronchopulmonary dysplasia (BPD) and Wilson-Mikity syndrome, which the author believes to be part of a continuum of lung pathology. Under this term, one might also place chronic pulmonary insufficiency of prematurity. Perhaps the common feature of all these disorders is another term applied to the first two disorders, pulmonary fibroplasia.

ETIOLOGY AND PATHOPHYSIOLOGY

The features of the three disorders are summarized in Table 9–1. Exposure of the neonatal lung to oxygen in high concentration and the use of assisted ventilation using a positive pressure machine may certainly produce the changes that have been labeled bronchopulmonary dysplasia. The role of the endotracheal tube, the underlying disease, and other factors are not clearly understood, but changes seem more likely to occur in immature lungs in a shorter time. High peak airway pressure may be important in BPD. The role of vitamin E

TABLE 9–1. DISTINGUISHING FEATURES OF CHRONIC LUNG DISEASES OF PREMATURITY

Feature	BPD	W-MS	CPIP
Associated Antecedents			
RDS	+ +	−	−
Positive pressure via assisted ventilation	+ +		
Increased oxygen concentration	+ +	±	±
Extreme prematurity	+	+ + +	+ +
Age at Onset	4–7 days	10–14 days	4–7 days
Chest x-ray study findings			
Bubbly or honeycomb lung	+ + +	+ + +	−
Hyperinflation and flat diaphragm	+ + +	+ +	±
White out	+ + (early)	±	±
Biochemistry			
pH ↓	+	±	±
pCO$_2$ ↑	+ +	+	+ +
Pathology			
Exudative change	+ + (early)	−	?
Pulmonary fibrosis	+ + +	+ + +	?
Dysplastic change	+ + +	±	?
Obstructive bronchiolitis	+ + +	+ +	?

BPD = bronchopulmonary dysplasia; CPIP = chronic pulmonary insufficiency of prematurity; RDS = respiratory distress syndrome; W-MS = Wilson-Mikity syndrome; + = quite common; + + = common; + + + = very common; ± = sometimes; − = rare.

(acting as an antioxidant) in preventing or ameliorating the changes of BPD is disputed. Cytomegalovirus has also been implicated in chronic lung disease of later onset.

DIAGNOSIS

Differentiation of these conditions has primarily been made on the basis of clinical course, in conjunction with the chest radiograph (Figs. 9–7 and 9–8). BPD usually starts earlier in association with mechanical ventilation. Wilson-Mikity syndrome usually occurs in very premature infants who have had minimal exposure to increased inspired oxygen. Both have cystic changes on chest x-ray study—so-called bubbly lung. Chronic pulmonary insufficiency of prematurity, like Wilson-Mikity syndrome, has an insidious onset and occurs in very premature infants. The chest x-ray study shows a diffuse haziness, reminiscent of the exudative phase of BPD, or it may be normal. In all of these conditions, tachypnea and dyspnea occur, with increasing oxygen dependency and retention of carbon dioxide.

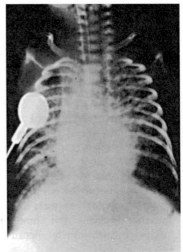

FIGURE 9–7. Bronchopulmonary dysplasia, showing hyperexpansion of both lungs, particularly at the left base, and scattered cystic lesions.

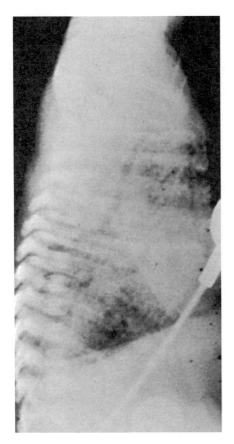

FIGURE 9–8. A lateral radiograph of the baby in Figure 9–7, showing cystic lesions in the region above the diaphragm.

MANAGEMENT

Supportive management with oxygen, possibly chest physiotherapy, and intravenous fluids is usually indicated. Cor pulmonale may ensue and is often responsive to digoxin and diuretics, although severe cases may result in death. Corticosteroids may be valuable for severe cases of BPD to aid in the weaning process from mechanical ventilation. If these babies can be supported through the first months of life, the long-term prognosis appears to be good, although some recent extended experience suggests that some infants have prolonged difficulty with bronchial hyperreactivity. Because these children are often exquisitely sensitive to oxygen, they should be handled as gently as possible. Prolonged hospitalization may be avoided in some cases by providing oxygen by nasal cannula and treating the child at home. Home oxygen therapy may be facilitated by using transcutaneous pO_2 (or O_2 saturation) monitoring.

Another problem encountered in infants with BPD is intermittent fever. The cause is frequently elusive, although it may be related to atelectasis. It is difficult not to investigate these infants for superimposed infection, but it is found rarely.

SUMMARY

Very premature babies may develop a chronic picture of tachypnea, dyspnea, and oxygen dependency, with radiographic features of cystic changes or diffuse haziness. The immature lung may only be capable of reacting in a limited number of ways to different noxious stimuli (including mechanical ventilation and high inspired oxygen concentration). Treatment is symptomatic and may include management of cor pulmonale. The long-term prognosis appears to be good if babies survive the first months of life.

RESPIRATORY DISORDERS AMENABLE TO SURGERY

The following disorders have been discussed earlier: diaphragmatic hernia (p. 91), tracheoesophageal fistula (p. 89), and pneumothorax (p. 119). Other disorders that should be mentioned follow.

CHOANAL ATRESIA

Choanal atresia varies from a web to a bony bridge at the back of the nose and prevents the usual obligatory nasal breathing of newborns, which may result in severe respiratory embarrassment in the delivery room with gasping respiration. If respiration is established, intermittent difficulty is likely to follow, particularly when the oral airway is occluded at feeding time (see also Chapter 24). It may be associated with other anomalies and a serious prognosis (including mental retardation). Together, these abnormalities have been listed under the acronym CHARGE association (coloboma, heart disease, atresia choanae, retarded growth and development, genital hypoplasia, and ear anomalies and/or deafness).

MICROGNATHIA AND GLOSSOPTOSIS

When the jaw is abnormally small (micrognathia), the tongue may tend to occlude the airway (glossoptosis). In association with cleft palate, this condition is called Pierre Robin syndrome. Suitable positioning may allow the tongue to fall forward. Although it occasionally was suggested that the tongue be surgically sutured to the lip, prolonged use of a nasopharyngeal airway seems to have been well tolerated. In a baby treated by the author, a palatal prosthesis seemed to produce marked improvement by restoring the nasal airway (see also Chapter 24).

CONGENITAL CYSTIC ADENOMATOID MALFORMATION

Congenital cystic adenomatoid malformation may be confused with diaphragmatic hernia on x-ray study, with multiple small cysts in an intrapulmonary mass. The abnormal lung may produce considerable compression of normal lung (often herniating to the opposite side).

CONGENITAL LOBAR EMPHYSEMA

Congenital lobar emphysema is the result of overdistension of one or more lobes of the lung (usually upper lobes or right-middle lobe). It presents more frequently after several weeks of life but may be noted soon after birth. There is inability of the lung to deflate normally, which results in compression of normal lung tissue. It may be the result of (1) congenital deficiency of bronchial cartilage, (2) partial intraluminal bronchial obstruction, or (3) extraluminal bronchial obstruction.

BIBLIOGRAPHY

Thibeault, D. W., and Gregory, G. A.: *Neonatal Pulmonary Care.* Addison-Wesley Publishing Company, Menlo Park, CA, 1979.

Respiratory Distress Syndrome

Gluck, L., and Kulovich, M. V.: Fetal lung development: Current concepts. *Pediatr. Clin. North Am.* 1973, 20:367.
Cowett, R. M., Unsworth, E. J., Hakanson, D. O., et al.: Foam-stability test on gastric aspirate and the diagnosis of respiratory-distress syndrome. *N. Engl. J. Med.* 1975, 293:413.
Usher, R. H., Saigal, S., O'Neill, A., et al.: Estimation of red blood cell volume in premature infants with and without respiratory distress syndrome. *Biol. Neonate* 1975, 26:241.

Gewolb, I. H., Lebowitz, R. L., and Taeusch, H. W. G.: Thymus size and its relationship to the respiratory distress syndrome. *J. Pediatr.* 1979, 95:108.

Heaf, D. P., Belik, J., Spitzer, A. R., et al.: Changes in pulmonary function during the diuretic phase of respiratory distress syndrome. *J. Pediatr.* 1982, 101:103–107.

Engle, W. D., Arant, B. S., Jr., Wiriyathian, S., and Rosenfeld, C. R.: Diuresis and respiratory distress syndrome: Physiologic mechanisms and therapeutic implications. *J. Pediatr.* 1983, 102:912–917.

Kaapa, P., Lanning, P., and Koivisto, M.: Early closure of patent ductus arteriosus with indomethacin in preterm infants with idiopathic respiratory distress syndrome. *Acta Paediatr.* 1983, 72:179–184.

Turkel, S. B., and Mapp, J. R.: A ten-year retrospective study of pink and yellow neonatal hyaline membrane disease. *Pediatrics* 1984, 104:240.

Avery, M. E.: The argument for prenatal administration of dexamethasone to prevent respiratory distress syndrome. *J. Pediatr.* 1984, 104:240.

Yeh, T. F., Shibli, A., Leu, S. T., et al.: Early furosemide therapy in premature infants (<2000 gm) with respiratory distress syndrome: A randomized controlled trial. *J. Pediatr.* 1984, 105:603–609.

White, E., Shy, K. K., and Daling, E. R.: An investigation of the relationship between Cesarean section birth and respiratory distress syndrome of the newborn. *Am. J. Epidemiol.* 1985, 121:651–663.

Speer, C. P., Robertson, B., Curstedt, T., et al.: Randomized European multicenter trial of surfactant replacement therapy for severe neonatal respiratory distress syndrome: Single versus multiple doses of Curosurf. *Pediatrics* 1992, 89:13–20.

Corbet, A.: Clinical trials of synthetic surfactant in the respiratory distress syndrome of premature infants. *Clin. Perinatol.* 1993, 20:737–760.

Jobe, A. H., Mitchell, B. R., and Gunkel, J. H.: Beneficial effects of the combined use of prenatal corticosteroids and postnatal surfactant on preterm infants. *Am. J. Obstet. Gynecol.* 1993, 168:508–513.

Mercier, C. E., and Soll, R. F.: Clinical trials of natural surfactant extract in respiratory distress syndrome. *Clin. Perinatol.* 1993, 20:711–736.

Pneumonia

Oliver, T. K., Jr., Smith, B., and Clatworthy, H. W., Jr.: Staphylococcal pneumonia. *Pediatr. Clin. North Am.* 1959, 6:1043.

Kuhn, J. P., and Lee, S. B.: Pneumatoceles associated with *Escherichia coli* pneumonias in the newborn. *Pediatrics* 1973, 51:1008.

Papegeorgiou, A., Bauer, C. R., Fletcher, B. D., and Stern, L.: *Klebsiella pneumoniae* with pneumatocele formation. *Can. Med. Assoc. J.* 1973, 109:1217.

Hammerschlag, M. R.: Chlamydial pneumonia in infants (Editorial). *N. Engl. J. Med.* 1978, 298:1083.

Menke, J. A., Giacoia, G. P., and Jackia, H.: Group B beta hemolytic streptococcal sepsis and the idiopathic respiratory distress syndrome: A comparison. *J. Pediatr.* 1979, 94:467.

Jacob, J., Edwards, D., and Gluck, L.: Early-onset sepsis and pneumonia observed as respiratory distress syndrome. Assessment of lung maturity. *Am. J. Dis. Child.* 1980, 134:766–768.

Sherman, M. P., Goetzman, B. W., Ahlfors, C. E., and Wennberg, R. P.: Tracheal aspiration and its clinical correlates in the diagnosis of congenital pneumonia. *Pediatrics* 1980, 65:258.

Yoder, P. R., Gibbs, R. S., Blanco, J. D., et al.: A prospective, controlled study of maternal and perinatal outcome after intra-amniotic infection at term. *Am. J. Obstet. Gynecol.* 1983, 145:695–701.

Philip, A. G. S.: Response of C-reactive protein in neonatal group B streptococcal infection. *Pediatr. Infect. Dis.* 1985, 4:145–148.

Aspiration Syndromes

Matsaniotis, N., Karpouzas, J., Tzortzatou-Vallianou, M., and Tsagournis, E.: Aspiration due to difficulty in swallowing. *Arch. Dis. Child.* 1971, 46:788.

Applebaum, P. C., Holloway, Y., Ross, S. M., and Duphelia, I.: The effect of amniotic fluid on bacterial growth in three population groups. *Am. J. Obstet. Gynecol.* 1977, 128:868.

Yeh, T. F., Srinivasan, G., Harris, V., and Pildes, R. S.: Hydrocortisone therapy in meconium aspiration syndrome: A controlled study. *J. Pediatr.* 1977, 53:74.

Lucas, A., Christofides, N. D., Adrian, T. E., et al.: Fetal distress, meconium, and motilin. *Lancet* 1979, i:718.

Gage, J. E., Taeusch, H. W., Jr., Treves, S., and Caldicott, W.: Suctioning of upper airway meconium in newborn infants. *J.A.M.A.* 1981, 246:2590–2592.

Meis, P. J., Hobel, C. J., and Ureda, J. R.: Late meconium passage in labor—a sign of fetal distress? *Obstet. Gynecol.* 1982, 59:332–335.

Murphy, J. D., Vawter, G. F., and Reid, L. M.: Pulmonary vascular disease in fatal meconium aspiration. *J. Pediatr.* 1984, 104:758–762.

Wiswell, T. E., Tuggle, J. M., and Turner B. S.: Meconium aspiration syndrome: Have we made a difference? *Pediatrics* 1990, 85:715–721.

Retained Lung Fluid Syndromes

Avery, M. E., Gatewood, O. B., and Brumley, G.: Transient tachypnea of the newborn. *Am. J. Dis. Child.* 1966, 111:380.

Sundell, H., Garrott, J., Blankenship, W. J., et al.: Studies of infants with type II respiratory distress syndrome. *J. Pediatr.* 1971, 78:754.

Patel, D. M., Donovan, E. F., and Keenan, W. J.: Transient respiratory difficulty following cesarean delivery. *Biol. Neonate* 1983, 43:146–151.

Rawlings, J. S., and Smith, F. R.: Transient tachypnea of the newborn: An analysis of neonatal and obstetric risk factors. *Am. J. Dis. Child.* 1984, 138:869–871.

Pneumothorax and Pneumomediastinum

Ogata, E. S., Gregory, G. A., Kitterman, J. A., et al.: Pneumothorax in the respiratory distress syndrome: Incidence and effect on vital signs, blood gases and pH. *Pediatrics* 1976, 58:177.

Bashour, B. N., and Balfe, J. W.: Urinary tract anomalies in neonates with spontaneous pneumothorax and/or pneumomediastinum. *Pediatrics* 1977, 59(Suppl):1048.

Noack, G., and Freyschuss, U.: The early detection of pneumothorax with transthoracic impedance in newborn infants. *Acta Paediatr.* 1977, 66:677.

Allen, R. W., Jr., Jung, A. L., and Lester, P. D.: Effectiveness of chest tube evacuation of pneumothorax in neonates. *J. Pediatr.* 1981, 99:629–634.

Rothberg, A. D., Marks, K. H., and Maisels, M. J.: Understanding the Pleurevac. *Pediatrics* 1981, 67:482–484.

Cooke, R. W. I., Rennie, J. M., and Lerman, S. I.: Pancuronium and pneumothorax. *Lancet* 1984, i:286–287.

Pulmonary Interstitial Emphysema

Dickman, G. L., Short, B. L., and Krauss, D. R.: Selective bronchial intubation in the management of unilateral pulmonary interstitial emphysema. *Am. J. Dis. Child.* 1977, 131:365.

Primhak, R. A.: Factors associated with pulmonary air leak in premature infants receiving mechanical ventilation. *J. Pediatr.* 1983, 102:764–768.

Dear, P. R. F., and Conway, S. P.: Treatment of severe bilateral interstitial emphysema in a baby by artificial pneumothorax and pneumonotomy. *Lancet* 1984, i:273–275.

Greenough, A., Dixon, A. K., and Roberton, N. R. C.: Pulmonary interstitial emphysema. *Arch. Dis. Child.* 1984, 59:1046–1051.

Persistent Pulmonary Hypertension

Murphy, J. D., Rabinovitch, M., Goldstein, J. D., and Reid, L. M.: The structural basis of persistent pulmonary hypertension of the newborn infant. *J. Pediatr.* 1981, 98:962–967.

Brett, C., Dekle, M., Leonard, C. H., et al.: Developmental follow-up of hyperventilated neonates: Preliminary observations. *Pediatrics* 1981, 68:588–591.

Drummond, W. H., Gregory, G. A., Heymann, M. A., and Phibbs, R. H.: Independent effects of hyperventilation, tolazoline and dopamine on infants with persistent pulmonary hypertension. *J. Pediatr.* 1981, 98:603–611.

Stenmark, K. R.: Leukotriene C_4 and D_4 in neonates with hypoxemia and pulmonary hypertension. *N. Engl. J. Med.* 1983, 309:77–80.

Goldberg, R. N., Suguihara, C., Steitfield, M. M., et al.: Effects of leukotriene antagonist FPL 57231 on early hemodynamic manifestations of group b beta streptococcal sepsis in piglets. *Pediatr. Res.* 1985, 19:342A.

Kinsella, J. P., Neish, S. R., Ivy, D. D., et al.: Clinical responses to prolonged treatment of persistent pulmonary hypertension of the newborn with low doses of inhaled nitric oxide. *J. Pediatr.* 1993, 123:103–108.

Walsh-Sukys, M. C.: Persistent pulmonary hypertension of the newborn: The black box revisited. *Clin. Perinatal.* 1993, 20:127–144.

Kanto, W. P., Jr.: A decade of experience with neonatal extracorporeal membrane oxygenation. *J. Pediatr.* 1994, 124:335–347.

Pulmonary Hypoplasia

Fliegner, J. R., Fortune, D. W., and Eggers, T. R.: Premature rupture of the membranes, oligohydramnios and pulmonary hypoplasia. *Aust. N.Z. J. Obstet. Gynaecol.* 1981, 21:77–81.

Hislop, A., and Fairweather, D. V. I.: Amniocentesis and lung growth: An animal experiment with clinical implications. *Lancet* 1982, i:1271–1272.

Wigglesworth, J. S., and Desai, R.: Is fetal respiratory function a major determinant of perinatal survival? *Lancet* 1982, i:264–267.

Blott, M., Greenough, A., and Nicolaides K. H.: Fetal breathing movements in pregnancies complicated by premature membrane rupture in the second trimester. *Early Hum. Dev.* 1990, 21:41–48.

Chronic Lung Disease

Krauss, A. N., Klain, D. S., and Auld, P. A. M.: Chronic pulmonary insufficiency of prematurity (CPIP). *Pediatrics* 1975, 55:55.

Philip, A. G. S.: Oxygen plus pressure time: The etiology of bronchopulmonary dysplasia. *Pediatrics* 1975, 55:44.

Saunders, R. A., Milner, A. D., and Hopkin, I. E.: Longitudinal studies of infants with the Wilson-Mikity syndrome. Clinical, radiological and mechanical correlations. *Biol. Neonate* 1978, 33:90.

Ballard, R. A., Drew, W. L., Hufnagle, K. G., and Riedel, P. A.: Acquired cytomegalovirus infection in preterm infants. *Am. J. Dis. Child.* 1979, 133:482.

O'Brodovich, H. M., and Mellins, R. B.: Bronchopulmonary dysplasia: Unresolved neonatal acute lung injury. *Am. Rev. Respir. Dis.* 1985, 132:694–709.

Cummings, J. J., D'Eugenio, D. B., and Gross, S. J.: A controlled trial of dexamethasone in preterm infants at high risk for bronchopulmonary dysplasia. *N. Engl. J. Med.* 1989, 320:1505–1510.

Northway, W. H., Jr., Moss, R. B., Carlisle, K. B., et al.: Late pulmonary sequelae of bronchopulmonary dysplasia. *N. Engl. J. Med.* 1990, 323:1793–1799.

Bronchopulmonary dysplasia. *Clin. Perinatal.* 1992, 19:489–700.

Singer, L., Martin, R. T., Hawkins, S. W., et al.: Oxygen desaturation complicates feeding in infants with bronchopulmonary dysplasia after discharge. *Pediatrics* 1992, 90:380–384.

Disorders Amenable to Surgery

DeLuca, F. G. K., and Wesselhoeft, C. W.: Surgically treatable causes of neonatal respiratory distress. *Clin. Perinatol.* 1978, 5:377.

Nishibayashi, S. W., Andrassy, R. J., and Wooley, M. M.: Congenital cystic adenomatoid malformation: A 30 year experience. *J. Pediatr. Surg.* 1981, 16:704–706.

Pagon, R. A., Graham, J. M., Jr., Zonana, J., and Yong, S-L.: Coloboma, congenital heart disease and choanal atresia with multiple anomalies: CHARGE association. *J. Pediatr.* 1981, 99:223–227.

Heaf, D. P., Helms, P. J., Dinwiddie, R., and Matthew, D. J.: Nasopharyngeal airways in Pierre-Robin syndrome. *J. Pediatr.* 1982, 100:698–703.

Man, D. W. K., Hamdy, M. H., Hendry, G. M. A., et al.: Congenital lobar emphysema: Problems in diagnosis and management. *Arch. Dis. Child.* 1983, 58:709–712.

10
BILIRUBIN METABOLISM AND JAUNDICE

Jaundice is present in a large number of newborn infants. When the level of bilirubin is greatly elevated, a large variety of disorders may be implicated. Almost all infants with mild elevations in bilirubin level either are not investigated or their jaundice is dismissed as physiologic. A good understanding of the mechanisms that contribute to normal bilirubin metabolism is important in the consideration of both physiologic and pathologic jaundice. Such considerations are probably second in frequency only to consideration of respiratory difficulty.

BASIC BILIRUBIN METABOLISM

Unconjugated bilirubin is derived from the breakdown of hemoglobin from red blood cells. This process may occur more rapidly in starvation, under the influence of heme oxygenase. Approximately 35 mg of bilirubin is generated by 1 g of hemoglobin (the tetrapyrrole ring of hemoglobin being converted to a tetrapyrrole chain).

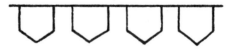

Unconjugated bilirubin is fat soluble and is converted to the water-soluble conjugated bilirubin (diglucuronide) by the following reaction:

uridine diphosphoglucuronic acid + bilirubin →
$$\text{bilirubin GA} + \text{uridine diphosphate}$$

under the influence of glucuronyl transferase in the liver cell. A sulfate pathway may also be used.

Transport of unconjugated bilirubin in the blood is achieved by binding to albumin. There appear to be primary and secondary binding sites. When all such binding sites are filled, the bilirubin is no longer bound but is now free.

This fat-soluble free unconjugated bilirubin can then be deposited in fatty areas, including the brain. Such deposition of bilirubin in the basal nuclei of the brain may result in the condition called kernicterus.

For unconjugated bilirubin to enter the liver cell, an active transport mechanism is necessary (Fig. 10–1). This mechanism consists of transport proteins labeled Y and Z proteins (sometimes called ligandins).

After conjugation, bilirubin diglucuronide is excreted into the biliary system and hence into the gut. Whether or not another transport mechanism is implicated is unclear. After it is excreted into the gut, it may be acted on by a β-glucuronidase, which releases unconjugated bilirubin, and this may be reabsorbed (via the enterohepatic circulation).

One additional concept has received considerable attention in recent years: photobilirubin. During any light exposure, particularly phototherapy (discussed later, p. 392), bilirubin is photoisomerized into four isomers of bilirubin, which appear to be nontoxic. The structural isomers (called lumirubin) are water soluble and can be excreted in urine. These isomers can also be excreted into bile without the need for conjugation. The picture becomes more confused because usual methods of measuring plasma bilirubin do not distinguish natural unconjugated bilirubin (potentially toxic) from photobilirubin (apparently nontoxic).

ALBUMIN-BILIRUBIN BINDING

It has been suggested that bilirubin binds to certain sites on albumin (primary sites) more strongly than to others (secondary sites). The total amount

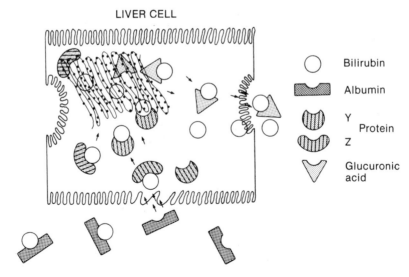

FIGURE 10–1. A schematic representation of the liver cell, showing the essentials of bilirubin metabolism.

of bilirubin that can be bound at any one time depends not only on the total amount of albumin available but also on (1) the presence of substances that may be competing for binding sites, including naturally occurring substances (e.g., free fatty acids, steroid hormones) and exogenous substances (e.g., long-acting sulfonamides, benzoates, salicylates); and (2) factors that alter the binding tightness (e.g., decreasing pH decreases binding).

Under certain circumstances (apparently prolonged cholestasis), very firm binding can occur, which seems to be quite different from usual binding. Whether or not this phenomenon occurs in the neonate is uncertain.

PHYSIOLOGIC JAUNDICE

INTRODUCTION

A great many babies, both term and preterm, demonstrate clinical jaundice (appear yellow). The diagnosis of physiologic jaundice should probably be one of exclusion, but in clinical practice if the day of onset is appropriate, if the height of bilirubin does not exceed certain limits, and if the baby appears vigorous and is feeding well, an extensive series of investigations is usually unnecessary.

PATHOPHYSIOLOGY

From the preceding discussion on bilirubin metabolism, one may deduce that several reasons may exist for the physiologic development of an elevated bilirubin level. For many years, it was considered to be solely the result of a transient deficiency of the enzyme glucuronyl transferase. With a rising bilirubin level (unconjugated), substrate stimulation of the enzyme occurs, which soon accommodates to the rising bilirubin load, although the enzyme may take a little longer to be "turned on" in the preterm infant.

Almost certainly, two other mechanisms are involved, the first being a relative deficiency of the acceptor proteins (the transport proteins, Y and Z), and the second being an increase in the amount of glucuronidase present in the gut, which allows unconjugated bilirubin to be recycled. If a delay in the passage of meconium occurs, the levels of bilirubin are higher because more time exists for glucuronidase to act.

DIAGNOSIS

Physiologic jaundice normally should not be considered in the diagnosis in babies younger than 48 hours (although it occasionally seems to occur before 48 hours). Jaundice is usually noted first on the face and then spreads in a caudal direction. In all other respects, the baby appears to be well. When jaundice is only over the face and neck, the level of bilirubin is approximately 4 to 8 mg/dl. When the upper trunk is involved, the level may range from 5 to 12 mg/dl in term babies. The level at which jaundice appears is somewhat lower in preterm infants. Most authors would accept unconjugated bilirubin levels of 12 mg/dl in the term baby and 15 mg/dl in the preterm baby as the upper limits resulting from physiologic mechanisms. (NOTE: This does not imply that such limits are safe for the preterm infant.) The ability to obtain more rapid estimates of bilirubin levels using transcutaneous bilirubinometers means that a "number" can be obtained more rapidly. This can minimize the need to determine serum bilirubin levels.

MANAGEMENT

Most infants with physiologic jaundice require no specific treatment. Early feeding may help to prevent it. Mothers of infants who are obviously jaundiced over the whole trunk on the third or fourth day should have a review of their blood group. The baby's blood group and the results of a Coombs test, together with a complete blood count (including a smear of cells for morphology), should be determined, and a total and fractionated (direct and indirect) bilirubin level should be obtained. A total protein level determination (as an indicator of albumin concentration) may also be helpful. In babies born at term, if the unconjugated (indirect) bilirubin level is higher than 15 mg/dl, it has been customary to start phototherapy (see p. 392) to prevent levels from exceeding 20 mg/dl. However, the "magic number" of 20 mg/dl was derived from studies in infants with hemolytic disease of the newborn. Information has been available for a number of years that suggests that considerably higher levels of bilirubin can be tolerated by term neonates who do not demonstrate hemolysis. This information was recently brought to the attention of pediatricians, with commentary suggesting that this is needless "vigintiphobia" (or more correctly, "eikosiphobia"). The whole subject of what constitutes a dangerous level is very confused, particularly for the preterm infant who is sick (see Lucey, 1982). In preterm babies, it is our practice to begin phototherapy if the unconjugated bilirubin level approaches or exceeds 10 mg/dl (see next section).

Guidelines for the management of the healthy term newborn with hyperbilirubinemia have been published (Table 10–1).

SUMMARY

Physiologic jaundice occurs after 48 hours of age and is seen commonly in most nurseries around the world. The principal mechanism implicated is probably a transient deficiency of the enzyme glucuronyl transferase, but deficiency of acceptor proteins and recycling via the enterohepatic circulation are also involved. No specific treatment is usually required, but occasionally phototherapy is needed after baseline investigations have been performed.

TABLE 10-1. MANAGEMENT OF HYPERBILIRUBINEMIA IN THE HEALTHY TERM NEWBORN*

	Total Bilirubin Level, mg/dl (μmol/l)			
Age (Hours)	Consider Phototherapy†	Phototherapy	Exchange Transfusion if Intensive Phototherapy Fails‡	Exchange Transfusion and Intensive Phototherapy
≤24‖	—	—	—	—
25–48	≥12 (170)	≥15 (260)	≥20 (340)	≥25 (430)
49–71	≥15 (260)	≥18 (310)	≥25 (430)	≥30 (510)
>72	≥17 (290)	≥20 (340)	≥25 (430)	≥30 (510)

*Modified from American Academy of Pediatrics: Management of hyperbilirubinemia in the healthy term newborn. *Pediatrics* 1994, 94:558–565.
†Phototherapy at these levels is a clinical option, to be used on the basis of individual clinical judgment.
‡Intensive phototherapy should produce a decline of total bilirubin of 1 to 2 mg/dl within 4 to 6 hours, and the level should continue to fall and remain below the threshold level for exchange transfusion.
‖Term infants who are clinically jaundiced at ≤24 hours old are not considered healthy and require further evaluation.

BILIRUBIN AND THE BREASTFED INFANT

In recent years, there has been greater acceptance of the idea that breast-fed infants are more likely to experience jaundice than are bottle (formula)–fed infants. The jaundice seems to be of two types: that seen early, which is usually designated jaundice associated with breast feeding, and that seen late (after 7 days), which may be designated "breast milk jaundice." The latter term suggests something specific is in the milk that interferes with bilirubin metabolism. When originally described, the substance inhibiting glucuronyl transferase was thought to be 3α,20β-pregnanediol, but then the inhibitor seemed to be an increase in either lipoprotein lipase or nonesterified fatty acids. More recently, it has been suggested that breast milk jaundice is due to an increase in breast milk β-glucuronidase with increased enterohepatic recycling rather than due to glucuronyl transferase inhibition. It seems possible that some cases of early jaundice are associated with increased levels of β-glucuronidase in breast milk.

The incidence of high levels of serum bilirubin is greater in breast-fed infants, with the levels in approximately 9% of breast-fed infants exceeding 12.9 mg/dl, compared with 2% of formula-fed infants. In healthy breast-fed infants, investigations for hyperbilirubinemia may not be indicated unless serum bilirubin levels exceed approximately 15 mg/dl, compared with 12 mg/dl in bottle-fed infants. For those who exceed 17 mg/dl, several treatment options can be offered to parents, including continuing or discontinuing breast feeding, with or without phototherapy. However, such interruption of breast feeding may result in earlier termination of breast feeding and possible development of the vulnerable child syndrome.

BILIRUBIN AND THE PREMATURE INFANT

For many reasons, the premature (preterm) infant is at special risk as far as bilirubin toxicity is concerned. Kernicterus has been observed in premature infants who died after having unconjugated bilirubin levels that did not exceed 12 mg/dl. However, it is not clear whether or not this phenomenon would occur in the absence of asphyxia and/or acidosis. Bilirubin staining of the brain has occurred in the presence of asphyxia by apparent leakage of blood vessels. Whether or not this condition is kernicterus is debatable because the "kerns" (nuclei) are not selectively affected. This type of kernicterus may be reflected in an increased frequency of yellow (rather than pink) hyaline membranes at necropsy. In addition to these postmortem findings, poor outcome in some preterm infants was correlated with only minor increases in bilirubin levels. It is now known that infants with intraventricular or periventricular hemorrhage (and presumably associated ischemia) tend to have higher levels of bilirubin, as with other forms of enclosed hemorrhage (see p. 144). Thus, what is the cause of long-term deficit remains a matter for conjecture. Nevertheless, the following special concerns should be taken into consideration.

Total protein (and albumin) level rises with advancing gestational age, but the range at any given gestational age is quite broad (approximately 2 g/dl). Although the amount of albumin available is obviously important in estimating how much bilirubin can be bound, there is great variability in the bilirubin to albumin molar ratio. There now is still no uniformity of opinion about the value of a large number of albumin-bilirubin binding tests. An approximation of the dangerous level of unconjugated bilirubin was made by Odell (1969) (total protein [g/dl] × 3.7).

Such numbers are merely approximations, and other factors must be taken into consideration, particularly the clinical status of the baby.

Premature infants (indeed, all low-birth-weight infants) are more likely to be subjected to cold stress, with release of free fatty acids in large quantities. These acids compete for binding sites on albumin and may displace bilirubin.

Acidosis is more likely to be seen in association with sepsis and the respiratory disorders seen in premature infants. The associated drop in pH may affect the affinity of bilirubin to bind to albumin. This problem may be further compounded by the tendency of cooling to produce acidosis.

Physiologic mechanisms are exaggerated in the premature infant. It may take longer to stimulate glucuronyl transferase to turn on. The acceptor proteins (Y and Z) are probably present in smaller quantities. β-Glucuronidase seems to be present in greater quantities in premature infants, and, in addition, such infants may not be fed enterally for several days.

Total body fat, particularly subcutaneous fat, may act as a sort of reservoir into which bilirubin flows. When the reservoir is full, the risk of kernicterus increases. Preterm infants are markedly deficient in fat stores, which accumulate in the last 2 to 3 months of gestation.

HEMOLYTIC DISEASE OF THE NEWBORN (ERYTHROBLASTOSIS FETALIS)

Among the many disorders contributing to increased levels of bilirubin, several blood group incompatibilities play an important role. Together, these conditions are designated as hemolytic disease of the newborn because the underlying problem is the hemolysis of red blood cells by antibody transferred to the baby from the mother across the placenta (and therefore known to be in the immunoglobulin G group).

By far, the most important of these hemolytic conditions is rhesus incompatibility. Erythroblastosis (an excess of circulating nucleated red blood cells) is frequently encountered and accounts for the older (but less accurate) term erythroblastosis fetalis. ABO incompatibility accounts for an increasingly higher percentage of all cases of hemolytic disease of the newborn, but less common blood types (e.g., Kell, Duffy) may also produce significant clinical disease.

RHESUS INCOMPATIBILITY

Introduction and Incidence

One of the most dramatic stories in medicine in the past 20 years is the remarkable decrease in the number of Rh-negative mothers who have become sensitized during pregnancy involving an Rh-positive fetus, with a consequent decrease in the number of affected infants. This situation resulted from the use of anti-D globulin (Rh_o[D] immune globulin [RhoGAM]). In the 3 years from 1970 to 1973, the prevalence of Rh hemolytic disease fell from 45 in 10,000 live births to 27 in 10,000 live births in the United States. It was originally predicted that this disease would be virtually eliminated by this time. However, for several reasons, not all of which are preventable, this problem is still encountered from time to time. Prenatal administration of anti-D globulin (at about 28 weeks' gestation) has been recommended by numerous authorities, but the cost/benefit ratio is still debated.

Pathophysiology

This type of hemolytic disease of the newborn provides the basic mechanism for the whole group. It is known that a few fetal red blood cells cross the placenta and enter the maternal bloodstream at intervals during pregnancy. If the fetus has Rh-positive red cells and the mother is Rh negative, it is possible that enough red cells will cross the placenta to stimulate the production of antibody. The Rh-negative mother is usually designated as d, whereas the Rh-positive fetus is designated as D. The antibody that is produced is therefore endogenous anti-D.

Usually, the number of cells crossing the placenta is not sufficient to induce this production of antibody during pregnancy. However, in some cases, this phenomenon does seem to happen and may account for some of the failures with postpartum administration of anti-D globulin. (For this reason, more widespread adoption of administration of anti-D globulin early in the third trimester has recently occurred.) More typically, with separation of the placenta at the time of delivery, a shower of fetal red cells may be released into the maternal circulation. Unless exogenous anti-D is present in the next few days (or earlier, if transplacental passage of red cells has occurred), endogenous anti-D is likely to be produced. Because this material is IgG, it is free to pass the placental barrier in any subsequent pregnancy and may then hemolyze fetal red cells, with various clinical results.

Diagnosis

Whenever a mother is found to be Rh negative, she should be observed at intervals during the pregnancy to determine whether or not a rise in antibody (particularly anti-D) titers has occurred. In the presence of a rising titer or initially elevated titers (greater than 1:16), samples of amniotic fluid may be tested for elevated levels of bilirubin (which normally drop as pregnancy progresses). Serial samples can be plotted against various curves (e.g., Liley's curves) used to predict the outcome of pregnancy. When elevated levels are detected, the diagnosis of Rh incompatibility can be predicted with a high degree of probability. The outcome may be one of several different clinical pictures originally described as different conditions but now known to be part of a clinical continuum. These conditions are (1) hemolytic anemia of the newborn, (2) icterus gravis neonatorum (deep jaundice of the newborn), and (3) hydrops fetalis.

Hydrops fetalis may result from other conditions (e.g., α-thalassemia, fetomaternal hemorrhage [see p. 244], congenital syphilis) but is almost invariably the result of profound anemia with lowered serum protein levels, which results in accumulation of fluid in all body spaces (including massive ascites) (Fig. 10–2). True hydrops fetalis almost always results in death (Fig. 10–3). The state of prehydrops may be reversible.

Diagnosis of the affected newborn of an Rh-negative mother is confirmed by finding an Rh-positive infant with positive results on a direct Coombs test, an elevated cord blood bilirubin level or rapidly rising bilirubin levels, and anemia. In more severely affected infants, hepatosplenomegaly is the rule, and petechiae and purpura (with or without thrombocytopenia) may be present. Infections included in the TORCH syndrome may present a similar picture without the incompatible blood groups (see p. 192). The peripheral blood smear shows nucleated red cells and reticulocytosis.

In some severely affected infants, hepatocellular swelling produces an obstructive element and a combined elevation of conjugated (direct) and unconjugated (indirect) bilirubin. Another interesting feature, in the most severe cases, is hypoglycemia, which may be correlated with hyperplasia of the islets of Langerhans.

Management

Depending on the evaluation during pregnancy, the obstetrician may elect to deliver an affected baby several weeks early, 1 or 2 weeks early, or at term. In severely affected cases detected by amniocentesis in midpregnancy, it may be necessary to give the fetus a blood transfusion. This was originally performed by instilling red cells into the fetal peritoneal cavity (intrauterine transfusion). However, current methodology is to give the red cells directly into the umbilical cord of the fetus, using cordocentesis. It was suggested that oral Rh treatment

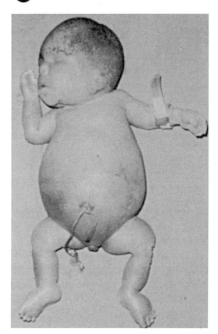

FIGURE 10–2. Hydrops fetalis in a baby with hemolytic disease due to Rh incompatibility. Generalized edema is seen in addition to marked abdominal distension.

FIGURE 10–3. Postmortem examination of another baby with hydrops fetalis showing massive enlargement of the liver.

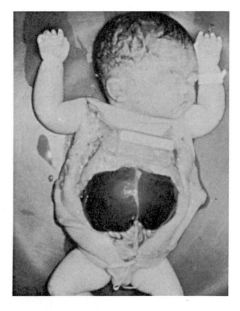

might ameliorate these severe cases, but recent experience does not support this idea. Other infants require immediate transfusion of packed red blood cells in the delivery room if profound anemia is noted. Most frequently, the treatment of choice is exchange transfusion (see p. 386) with whole blood in the intensive care nursery. However, despite widespread use of the Allen and Diamond curves, it is extremely difficult to predict the severity of hyperbilirubinemia based on the cord blood values of hematocrit and bilirubin. Lesser degrees of sensitization may be treated with phototherapy but may require simple transfusion later.

Summary

Since the advent of anti-D globulin, Rh incompatibility is a rapidly declining problem that may eventually be eliminated. Fetal red cells may sensitize the Rh-negative mother and stimulate production of antibody, which affects subsequent infants. The problem varies from mild anemia to intrauterine death from hydrops fetalis. Treatment is by intrauterine or extrauterine blood transfusion.

ABO INCOMPATIBILITY

Introduction and Incidence

In contrast to Rh incompatibility, this disorder is frequently encountered in first pregnancies. Some of the other differences are displayed in Table 10–2. Incidence is approximately 1 in 200 deliveries. Girls may be affected more frequently than boys.

Etiology

The mechanism involved in ABO incompatibility is not as straightforward as that for Rh incompatibility. The most common circumstance is a mother with

TABLE 10–2. CONTRAST BETWEEN Rh AND ABO INCOMPATIBILITY

	Rh Incompatibilty	ABO Incompatibility
Rh-negative mother	+	−
First pregnancy affected	Rare	Often
Cord bilirubin elevated	+	±
Early anemia prominent	+	−
Jaundice in first 24 hours	+ +	+
Nucleated red blood cells	+ + +	+
Spherocytes	±	+ +
Reticulocytosis	+ +	+ to + +
Direct Coombs' test	+ + +	− to ±
Indirect Coombs' test	Not necessary	+

+ = quite common; + + = common; + + + = very common; ± = sometimes; − = absent.

blood group O and a baby with blood group A or B. The mother has naturally occurring anti-A and anti-B, which are primarily immunoglobulin M and therefore do not cross the placenta. In a significant number of cases there is a considerable amount of immune (IgG) anti-A and anti-B, which may be stimulated by exogenous sources (e.g., helminthic infection). Apparently, the more usual reason for stimulation of this immune antibody is passage of the baby's A or B cells across the placenta. As gestation progresses, the antigenicity of these cells also seems to increase, which helps explain why most infants are not severely affected at birth and why preterm infants are infrequently affected. The antibody produced is capable of crossing the placenta to affect the fetus. The amount transferred is variable, but hemolysis is not usually severe, and consequently anemia is not commonly a major problem. The reason that subsequent pregnancies are not increasingly more severely affected is probably the result of suppression of the stimulus to produce IgG (immune)–type anti-A or anti-B by naturally occurring IgM-type anti-A or anti-B.

Diagnosis

With an O-positive mother and a baby with blood group A or B, diagnosis may be based on the features listed in Table 10–2. Spherocytosis is usually prominent, whereas results of the direct Coombs' test are most frequently negative, although the yield is higher with cord blood. An increase in the erythrocyte sedimentation rate has also been described in infants with ABO incompatibility. Although the test is infrequently performed, a decrease in the level of erythrocyte acetyl cholinesterase may also be seen with this disorder.

Management

With the early use of phototherapy, it is now uncommon to have to resort to exchange transfusion for hyperbilirubinemia in this disorder. Some investigators have advocated the use of phenobarbital, which stimulates the production of liver enzymes and, in particular, glucuronyl transferase. Conflicting information exists about the value of cord blood bilirubin levels in predicting subsequent levels.

Summary

ABO incompatibility may occur in the firstborn, usually when the mother's blood group is O and baby's group is A or B. Hyperbilirubinemia, spherocytosis, and positive results on an indirect Coombs' test are the prominent findings. If treatment is required, phototherapy is usually effective in preventing toxic levels of bilirubin.

JAUNDICE SECONDARY TO ENCLOSED HEMORRHAGE

In the presence of cephalhematoma (traumatic delivery) or diffuse subcutaneous ecchymoses (bruising), as seen in some breech and premature deliveries, the amount of hemoglobin available to be degraded to bilirubin may be quite large. Particularly in the small premature infant, hyperbilirubinemia should be anticipated, and phototherapy should always be considered early. Another form of enclosed hemorrhage that should be kept in mind is adrenal hemorrhage. As mentioned earlier, the preterm infant with periventricular hemorrhage may also have a large amount of degradable hemoglobin.

A rough idea of how much bilirubin may be released can be obtained by remembering that 1 g of hemoglobin generates 35 mg of bilirubin. Given a hemoglobin level of 20 g/dl, 1 g of hemoglobin is contained in 5 ml of blood. Enclosed hemorrhage of 10 ml could generate 70 mg of bilirubin over several days.

KERNICTERUS (BILIRUBIN ENCEPHALOPATHY)

INTRODUCTION

The concern about elevated levels of unconjugated bilirubin relates to the possibility of producing brain damage (or toxic encephalopathy).

PATHOPHYSIOLOGY

A complete understanding of the precise mechanism of action of bilirubin in producing brain injury is still lacking. As stated earlier, unconjugated bilirubin may become free when all binding sites on albumin are filled. This free fraction may be deposited in fatty areas, including the basal nuclei. At this level, it appears to disrupt the function of certain enzymes, resulting in a clearly distinguishable clinical picture. A specific level above which toxicity occurs cannot be stated. The factors making premature infants more susceptible to toxicity should be reviewed (earlier in this chapter), with the understanding that not everything that is called kernicterus is necessarily consistent with the original description. The gross (widespread) bilirubin staining of the neonatal brain, which can be seen without hyperbilirubinemia or specific microscopic changes, is probably not the same clinicopathologic entity as classic kernicterus.

DIAGNOSIS

If appropriate measures are not taken to limit the amount of circulating bilirubin, the jaundiced baby is likely to become increasingly more lethargic or irritable, to feed poorly, to begin to adopt a position of hyperextension of the head and finally frank opisthotonus (Fig. 10–4), and may become apneic. If appropriate treatment is not instituted before such signs are advanced, it is likely that the long-term sequelae of mental retardation, choreoathetosis, and deafness will result. The frequency of kernicterus rises with increasing levels of bilirubin, but (for the reasons mentioned earlier) it is impossible to say that above or below a specific level an infant will or will not display evidence of

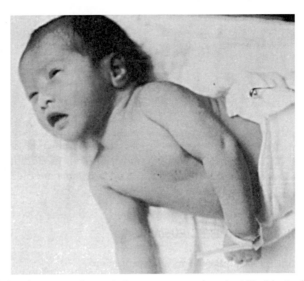

FIGURE 10–4. Baby demonstrating opisthotonos secondary to bilirubin toxicity (kernicterus).

kernicterus. Lack of overt manifestations is not a guarantee that minor neurologic abnormalities will be absent later in life. However, in a follow-up study of survivors of Rh-hemolytic disease, only 4 of 1476 had kernicterus, and all had a bilirubin level above 25 mg/dl. It seems even less likely that infants without evidence of hemolysis will develop kernicterus.

MANAGEMENT

Although prevention is the goal, some older clinical evidence supports the belief that if exchange transfusion is carried out soon after the signs become obvious, toxicity may be prevented. There is also some recent evidence from altered brain stem auditory evoked potentials in the presence of elevated bilirubin levels. These changes were reversed by exchange transfusion.

SUMMARY

With the advent of exchange transfusion and the use of phototherapy, toxic encephalopathy due to bilirubin should never be seen. Lethargy, irritability, poor feeding, apnea, or opisthotonus in the jaundiced infant may dictate treatment by exchange transfusion, but the prognosis would remain uncertain.

PHARMACOLOGIC MANAGEMENT OF HYPERBILIRUBINEMIA

The primary methods of managing high levels of bilirubin have been exchange transfusion and phototherapy. However, other methods of trying to prevent hyperbilirubinemia exist. The pharmacologic approach to prevention has been by two main pathways. The first is the use of phenobarbital to accelerate the excretion of bilirubin. This treatment seems to work primarily by stimulating glucuronyl transferase activity and is more successful when given antenatally, but it remains a successful strategy with postnatal therapy. Countries with a high incidence of hyperbilirubinemia secondary to glucose-6-phosphate dehydrogenase deficiency have considerable experience with phenobarbital therapy. The treatment may also distinguish between certain types of inherited glucuronyl transferase deficiency (Crigler-Najjar syndrome) and may be valuable before the delivery of very-low-birth-weight infants.

Phenobarbital has also been used postnatally in some cases of conjugated hyperbilirubinemia because it also seems to enhance the excretion of conjugated bilirubin.

The other major approach, which has gathered impetus in recent years, is the inhibition of the enzyme heme oxygenase, which is responsible for converting heme to bilirubin. The inhibiting substances that have been used are synthetic metalloporphyrins (tin-protoporphyrin, tin-meso porphyrin and zinc-protoporphyrin). Interestingly, heme does not accumulate, because biliary excretion of heme is enhanced.

Although it seems wise to prevent bilirubin levels from rising too high, bilirubin may play an important role in the body's natural defense mechanisms. Bilirubin is a potent antioxidant and may protect against organic free radicals.

OTHER CAUSES OF HYPERBILIRUBINEMIA

Numerous other disorders may result in jaundice and are discussed further in Chapter 25. Figure 10–5 gives an approximation of the most important days of onset for different disorders. In addition to the problems already mentioned, the following problems are more likely to be occasionally encountered.

UNCONJUGATED HYPERBILIRUBINEMIA

1. Jaundice secondary to oxytocin infusion
2. Inherited defects of red blood cells
3. Exposure to phenolic disinfectant
4. Metabolic problems (e.g., congenital hypothyroidism)

It has been suggested that induction of labor with oxytocin, rather than augmentation, is responsible for the observed association. Disorders of red blood cells usually involve red blood cell enzymes. The most common disorder is a deficiency of glucose-6-phosphate dehydrogenase. This deficiency is a common cause of jaundice in Greece, Sardinia, and the Far East, and in Sephardic Jews.

	Day	1	2	3	4	5	6	7	14	21
Blood group incompatibility										
Sepsis and viral infections										
"Physiologic jaundice"										
Inherited r.b.c. defect										
Congenital biliary atresia										
"Breast-milk jaundice"										
"Enclosed" hemorrhage										

FIGURE 10–5. Differential diagnosis of prominent jaundice by age of onset.

Epidemics of hyperbilirubinemia have occurred in some nurseries when the concentration of phenolic detergents, used for cleaning bassinets and incubators, was too high.

CONJUGATED HYPERBILIRUBINEMIA

1. Congenital biliary atresia (versus hepatitis)
2. α_1-Antitrypsin deficiency
3. Choledochal cyst
4. Cholestasis due to parenteral nutrition

The major difficulty has been distinguishing congenital biliary atresia, which occurs with a frequency of 1 in 15,000 live births, from (viral) hepatitis. For many years, debate has existed about the etiology of biliary atresia, and there now seems little doubt that in some cases biliary atresia starts as neonatal hepatitis. The estimation of the level of α-fetoprotein may be helpful in distinguishing between the two. With neonatal hepatitis, α-fetoprotein levels are usually higher than 35 μg/ml. A peak level of higher than 40 μg/ml probably indicates a baby who will not develop biliary atresia. Levels lower than 10 μg/ml have been observed with biliary atresia or other hepatic pathology. Absence of biliary obstruction may be detected if visual evidence exists of bilirubin pigment in duodenal fluid obtained during a 24-hour collection. Recently, the use of ultrasound, in conjunction with more traditional methods in nuclear medicine (^{131}I rose bengal or technetium-99 scans), has helped in differentiation. Biliary atresia is virtually ruled out either if radionuclide passes into the intestine or if ultrasound demonstrates a normal gallbladder. In the absence of these findings, hepatic biopsy and exploration are mandatory. A decision about surgery (Kasai's procedure) should be made before 2 months of age.

In a significant number of cases, prolonged obstructive jaundice results from α_1-antitrypsin deficiency. Thus, it is always worthwhile to perform an α_1-antitrypsin level determination under such circumstances. Routine screening does not seem practical, but in one large study, 11% of babies with a severe deficiency (PiZ phenotype) developed prolonged obstructive jaundice.

Confusion may arise when the obstruction is produced by a choledochal cyst. With this condition, considerable fluctuation may exist in the level of jaundice (and bilirubin levels). Consequently, it is unusual to make a diagnosis in the neonatal period, but it is possible to do so if the diagnosis is kept in mind.

With the increasing use of total parenteral nutrition in many preterm or sick infants, cholestasis has been observed more frequently. The culprit seems to be the amino acid component (rather than the lipid), but it is unusual for this phenomenon to occur when amino acid infusions are given for less than 1 week. Conjugated hyperbilirubinemia also occurs frequently in patients treated with extracorporeal membrane oxygenation.

BIBLIOGRAPHY

Maisels, M. J. (ed.): Neonatal Jaundice. *Clin. Perinatal.* 1990, 17:245–511.

Bilirubin Metabolism

Valaes, T., and Hyte, M.: Effect of exchange transfusion on bilirubin binding. *Pediatrics* 1977, 59:881.
Levine, R. L.: Bilirubin: Worked out years ago? *Pediatrics* 1979, 64:380.
McDonagh, A. F.: Phototherapy: A new twist to bilirubin. *J. Pediatr.* 1981, 99:909–911.
McDonagh, A. F., and Lightner, D. A.: "Like a shrivelled blood orange"—Bilirubin, jaundice, and phototherapy. *Pediatrics* 1985, 75:443–455.
Spivak, W.: Bilirubin metabolism. *Pediatr. Ann.* 1985, 14:451–457.

Physiologic Jaundice

Rosta, J., Makoi, A., and Kertesz, A.: Delayed meconium passage and hyperbilirubinemia. *Lancet* 1968, iis:1138.
Kramer, L. I.: Advancement of dermal icterus in the jaundiced newborn. *Am. J. Dis. Child.* 1969, 118:454.
Lucey, J. F.: Bilirubin and brain damage: A real mess. *Pediatrics* 1982, 69:381.
Watchko, J. F., and Oski, F. A.: Bilirubin 20 mg/dl = vigintiphobia. *Pediatrics* 1983, 71:660–663.
Strange, M., and Cassady, G.: Neonatal transcutaneous bilirubinometry. *Clin. Perinatol.* 1985, 12:51–62.
Knudsen, A., Kruse, C., and Ebbesen, F.: Detection of hyperbilirubinemia by skin color measurements in icteric newborn infants at 5 to 14 days of age. *Acta Paediatr. Int. J. Paediatr.* 1993, 82:510–513.
American Academy of Pediatrics: Practice Parameter: Management of hyperbilirubinemia in the healthy term newborn. *Pediatrics* 1994, 94:558–565.

Bilirubin and the Breastfed Infant

Gourley, G. R., and Arend, R. A.: β-glucuronidase and hyperbilirubinemia in breast-fed and formula-fed babies. *Lancet* 1986, i:644–646.

Lascari, A. D.: "Early"—breast-feeding jaundice: Clinical significance. *J. Pediatr.* 1986, 108:156–158.

Maisels, M. J., and Gifford, K.: Normal serum bilirubin levels in the newborn and the effect of breast-feeding. *Pediatrics* 1986, 78:837–843.

Kemper, K., Forsyth, B., and McCarthy, P.: Jaundice, terminating breast-feeding and the vulnerable child. *Pediatrics* 1989, 84:773–778.

Martinez, J. C., Maisels, M. J., Otheguy, L., et al.: Hyperbilirubinemia in the breast-fed newborn: A controlled trial of four interventions. *Pediatrics* 1993, 91:470–473.

Bilirubin in the Premature Infant

Odell, G. B., Cohen, S. N., and Kelly, P. C.: Studies in kernicterus II: The determination of the saturation of serum albumin with bilirubin. *J. Pediatr.* 1969, 74:214.

Zamet, P., Nakamura, H., Perez-Robles, S., et al.: The use of critical levels of birth-weight and "free" bilirubin as an approach for prevention of kernicterus. *Biol. Neonate* 1975, 26:274.

Lee, K. S., Gartner, L. M., and Vaisman, S. L.: Measurement of bilirubin-albumin binding: I. Comparative analysis of four methods and four human serum albumin preparations. *Pediatr. Res.* 1978, 12:301.

Van de Bor, M., Ens-Dokkum, M., Schreuder, A. M., et al.: Hyperbilirubinemia in low birth weight infants and outcome at 5 years of age. *Pediatrics* 1992, 89:359–364.

Rhesus Incompatibility

Wennberg, R. P., Depp, R., and Heinrichs, W. L.: Indications for early exchange transfusion in patients with erythroblastosis fetalis. *J. Pediatr.* 1978, 92:789.

Frigoletto, F. D., Jr.: Intrauterine fetal transfusion in 365 fetuses during fifteen years. *Am. J. Obstet. Gynecol.* 1981, 139:781–790.

Bowell, P., Wainscoat, J. S., Peto, T. E. A., and Gunson, H. H.: Rhesus hemolytic disease of the newborn. *B.M.J.* 1982, 285:327–329.

Editorial: Low-dose rhesus immunoprophylaxis. *Lancet* 1982, ii:1028.

Tovey, L. A. D., Townley, A., Stevenson, B., et al.: The Yorkshire antenatal anti-D immunoglobulin trial in primigravidae. *Lancet* 1983, ii:244–245.

Chavez, G. F., Mulinare, J., and Edmonds, L. D.: Epidemiology of Rh hemolytic disease of the newborn in the United States. *J.A.M.A.* 1991, 265:3270–3274.

ABO Incompatibility

Peevy, K. J., and Wiseman, H. J.: ABO hemolytic disease of the newborn: Evaluation of management and identification of racial and antigenic factors. *Pediatrics* 1978, 61:475.

Zipursky, A., Chinta, C., Brown, E., and Brown, E. J.: The quantitation of spherocytes in ABO hemolytic disease. *J. Pediatr.* 1979, 94:965.

Grundbacher, F. J.: The etiology of ABO hemolytic disease of the newborn. *Transfusion* 1980, 20:563–568.

Brouwers, H. A. A., Van Ertbruggen, I., Alsbach, G. P. J., et al.: What is the best predictor of the severity of ABO-haemolytic disease of the newborn? *Lancet* 1988, ii:641–644.

Enclosed Hemorrhage

Dickerman, J. D., and Tampas, J. P.: Adrenal hemorrhage in the newborn. *Clin. Pediatr.* 1977, 16:314.

Kernicterus

Broderson, R.: Bilirubin transport in the newborn infant, reviewed with relation to kernicterus. *J. Pediatr.* 1980, 96:349.

Cashore, W. J., and Stern, L.: Neonatal hyperbilirubinemia. *Pediatr. Clin. North Am.* 1982, 29:1191–1203.

Turkel, S. B., Miller, C. A., Guttenberg, M. E., et al.: Clinical pathological reappraisal of kernicterus. *Pediatrics* 1982, 69:267–272.

Newman, T. B., and Klebanoff, M. A.: Neonatal hyperbilirubinemia and long-term outcome: Another look at the collaborative perinatal project. *Pediatrics* 1993, 92:651–657.

Pharmacologic Management of Hyperbilirubinemia

Rayburn, W., Donn, S., Piehl, E., and Compton, A.: Antenatal phenobarbital and bilirubin metabolism in the very low birth weight infant. *Am. J. Obstet. Gynecol.* 1988, 159:1491–1493.

Valaes, T., Petmezaki, S., Henschke, C., et al.: Control of jaundice in preterm newborns by an inhibitor of bilirubin production: Studies with tin-mesoporphyrin. *Pediatrics* 1994, 93:1–11.

Unconjugated Hyperbilirubinemia

Drew, J. H., and Kitchen, W. H.: Jaundice in infants of Greek parentage: The unknown factor may be environmental. *J. Pediatr.* 1976, 89:248.

Wysowski, D. K., Flynt, J. W., Goldfield, M., et al.: Epidemic neonatal hyperbilirubinemia and use of a phenolic disinfectant detergent. *Pediatrics* 1978, 61:165.

Kaplan, M., and Abramov, A.: Neonatal hyperbilirubinemia associated with glucose-6-phosphate dehyrogenase deficiency in Sephardic-Jewish neonates: Incidence, severity and the effect of phototherapy. *Pediatrics* 1992, 90:401–405.

Conjugated Hyperbilirubinemia

Barlow, B., Tabor, E., Blanc, W. A., et al.: Choledochal cyst—review of 19 cases. *J. Pediatr.* 1976, 89:934.

Anderson, K. D.: Biliary atresia. *Clin. Perinatol.* 1978, 5:19.

Zeltzer, P. M.: Alpha-fetoprotein in the differentiation of neonatal hepatitis and biliary atresia: Current status and implications for the pathogenesis of these disorders. *J. Pediatr. Surg.* 1978, 13:381.

Greene, H. L., Helinek, G. L., Moran, R., and O'Neill, J.: A diagnostic approach to prolonged obstructive jaundice by 24-hour collection of duodenal fluid. *J. Pediatr.* 1979, 95:412.

Majd, M., Reba, R. C., and Altman, R. P.: Hepatobiliary scintigraphy with [99m]TcPIPIDA in the evaluation of neonatal jaundice. *Pediatrics* 1981, 67:140–145.

Wright, K., and Christie, D. L.: Use of γ-glutamyl transpeptidase in the diagnosis of biliary atresia. *Am. J. Dis. Child.* 1981, 135:134–136.

Abramson, S. J., Treves, S., and Teele, R. S.: The infant with possible biliary atresia: Evaluation by ultrasound and nuclear medicine. *Pediatr. Radiol.* 1982, 12:1–5.

Nemeth, A., and Strandvik, B.: Natural history of children with alpha-1-antitrypsin deficiency and neonatal cholestasis. *Acta Paediatr.* 1982, 71:993–999.

Gartner, L. M.: Cholestasis of the newborn (obstructive jaundice). *Pediatr. Rev.* 1983, 5:163–171.

Lilly, J. R., Hall, R. J., and Altman, R. P.: Liver transplantation and Kasai operation in the first year of life: Therapeutic dilemma in biliary atresia. *J. Pediatr.* 1987, 110:561–562.

Rosenthal, P., and Sinatra, F.: Jaundice in infancy. *Pediatr. Rev.* 1989, 11:79–86.

Waneck, E. A., Karrer, F. M., Brandt, C. T., and Lilly, J. R.: Biliary atresia. *Pediatr. Rev.* 1989, 11:57–62.

Walsh-Sukys, M. C., Cornell, D. J., and Stork, E. K.: The natural history of direct hyperbilirubinemia associated with extracorporeal membrane oxygenation. *Am. J. Dis. Child.* 1992, 146:1176–1180.

Moss, R. L., Das, J. B., Raffensperger, J. G., et al.: Total parenteral nutrition-associated cholestasis: Clinical and histopathologic correlation. *J. Pediatr. Surg.* 1993, 28:1270–1275.

11
FEEDING

BREAST-FEEDING

Human breast milk is the natural food of human babies and has successfully nourished millions of infants. It is strongly recommended for feeding all babies when it is available. In the absence of an available friend or relative who successfully breast-fed her offspring, the providers of perinatal care must be prepared to give good advice and answer questions sensibly. The ability to do this requires more information than can be easily summarized. The following discussion should be considered as an introduction, and the references should be consulted for further guidance.

PHYSIOLOGY

As pregnancy progresses, the breasts become more vascular in preparation for milk production, which occurs primarily in the acini. Under the influence of the suckling stimulus to the nipple, prolactin is produced, and the posterior pituitary releases oxytocin. This action stimulates milk formation and produces contraction of the myoepithelial cells, forcing milk into the lacteal sinuses. The lacteal sinuses are rhythmically compressed by the baby's gums, squeezing milk into the posterior oropharynx. When this mechanism is well established, the contractility may be great enough to force milk to spurt out. This is then termed the letdown, or draught, reflex.

The composition of human milk is roughly 1.25% protein (0.75% lactalbumin, 0.5% caseinogen), 7.5% carbohydrate, and 3.5% fat, providing approximately 8, 42, and 50%, respectively, of the calories (67 cal/100 ml of milk). Cows' milk has more protein and less carbohydrate than human milk, and the quality of the protein is different.

In the first few days of the baby's life, the mother's breasts produce colostrum, which resembles yellowish milk but has a lower caloric content. Gradually, the milk becomes apparently more watery, with a bluish hue, and achieves the typical composition and caloric content stated previously. Considerable variation may exist in the composition from one woman to another, and from one time to another in the same woman.

Preparation may be the most important part of breast-feeding, and the decision to breast-feed should be discussed weeks or months before delivery.

For example, it is important that the nipple is not retracted. The normal nipple is capable of great protractility as sucking takes place, so that although the gums are on the areola, the tip of the nipple is at the back of the tongue. Obviously, it is difficult for the retracted nipple to become protractile.

Explaining that breast size has no bearing on the ability to successfully breast-feed may provide considerable reassurance. Antenatal expression of colostrum by manual compression of the breast helps to clear ducts of inspissated secretions and reduce postpartum engorgement.

After delivery, the mother should be counseled not to have unrealistic expectations. Most babies do not feed ravenously during the first few days. The rooting reflex may allow the baby to locate the nipple, but a little help in directing the nipple into the baby's mouth (while preventing the gums from clamping down on it) is often appreciated. To stimulate milk production and prevent engorgement, the baby should be fed at both breasts at each feeding (at least in the first several days). Duration of feedings should initially be limited to about 5 minutes on each breast. Later, the feeding time may last for 15 to 20 minutes. Feedings should start on alternate breasts. Most milk is obtained in the first 5 or 10 minutes, and the rest of the time is frequently spent satisfying the baby's desire to suck. Although a little "playing" is permissible, prolonged feedings (longer than 30 minutes) are to be discouraged because they are more likely to result in fissures, excoriation, or painful breasts. For the neurohormonal mechanism to be most effective in milk production, the mother should be encouraged to adopt a relaxed attitude (often easier said than done).

A modified-demand schedule seems preferable to a rigid schedule that limits feeding to specified times (usually every 4 hours). A modified-demand schedule of 3 to 5 hours (2½ to 4 hours for babies weighing < 2500 g) means that the baby should not be put to the breast again until approximately 3 hours after the last feeding but that he or she should be fed within 5 hours. This schedule is primarily to prevent maternal problems of undue trauma to the nipples or engorgement. Some women have no difficulty with a demand schedule, putting the baby to the breast whenever he or she appears hungry. After the first 1 or 2 weeks, the maximum duration between feedings may be extended to "as long as the baby will sleep." It usually takes several weeks before a baby sleeps 6 to 8 hours at night.

Occasionally, breast-fed infants become malnourished because they have a poor suck, feed slowly at extended intervals, sleep a great deal, or do not appear hungry. Mothers may not realize that anything is wrong, because the baby appears content. The decreased milk (fluid) intake may result in hypernatremic dehydration, which may also be caused by a marked increase in breast-milk sodium. Early reevaluation after hospital discharge is recommended for breast-fed infants.

ADVANTAGES

Breast-feeding has several advantages that may be expressed to mothers:

1. Breast-feeding is sterile and convenient.

2. Breast-feeding is psychologically beneficial to both infant and mother.
3. Breast milk is easily assimilated and digested.
4. Breast milk provides host resistance factors.
5. Breast milk provides more physiologic intestinal flora than formula.

CONTRAINDICATIONS

Few absolute contraindications to breast-feeding exist, and prematurity is not one of them. Mothers of premature infants should be encouraged to express milk either manually or by use of a breast pump. The content of such preterm milk may have special advantages. It can be given to the baby via gavage tube until he or she is able to suck effectively on a bottle or at the breast. Some supplementation (e.g., calcium) may be necessary in the very premature baby. The following are considered contraindications to breast feeding: (1) active tuberculosis, (2) severe cleft palate, (3) anticancer and some antithyroid medications given to the mother, (4) postpartum psychosis (temporary), and (5) maternal sepsis (temporary).

Great variability exists in the excretion of drugs in breast milk (see Chapter 21), and it may be necessary to temporarily stop breast-feeding when certain drugs are being given.

PRACTICAL CONSIDERATIONS

1. Some discomfort is generally experienced at the first few feedings.
2. The baby may be prevented from biting on the nipple by insertion of the mother's finger between the gums.
3. Milk may spurt from the breasts when the baby cries before feeding or from the opposite breast at the start of feeding (letdown reflex). Pads may be placed inside the brassiere to absorb the ejected milk.
4. The nipples are best cleaned with water because soap and alcohol may cause drying and cracking.
5. Breast engorgement may not permit the baby to accept the nipple into the mouth. Manual expression of some milk may overcome the problem.
6. Because babies are obligatory nasal breathers for the first 2 or 3 months, it is difficult for them to feed if nasal obstructions exists.
7. Bowel movements may be quite loose and also quite frequent (as often as 10 times per day). If the stool is yellow and has some formed material, it is unlikely to be a problem. Bowel movements at the beginning and end of a feeding constitute one bowel movement. Occasionally, absorption seems to be so efficient that bowel movements are quite infrequent.
8. Relaxation of the mother is the key to successful breast-feeding. If she is worrying that she does not have enough milk for the next feeding, formula may be offered, either in place of the breast (supplementary) or in addition to it (complementary). This method may relieve anxiety so quickly that repeating the procedure is rarely required. This policy is not to be encouraged during the first 2 weeks, when suckling is so important for stimulation of milk production.

9. If milk is to be stored, macrophage activity is lost, but antimicrobial proteins persist with freezing. The same proteins do not survive heating. In the premature infant, it is preferable to use fresh breast milk, but it is frequently impractical.

10. With preterm breast milk, it may be necessary to add fortifier, primarily to provide additional calcium and phosphorus.

ARTIFICIAL (BOTTLE) FEEDING

Despite a recent increase in breast-feeding, more babies are bottle-fed than breast-fed. The ability of manufacturers to produce milk formula that closely resembles human breast milk and is packaged ready to use says more for their skill than for the common sense of the public. Most full-term babies can accept full-strength (67 cal/100 ml) formula shortly after delivery and thrive on it. Because of modifications, such formula is unlikely to be associated with problems frequently encountered in the past (e.g., high phosphate content could not be excreted, and such a load produced late hypocalcemia).

The principles of timing of bottle-feeding are the same as those for breast-feeding. The quantity is limited by gastric capacity and is best calculated (in term infants) on the basis of 5 ml/kg per feeding on the first day, 10 ml/kg on the second day, and 15 ml/kg on the third day. Another method of calculation suggests that by the 10th day of life, gastric capacity is approximately 3% of the baby's weight. In other words, mothers should be warned not to expect too much of their babies. Most infants limit themselves to 15 to 30 ml/feeding on the first and second days. Thereafter, an intake of 150 to 180 ml/kg (100 to 120 cal/kg) per day is required for steady growth.

The bottle should be held so that only milk (not air) is in the nipple. Nevertheless, some air is swallowed, and the baby should be burped at the end of a feeding (either breast or bottle) or after 60-ml increments. Babies are burped by placing them on the shoulder, or in a sitting forward position, and patting or stroking the back gently. The prone and right lateral positions are most conducive to gastric emptying. In the term baby, emptying follows an exponential pattern, with a half-life of about 90 minutes (preterm may be faster).

Although a ready-to-use formula is obviously most convenient, both powdered and evaporated milks are less expensive. The former costs less and is less bulky, but the latter may be easier to prepare (by dilution). Mistakes in preparations are not common but may produce devastating effects (e.g., hypernatremia). All mothers should be familiar with the particular formula they plan to use. Instruction in the sterilization of bottles is required, except when ready-to-use formula is used. Another problem to be anticipated is the appropriate hole size in the nipple. This hole should be sufficiently large to allow a slow steady stream of drops to fall when the bottle is inverted. If the hole is too small, the baby has to work hard to get the milk and usually swallows a lot of air, whereas if the hole is too large, the baby may not be able to swallow fast enough and may choke.

GAVAGE FEEDING

Babies younger than 32 weeks' gestation do not suck and always require gastric feeding by artificial means. Most babies older than 34 weeks' gestation can coordinate suck and swallow and take nipple feedings, but tube (gavage) feeding may be required in several categories of sick infants (e.g., those recovering from respiratory problems or those with central nervous problems) who are close to term gestation. Most gavage feeding is started more cautiously than is bottle feeding, with intravenous or intraarterial infusions being gradually replaced as the volume is increased. The usual regimen for intermittent gavage feeding in premature infants is 2 to 3 ml/kg of sterile water at the first feeding, followed by 3 ml/kg of breast milk or 44 cal/100 ml (13 cal/ounces) formula for 12 to 24 hours, followed by 3 to 4 ml/kg of breast milk or 67 cal/100 ml (20 cal/ounces) formula for another 12 to 24 hours, with continued increments of 1 to 2 ml added at each subsequent feeding until approximately 15 ml/kg maximum is attained. Current formulas for extremely preterm infants may provide 80 cal/100ml (24 cal/ounces) and contain higher amounts of calcium and phosphorus to minimize the risk of rickets of prematurity. For the composition of some formulas, see Table 11–1. The gastric content is aspirated before each feeding, and if it is more than 2 or 3 ml, the volume is not increased. Feedings may be given every 2 or 3 hours, depending on the size of the baby and the demonstrated gastric capacity (the volume tolerated easily). Intermittent gavage feedings should be given by gravity flow to avoid the potential dangers of overdistension that may result when formulas are injected. Gastric emptying is slower in preterm babies in the first day or so, but emptying rapidly increases by the end of the second day.

In some babies (those weighing < 1500 g, especially < 1000 g), continuous gavage feeding is sometimes more convenient and better tolerated than intermittent feeding. Continuous feeding is accomplished using a constant infusion pump, with starting rates of 1 to 2 ml/kg/hr. Occasional aspiration of gastric contents (for quantity) is needed to avoid missing retention. We prefer to use the orogastric route rather than the nasogastric route to maintain patency of the preferred airway in these obligatory nasal breathers. It may also be valuable to allow nonnutritive sucking during gavage feeds to enhance growth.

Even in the sickest infants, it has been suggested that stimulating gut enzymes by using very small amounts of enteral feeding may be important. This idea of minimal enteral feeding, or gut priming, using 0.5 to 1.0 ml/hr of continuous gavage feeding may allow more rapid advancement of feedings later.

Gavage feeding is possible even in babies who have an endotracheal tube in place (Fig. 11–1), but it should be intermittent because of the theoretical risk of crushing tissue between two indwelling tubes, which become hard after a few days. A recent study suggests that aspiration may be more common than we formerly believed, even with endotracheal tubes in place.

In babies who are being treated with nasal prongs or face mask ventilation, there is a tendency toward gastric distension with air or oxygen. This problem is usually relieved with a decompressing orogastric tube. Gastric feeding then becomes impractical, and it may be necessary to resort to transpyloric feeding,

TABLE 11-1. COMPOSITION OF HUMAN MILKS AND SPECIAL PREMATURE FORMULAS*

Per dl	Term Human Milk (68 kcal)	Preterm Human Milk (71 kcal)	Enfamil Premature (81 kcal)	SMA Premie (81 kcal)	Similac Special Care (81 kcal)
Protein (g)	1.0	2.2	2.4	2.0	2.2
whey: casein	60:40	—	60:40	60:40	60:40
Fat (g)	4.0	3.5	4.1	4.4	4.4
MCT (%)	—	—	40	27.5	50
LCT (%)	—	—	60	72.5	50
Carbohydrate (g)	6.8	7.1	8.9	8.6	8.6
Lactose (%)	100	100	40	50	50
Glucose polymers (%)	0	0	60	50	50
Minerals					
Calcium (mg)	26	28	95	75	144
Phosphorus (mg)	12	14	48	40	72
Magnesium (mg)	3.0	3.3	8.5	7	10
Sodium (mEq)	0.7	2.0	1.4	1.4	1.7
Potassium (mEq)	1.0	1.7	2.3	1.9	2.9
Chloride (mEq)	1.2	2.2	1.9	1.5	2.0
Zinc (μg)	530	530	810	800	1200
Copper (μg)	72	83	130	70	200
Vitamins					
A (IU)	217	Similar	970	240	550
D (IU)	2.1	to term milk	260	48	120
E (IU)	0.2		3.7	1.5	3.0
C (mg)	3.8		29	7.0	30
B_1 (μg)	20		200	80	200
B_2 (μg)	34		290	130	500
Niacin (mg)	0.1		1.0	0.7	4.0
B_6 (μg)	20		200	50	200
B_{12} (μg)	0.1		0.3	0.2	0.5
Folic acid (μg)	4.9		29	10	30
K_1 (μg)	2.0		10	7	10
Osmolality					
mOsm/kg water	273	270	300	280	300

*Adapted from Tsang, R. C., and Nichols, B. L. (eds): Nutrition During Infancy. Philadelphia, PA, Hanley and Belfus, 1988.
LCT = long-chain triglyceride; MCT = medium-chain triglyceride.

usually by the orojejunal or nasojejunal route. This route may also be needed in other babies who seem intolerant of gastric feeding. This type of feeding is usually given by continuous infusion. With appropriate care, complications are few and largely preventable. Gavage (or tube) feeding may therefore be divided into (1) gastric or transpyloric, (2) continuous or intermittent, and (3) oral or nasal route.

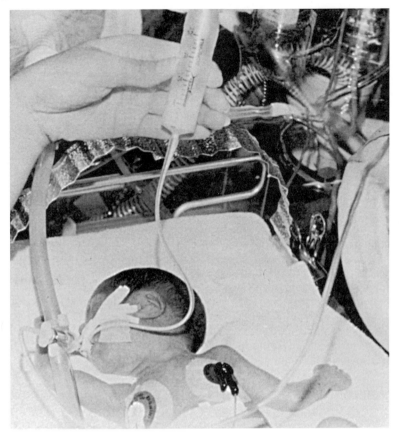

FIGURE 11–1. Tube (gavage) feeding by gravity flow in an infant with an endotracheal tube in place.

INFUSIONS

The parenteral route is chosen in a wide variety of circumstances that preclude enteral feeding, particularly respiratory difficulty. Infusions of various solutions may be given either intravenously or intraarterially (via umbilical artery catheter). Dextrose in a 10% solution is most frequently administered in the first 2 days of life, followed by electrolyte-containing solutions. Potassium levels are usually high in the first few days of life as a result of tissue and red cell breakdown, and frequently, metabolic acidosis is corrected in the sickest babies with sodium bicarbonate. Hence, sodium and potassium imbalance is unusual in the first few days of life but requires increasing attention thereafter. The approximate amounts of potassium and sodium required are 2 and 3 mEq/kg/day, respectively, but renal losses may demand more. Calcium supplements may also be required. Calculation of daily fluid requirements may be made on the following basis:

1. Maintenance fluids during first 2 days: about 70 ml/kg/day
2. Maintenance fluids after first 2 days: about 100 ml/kg/day
3. Maintenance fluids in babies with respiratory difficulty during first 2 days: about 100 ml/kg/day
4. Maintenance fluids in babies with respiratory difficulty after first 2 days: about 120 to 150 ml/kg/day

Additional fluids are required in extremely preterm infants (< 28 weeks' gestation) because of very thin skin and in babies under a radiant heat warmer or undergoing phototherapy. An additional 25 ml/kg/day should be added for each. Some babies may, therefore, need as much as 200 ml/kg/day, particularly in very preterm infants who have large amounts of insensible (transepidermal) loss. Other losses, such as through diarrhea or gastric suction, should be considered in the calculation of fluid requirements.

Perhaps the best way to determine if enough fluid is being given is to measure urine osmolality. One may approximate this by performing bedside urine specific gravity determinations by refractometer; the value should be kept below 1.008.

The less mature the baby, the greater the water content per kilogram of body weight. Therefore, on a per-kilogram basis, small premature babies may need higher estimated intakes.

A few small babies are intolerant of 10% dextrose and have significant glycosuria with a concomitant osmotic diuresis. This phenomenon is usually transient and is managed by reducing the infusion to 5% dextrose for 12 to 24 hours, after which a 7.5% or 10% solution is usually tolerated. With high volumes, it may be important to calculate glucose in mg/kg/min to determine what concentration of glucose will be tolerated. Occasionally glucose intolerance is more prolonged, and it may be necessary to use insulin (see Hyperglycemia section, p. 216). The use of a constant infusion pump provides accurate steady flow, which prevents fluctuations in caloric supply and prevents fluid overload.

In the smallest or sickest babies, it is not always possible to advance to enteral feedings in the first week of life. Because 10% dextrose provides approximately 40 cal/100 ml and because a minimum of 60 cal/100 ml is apparently needed to prevent tissue catabolism and produce growth, methods to improve caloric intake (supplemental or total parenteral nutrition) are often employed. The major additional sources of calories are amino acids and/or lipids. The former is usually increased slowly, but even 1.5 g/kg/day starting on day 1 may be well tolerated. The latter is in the form of a soybean emulsion (Intralipid) or is prepared from safflower oil (Liposyn) for intravenous use. Initially, central venous catheters were employed, but complications of this technique (notably sepsis) and the more recent availability of lipid have made peripheral vein infusions more popular. However, some infants with complicated courses, particularly those undergoing bowel resection, require total parenteral nutrition using central venous catheters (e.g., Broviac). Both premature and small-for-gestational age babies seem to be less tolerant of Intralipid and Liposyn than are term babies of appropriate weight for gestation. The use of supplemental or total parenteral nutrition should be confined to special care nurseries because other special problems may arise (e.g., metabolic acidosis, hyperlipidemia, platelet problems).

Although nutrition is important to brain growth, the need to mimic intrauterine growth rates is questioned by many authors. Prolonged malnutrition is to be avoided, but the optimal postnatal rate of growth has yet to be defined. Critical periods of brain growth may not be as short as implied by some animal studies, and catch-up growth is possible in most babies who have not been chronically deprived of nutrition.

VITAMINS AND OTHER MICRONUTRIENTS

In general, infants who are breast-fed do not require supplementation with vitamins (but see Chapter 17). Most formulas have vitamins added to them in amounts that provide usual daily requirements. However, infants who receive total parenteral nutrition need to have vitamins and trace elements (e.g., zinc, copper, manganese) added to the mixture. These requirements are periodically revised.

BIBLIOGRAPHY

American Academy of Pediatrics Committee on Nutrition: Nutritional needs of low-birth-weight infants. *Pediatrics* 1985, 75:976–986.

Breast Feeding

Evans, T. J., Ryley, H. C., Neale, L. M., et al.: Effect of storage and heat on antimicrobial proteins in human milk. *Arch. Dis. Child.* 1978, 53:239.

Lucas, A., Lucas, P. J., and Baum, J. D.: Pattern of milk flow in breast-fed infants. *Lancet* 1979, ii:57.

Howie, P. W., Houston, M. J., Cook, A., et al.: How long should a breast feed last? *Early Hum. Dev.* 1981, 5:71–77.

Fransson, G. B., and Lonnerdal, B.: Zinc, copper, calcium, and magnesium in human milk. *J. Pediatr.* 1982, 101:504–508.

Rowland, T. W., Zori, R. T., Lafleur, W. R., and Reiter, E. D.: Malnutrition and hypernatremic dehydration in breast-fed infants. *J.A.M.A.* 1982, 247:1016–1017.

Dworsky, M., Yow, M., Stagno, S., et al.: Cytomegalovirus infection of breast milk and transmission in infancy. *Pediatrics* 1983, 72:295–299.

Gross, S. J.: Growth and biochemical response of preterm infant fed human milk or modified infant formula. *N. Engl. J. Med.* 1983, 308:237–241.

Jarvenpaa, A. L., Raiha, N. C. R., Rassin, D. K., and Gaull, G. E.: Preterm infants fed human milk attain intrauterine weight gain. *Acta Paediatr.* 1983, 72:239–243.

Lucas, A., and Hudson, G. J.: Preterm milk as a source of protein for low birthweight infants. *Arch. Dis. Child.* 1984, 59:831–836.

Lewis, M. A., and Smith, B. A. M.: High volume feeds for preterm infants. *Arch. Dis. Child.* 1984, 59:779–781.

Lemons, P., Stuart, M., and Lemons, J. A.: Breast-feeding the premature infant. *Clin. Perinatol.* 1986, 13:111–122.

Lawrence, R. A.: Breast-feeding. *Pediatr. Rev.* 1989, 11:163–171.

Cronenwett, L., Stukel, T., Kearney, M., et al.: Single daily bottle use in the early weeks postpartum and breast-feeding outcomes. *Pediatrics* 1992, 90:760–766.

American Academy of Pediatrics Committee on Drugs: The transfer of drugs and other chemicals into human milk. *Pediatrics* 1994, 93:137–150.

Artificial Feeding

Cavell, B.: Gastric emptying in preterm infants. *Acta Paediatr.* 1979, 68:725.
Blumenthal, I., and Lealman, G. T.: Effect of posture on gastro-oesophageal reflux in the newborn. *Arch. Dis. Child.* 1982, 57:555–556.
Lawrence, R. A.: Infant nutrition. *Pediatr. Rev.* 1983, 5:133–140.
Klish, W. J.: Special infant formulas. *Pediatr. Rev.* 1990, 12:55–62.
Romero, R., and Kleinman, R. E.: Feeding the very low-birth-weight infant. *Pediatr. Rev.* 1993, 14:123–132.

Gavage Feeding

Heicher, D., and Philip, A. G. S.: Orogastric supplementation in small premature infants requiring mechanical respiration. *Am. J. Dis. Child.* 1976, 130:282.
Gupta, M., and Brans, Y. W.: Gastric retention in neonates. *Pediatrics* 1978, 62:26.
Stocks, J.: Effect of nasogastric tubes on nasal resistance during infancy. *Arch. Dis. Child.* 1980, 55:17.
Pereira, G. R., and Lemons, J. A.: Controlled study of transpyloric and intermittent gavage feeding in the small preterm infant. *Pediatrics* 1981, 67:68–72.
Aynsley-Green, A., Adrian, T. E., and Bloom, S. R.: Feeding and the development of enteroinsular hormone secretion in the preterm infant: Effects of continuous gastric infusions of human milk compared with intermittent boluses. *Acta Paediatr.* 1982, 71:379–383.
Bernbaum, J. C., Pereira, G. R., Watkins, J. B., and Peckham, G. J.: Nonnutritive sucking during gavage feeding enhances growth and maturation in premature infants. *Pediatrics* 1983, 71:41–45.
Van Someren, V., Linnett, S. J., Stothers, J. K., and Sullivan, P. G.: An investigation into the benefits of resiting naso-enteric feeding tubes. *Pediatrics* 1984, 74:379–383.
Goodwin, S. R., Graves, S. A., and Haberkern, C. M.: Aspiration in intubated premature infants. *Pediatrics* 1985, 75:85–88.
Dunn, L., Hulman, S., Weiner, J., and Kliegman, R.: Beneficial effects of early hypocaloric enteral feeding on neonatal gastro-intestinal function: Preliminary report of a randomized trial. *J. Pediatr.* 1988, 112:622–629.
Koo, W. W. K., and Tsang, R. C.: Mineral requirements of low-birth-weight infants. *J. Am. Coll. Nutr.* 1991, 10:474–486.
Berseth, C. L.: Effect of early feeding on maturation of the preterm infant's small intestine. *J. Pediatr.* 1992, 120:947–953.

Infusions

Dobbing, J.: Later growth of the brain: Its vulnerability. *Pediatrics* 1974, 53:2.
Oh, W.: Disorders of fluid and electrolytes in newborn infants. *Pediatr. Clin. North Am.* 1976, 23:601.
Goldman, S. L., and Hirata, T.: Attenuated response to insulin in very low birth weight infants. *Pediatr. Res.* 1980, 14:50.
Batton, D. G., Maisels, M. J., and Applebaum, P.: Use of peripheral intravenous cannulas in premature infants: A controlled study. *Pediatrics* 1982, 70:487–490.
Dolcourt, J. L., Bose, C. L.: Percutaneous insertion of Silastic central venous catheters in newborn infants. *Pediatrics* 1982, 70:484–486.
Easton, L. B., Halata, M. S., and Dweck, H. S.: Parenteral nutrition in the newborn: A practical guide. *Pediatr. Clin. North Am.* 1982, 29:1171–1190.
Vileisis, R. A., Cowett, R. M., and Oh, W.: Glycemic response to lipid infusion in the premature neonate. *J. Pediatr.* 1982, 100:108–112.
American Academy of Pediatrics Committee on Nutrition: Commentary on parenteral nutrition. *Pediatrics* 1983, 71:547–551.
Griffin, E. A., Bryan, M. H., and Angel, A.: Variations in intralipid tolerance in newborn infants. *Pediatr. Res.* 1983, 17:478–481.

De Leeuw, R., Kok, K., De Vries, I. J., and Beganovic, N.: Tolerance of intravenously administered lipid in newborns. *Acta Paediatr.* 1985, 74:52–56.

Sedin, G., Hammarlund, K., Nilsson, G. E., et al.: Measurements of transepidermal water loss in newborn infants. *Clin. Perinatol.* 1985, 12:79–99.

Heird, W. C., Kashyap, S., and Gomez, M. R.: Parenteral alimentation of the neonate. *Semin. Perinatol.* 1991, 15:493–502.

Rivera, A., Jr., Bell, E. F., and Bier, D. M.: Effect of intravenous amino acids on protein metabolism of preterm infants during the first three days of life. *Pediatr. Res.* 1993, 33:106–111.

Vitamins and Other Micronutrients

Greene, H. L., Hambridge, K. M., Schanler, R., et al.: Guidelines for the use of vitamins, trace elements, calcium, magnesium and phosphorus in infants and children receiving total parenteral nutrition. *Am. J. Clin. Nutr.* 1988, 48:1324–1342.

12

PROBLEMS OF PREMATURITY

The infant born prematurely (preterm) is at an immediate disadvantage in many respects. Some of the problems that are exclusive to the premature newborn can quickly be overcome, but others persist despite the best possible management.

One of the first questions to be asked is, "Why was this baby born prematurely?" If no satisfactory explanation is rapidly apparent (e.g., placenta previa, incompetent cervix, multiple pregnancy), two other possibilities should be looked for. The first is the presence of congenital abnormalities because there is an almost linear increase in the prevalence of congenital abnormalities with decreasing gestational age. The second is the possibility of bacterial infection because it is apparent that infection frequently causes premature rupture of the membranes rather than being the result.

The next question to be answered is, "What are the chances that this baby will survive?" An approximate answer, and one which may be helpful in counseling parents, is provided in Appendix 9. The situation continues to change, particularly since 1990, when exogenous surfactants were introduced. Under some circumstances, such as with poor Apgar scores, the mortality risk for a given birth weight–gestational age category may be greatly increased. Parents should be provided with a realistic appraisal.

Immaturity of organ systems presents many problems. The most obvious of these is pulmonary immaturity and the lack of surfactant, which may predispose to respiratory distress syndrome and persistence of a patent ductus arteriosus (see Chapter 9). Renal immaturity may result in difficulties in fluid management, with a decreased glomerular filtration rate, and drugs excreted by this route may be administered less frequently in the preterm infant than in the infant and older child. In many cases, excessive excretion of both sodium and bicarbonate occurs, increasing urine pH and contributing to metabolic acidosis. Liver immaturity may accentuate the problem of bilirubin excretion. An immature gastrointestinal tract may impair the infant's ability to break down and absorb certain foodstuffs. The immature eye seems to be more susceptible to oxygen toxicity. Hyperoxemia-induced vasoconstriction or other reasons for ischemia (e.g., hypotension) may produce retinopathy of prematurity (retrolental fibroplasia). Vascular proliferation may lead to scarring or retinal detachment, with resultant loss of vision.

Almost all storage capabilities are functioning most effectively during the last 3 months of normal gestation. This means that the more premature the infant, the greater the deficiency of glycogen stores in the liver, subcutaneous fat, brown fat (to respond to cold stress), vitamins, and so on. This situation increases the tendency toward hypoglycemia and other metabolic problems (see Chapter 17).

For these reasons (deficient glycogen stores and so on), and because the smaller the object the greater the surface area to body weight ratio, the premature infant has difficulty with thermoregulation because of both decreased ability to produce heat and increased tendency to lose heat (cooling) (see Chapter 5).

Another deficiency of the newborn that is exaggerated in the premature infant is an increased susceptibility to infection, largely caused by ineffective defense mechanisms (see Chapter 15).

Feeding presents a special problem (discussed elsewhere) because of the very premature infant's inability to suck and swallow effectively (see Chapter 11). The problem is frequently compounded by the presence of respiratory difficulties and the tendency to develop necrotizing enterocolitis (see Chapter 18).

Oxygenation difficulties in the premature infant (secondary to pulmonary disease) are exaggerated at a tissue level because the premature infant is not able to give up oxygen as readily as a term infant, owing to a deficiency of 2,3-diphosphoglycerate. In other words, fetal blood picks up oxygen better than adult blood (because of increased affinity of fetal hemoglobin for oxygen) but gives it up to tissues more reluctantly.

As if this were not enough, the premature infant also has a deficiency in numerous coagulation factors and (because of some of the other problems) a greater tendency toward asphyxial insult. Taken in combination, these elements may explain the much higher incidence of intraventricular hemorrhage seen in premature infants (see Chapter 19).

The major problems of babies of low birth weight (LBW) are most easily remembered because most of them are commonly abbreviated (Table 12–1) with three letters, as in LBW (although to be fair, most of these problems occur most frequently in very low-birth-weight infants, i.e., those weighing less than 1500 g).

TABLE 12-1. MAJOR PROBLEMS ENCOUNTERED IN PREMATURE INFANTS

Abbreviation	Problem
RDS or HMD	Respiratory distress syndrome; hyaline membrane disease
BPD	Bronchopulmonary dysplasia
PIE	Pulmonary interstitial emphysema
PDA	Patent (persistent) ductus arteriosus
IVH or PVH	Intraventricular hemorrhage; periventricular hemorrhage
RLF or ROP	Retrolental fibroplasia; retinopathy of prematurity
NEC	Necrotizing enterocolitis
GBS	Group B streptococcal sepsis (and other infection)
TPN	Total parenteral nutrition (and its complications)
NTE	Neutral thermal environment (thermoregulation)

If a premature infant can survive the first critical days, unanticipated problems may still be ahead, including apnea of prematurity, Wilson-Mikity syndrome, chronic pulmonary insufficiency of prematurity, late metabolic ("feeding") acidosis, anemia of prematurity, and late edema of prematurity. Another problem that can be seen quite frequently in very-low-birth-weight infants is a hernia. Both umbilical and inguinal hernias are more common in premature infants than in term infants.

The miracle is that some premature infants have such a benign neonatal course that one hardly notices them, whereas others make their presence known by surviving from one problem to the next (Fig. 12–1). It is difficult to predict at birth with any degree of certainty into which of these two categories a premature infant will fall.

FOLLOW-UP OF THE LOW-BIRTH-WEIGHT INFANT

When changes in neonatal care resulted in improved survival for the low-birth-weight infant, questions about the wisdom of such success inevitably followed. Concern was raised regarding the quality of life of the survivors of intensive care nurseries. This concern was largely generated by the long-term follow-up studies conducted on premature infants who were born in the 1950s. These studies showed that many problems occurred in babies surviving the neonatal period who were born with a low birth weight (< 2500 g) and that

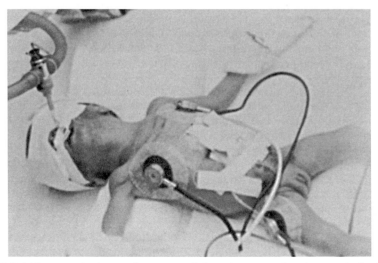

FIGURE 12–1. Photograph of a small premature infant, demonstrating the complexity (and problems) of modern neonatal intensive care. Chest and limb leads are attached to monitor heart and respiration rates. An orotracheal tube is attached to a respirator. An umbilical artery catheter monitors paO_2 (in particular) and provides fluid and calories via a constant infusion pump. The eyes are shaded to prevent damage from phototherapy used to prevent hyperbilirubinemia. The arms are restrained to prevent removal of any of these devices.

these problems were more striking in the very low-birth-weight infant ($<$ 1500 g). Overall, the decrease in mortality since that time has been accompanied by a decrease in morbidity, both short and long term. For instance, little difference exists between the neurologic evaluation of full-term infants and that of preterm infants at term conceptional age, although responses are weaker and some asymmetry may be present in preterm infants.

In the 1960s, considerable attention was paid to the regulation of temperature and oxygen and the administration of an adequate fluid and caloric input. The follow-up of these patients proved to be much more encouraging than the previous figures might have led one to expect. With the advent of assisted ventilation and the near-certainty that many babies who would formerly have died without such assistance were being saved, further concerns about the outcome for such babies have been expressed. Where formerly approximately 50% of all babies weighing less than 1500 g had significant neurologic deficit, the results of follow-up of babies born in the early 1970s weighing less than 1500 g showed that 75 to 85% of such babies are performing normally. Of the remainder, only 5 to 10% have any serious sequelae. These results have now been duplicated in babies weighing less than 1000 g, and most recently, the results of survivors in the 500- to 750-g birth weight group have also been encouraging (so much so that the limit of viability has become quite blurred). Good outcome is most likely to be associated with a relatively benign course and the absence of periventricular hemorrhage and ischemia.

Some discrepancy exists in the results with assisted ventilation. Most reports concerning survivors of assisted ventilation have been encouraging. This may be less true for very-low-birth-weight infants. One report of babies requiring assisted ventilation who weighed less than 1500 g suggests that many problems may indeed exist, but this cautionary report may relate to the quality of care delivered to such babies before they are admitted to the referral hospital. In other words, when a baby has to be transported long distances and receives sporadic or inadequate care before or during the transfer, the baby's condition may deteriorate. Reports from services in which most babies are inborn suggest that the long-term follow-up is not similarly compromised. In addition to these considerations, it is possible that the baby who is born small for gestational age may be at greater risk for long-term problems than the baby who is born appropriate for gestational age. Most of the evidence until recently has supported this contention, but some authors are now of the opinion that this finding is not always true. Nevertheless, it seems critical that continued long-term follow-up studies be carried out on all low-birth-weight babies to determine the risk/benefit ratio.

The latest figures on infants born in the late 1970s and early 1980s with extremely low birth weights ($<$ 1000 g in most studies, but $<$ 1250 g in some) provide information from the United Kingdom, the United States, Canada, and Australia to 8 years of age. These studies (based on treatment provided a decade earlier) suggest that we still need to be concerned about long-term follow-up of these tiny babies. Most severe disabilities are determined by the time the children are 2 years of age, but developmental delay at 2 years of age was not always associated with intellectual impairment at 8 years of age. On the other hand, one third of extremely low-birth-weight children do not perform in the normal range, and almost all show some disadvantage on every measure tested. Learning difficulties become more apparent with advancing age.

Many centers have observed an increase in the incidence of cerebral palsy, although some centers have not had this experience. This finding may relate to the development of cystic periventricular leukomalacia. Larger and more extensive cysts have been associated with quadriplegia.

CRITERIA FOR DISCHARGE

Some years ago, it was customary to wait until a certain weight had been achieved before the low-birth-weight infant was discharged. This weight was originally set at approximately 2500 g, later was decreased to about 2250 g, and currently (in most units) is not the prime consideration. More important than a specific weight is how well the baby is doing.

In general, a baby who is in room air, is able to take nipple feedings, can tolerate normal room temperatures, and is growing steadily (without apnea) is medically ready for discharge. It is also important to have parents who feel reasonably comfortable with the baby (almost all parents of preterm babies are nervous about taking the baby home). A few days of close contact with the baby (preferably rooming-in, or "nesting") are strongly recommended in the days immediately before discharge. (Referrals to appropriate community agencies should be made well in advance of discharge if possible.)

Most very-low-birth-weight babies can be weaned from the incubator at 1750 to 1800 g, and some who are small for gestational age can be weaned at much lower weight, roughly at 36 weeks' gestation. The author has discharged several babies who had weights of 1500 to 1600 g when all the criteria noted earlier were met. There are some circumstances in which not all criteria can be satisfied, but discharge is still possible. For example, some infants with bronchopulmonary dysplasia may be oxygen dependent but functioning well in other respects. Discharge with administration of oxygen at home may have many benefits, not the least of which is decreasing the cost of medical care (see also p. 128).

PROBLEMS AFTER DISCHARGE

In the section on follow-up, the discussion centers largely on neurodevelopmental follow-up, but clearly other problems may need to be dealt with by parents of preterm infants. As noted in Chapter 9, bronchopulmonary dysplasia is a fairly common problem in very-low-birth-weight infants and may necessitate supplemental oxygen at home. Such infants are particularly susceptible to infection with the respiratory syncytial virus.

Retinopathy of prematurity may have resolved before discharge, but in infants who require cryotherapy or laser therapy, careful follow-up to assess vision is needed. Other eye problems (e.g., strabismus) may also be more common in premature infants.

Hearing loss, which may result in poor articulation and delays in speech development, needs to be looked for in all infants with birth weights of less than 1500 g. Continued supplementation with multivitamins and iron are also needed. Despite this supplementation, many infants grow poorly and have more medical illnesses and surgical interventions than do infants with normal birth weights.

Most families experience considerable stress with the birth of a very preterm infant, which can exaggerate faulty interfamilial dynamics before and after the baby goes home. It may also result in the vulnerable child syndrome, with parents creating an overprotective environment. Intervention programs may prevent this phenomenon.

IMMUNIZATIONS

In the past it was common practice to defer immunization with DPT (diphtheria-pertussis-tetanus) vaccine, on the assumption that preterm infants would not have a suitable response until well beyond term gestation. It is now known that postnatal age (rather than post-conceptional age) is the prime determinant of response to DPT. Half-dose of DPT vaccine is not recommended because of poor serologic response.

Although the responses to hepatitis B vaccine and *Haemophilus influenzae* type B (HIB) vaccine are less reliable, the great majority of preterm infants have antibody production. It is therefore advised that postnatal schedules for immunization be used for preterm infants, except for the tiniest babies, who may not have enough muscle mass to tolerate injections.

Oral polio vaccine (a live virus vaccine) should be deferred until the day of discharge.

BIBLIOGRAPHY

Harper, R. G., Garcia, A., and Sia, C.: Inguinal hernia: Common problem of premature infants weighing 1,000 grams or less at birth. *Pediatrics* 1975, 56:112.

Vohr, B. R., Rosenfield, A. G., and Oh, W.: Umbilical hernia in the low-birth-weight infant (less than 1500 g). *J. Pediatr.* 1977, 90:807.

Davies, D. P.: The first feed of low birth-weight infants: Changing attitudes in the twentieth century. *Arch. Dis. Child.* 1978, 53:187.

Vohr, B. R., Oh, W., and Rosenfield, I. R.: The preterm small-for-gestational age infant: A two-year follow-up study. *Am. J. Obstet. Gynecol.* 1979, 133:425.

Alberman, E., Benson, J., and Evans, S.: Visual defects in children of low birth weight. *Arch. Dis. Child.* 1982, 57:818–822.

Lefebvre, F., Veilleux, A., and Bard, H.: Early discharge of low birthweight infants. *Arch. Dis. Child.* 1982, 57:511–513.

Lorenz, J. M., Kleinman, L. I., Kotagal, U. R., and Reller, M. D.: Water balance in very low birthweight infants: Relationship to water and sodium intake and effect on outcome. *J. Pediatr.* 1982, 101:423–432.

Ellison, R. C., Peckham, G. J., Lang, P., et al.: Evaluation of the preterm infant for patent ductus arteriosus. *Pediatrics* 1983, 71:364–372.

Hirata, T., Epcar, J. T., Walsh, A., et al.: Survival and outcome of infants 501 to 750 gm: A six-year experience. *J. Pediatr.* 1983, 102:741–748.

Rothberg, A. D., Maisels, M. J., and Bagnato, S.: Infants weighing 1,000 grams or less at birth: Developmental outcome for ventilated and non-ventilated infants. *Pediatrics* 1983, 71:599–602.

Committee Report: An international classification of retinopathy of prematurity. *Pediatrics* 1984, 74:127–133.

Koops, B. L.: Extreme immaturity: A frontier in neonatology. *Am. J. Dis. Child.* 1984, 138:713–714.

Laing, I. A., Glass, E. J., Hendry, G. M. A., et al.: Rickets of prematurity: Calcium and phosphorus supplementation. *J. Pediatr.* 1985, 106:265–268.

Koblin, B. A., Townsend, T. R., Muñoz, A., et al.: Response of preterm infants to diphtheria-tetanus-pertussis vaccine. *Pediatr. Infect. Dis. J.* 1988, 7:704–711.

Bernbaum, J., Daft, A., Samuelson, J., and Polin, R. A.: Half-dose immunization for diphtheria, tetanus, pertussis: Response of preterm infants. *Pediatrics* 1989, 83:471–476.

Bernbaum, J., Friedman, S., Hoffman-Williamson, M., et al.: Preterm infant care after hospital discharge. *Pediatr. Rev.* 1989, 10:195–206.

Pullan, C. R., and Hull, D.: Routine immunization of preterm infants. *Arch. Dis. Child.* 1989, 64:1438–1441.

Hack, M., Breslau, N., Weissman, B., et al.: Effect of very low birthweight and subnormal head size on cognitive abilities at school age. *N. Engl. J. Med.* 1991, 325:231–237.

Kitchen, W., Campbell, N., Carse, E., et al.: Eight-year outcome in infants with birth weight of 500 to 999 grams: Continuing regional study of 1979 and 1980 births. *J. Pediatr.* 1991, 118:761–767.

Saigal, S., Szatmari, P., Rosenbaum, P., et al.: Cognitive abilities and school performance of extremely low birth weight children and matched term regional children at age 8 years: A regional study. *J. Pediatr.* 1991, 118:751–760.

Flynn, J. T., Bancalari, E., Snyder, E. S., et al.: A cohort study of transcutaneous oxygen tension and the incidence and severity of retinopathy of prematurity. *N. Engl. J. Med.* 1992, 326:1050–1054.

Lau, Y.-L., Tam, A. Y. C., Ng, K. W., et al.: Responses of preterm infants to hepatitis B vaccine. *J. Pediatr.* 1992, 121:962–965.

Powell, P. J., Powell, C. V. E., Hollis, S., and Robinson, M. J.: When will my baby go home? *Arch. Dis. Child.* 1992, 67:1214–1216.

Robertson, C. M. T., Hrynchyshyn, G. J., Etches, P. C., and Pain, K. S.: Population-based study of the incidence, complexity and severity of neurologic disability among survivors weighing 500 through 1250 grams at birth: A comparison of two birth cohorts. *Pediatrics* 1992, 90:750–755.

Hack, M., Weissman, B., Breslau, N., et al.: Health of very low birth weight children during their first eight years. *J. Pediatr.* 1993, 122:887–892.

Hagberg, B., Hagberg, G., and Olow, I.: The changing panorama of cerebral palsy in Sweden: VI. Prevalence and origin during the birth year period 1983–86. *Acta Paediatr.* 1993, 82:387–393.

Marlow, N., Roberts, L., and Cooke, R.: Outcome at 8 years for children with birthweights of 1250g or less. *Arch. Dis. Child.* 1993, 68:286–290.

McCormick, M. C.: Has the prevalence of handicapped infants increased with improved survival of the very low birth weight infant. *Clin. Perinatol.* 1993, 20:263–277.

Page, J. M., Schneeweiss, S., Whyte, H. E. A., and Harvey, P.: Ocular sequelae in premature infants. *Pediatrics* 1993, 92:787–790.

Washburn, L. K., O'Shea, T. M., Gillis, D. C., et al.: Response to *Haemophilus influenzae* type B conjugate vaccine in chronically ill premature infants. *J. Pediatr.* 1993, 123:791–794.

Rogers, B., Msall, M., Owens, T., et al.: Cystic periventricular leukomalacia and type of cerebral palsy in preterm infants. *J. Pediatr.* 1994, 125:S1–8.

13
MULTIPLE PREGNANCIES

The prevalence of twin pregnancy used to be approximately 1 in 90 live births; triplets, 1:90 × 90, quadruplets, 1:90 × 90 × 90; and so on, but there has been a marked increase in the incidence of multiple pregnancies since the introduction of assisted reproduction techniques, such as hormonal therapy and in vitro fertilization. Determination of zygosity with reasonable certainty is not always as easy as it might appear, but twins of opposite sex are obviously dizygous. Examination of the placenta is the only way to arrive at a reasonable estimate of whether twins of the same sex are monozygous (identical) or dizygous (fraternal). With a monochorionic monoamnionic placenta, the twins are identical (but may be conjoined or "Siamese"); with a monochorionic diamnionic placenta, the twins are almost always identical, but with a dichorionic diamnionic placenta, there is less certainty that twins are fraternal. Even with two separate placentas, the possibility exists of monozygosity (Fig. 13–1). Extended blood and tissue typing may be needed to clarify uncertainty.

Very rarely, fertilization of two ova occurs at different times, and it is possible to have twins with two different fathers. This phenomenon is called superfetation and has been documented using human leukocyte antigen typing.

A rather unusual circumstance is the worldwide decline in dizygotic twinning. This has occurred despite widespread use of oral contraceptives, which, after recent discontinuance, doubles the frequency of dizygous twins. Recent advances in the treatment of infertility have contributed to an increase in other multiple births.

The problems of twins (triplets, and so on) relate mostly to being born prematurely (see Chapter 12) because there is a great tendency for twins to be delivered any time after the uterus contains a combined fetal weight of approximately 3.5 kg (in other words, the weight of an average term infant). In one study, the perinatal mortality for monozygotic twins was 2.7 times that for dizygotic twins. Problems were related to amniotic fluid infections and premature ruptures of membranes. Rest for the mother may prolong the pregnancy and increase the birth weight of the children significantly. There is usually a trend toward intrauterine growth retardation beyond 28 weeks' gestation. Sometimes, this phenomenon is limited to only one twin, and the result is twins who are discordant by weight (discordant twins). A discrepancy of 20 to 25% (or greater) of the weight of the larger twin has been used to designate discordance. The problems for the smaller twin are those of intrauterine growth retardation (see Chapter 16).

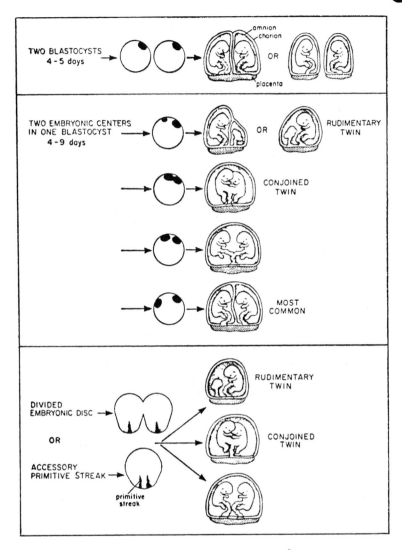

FIGURE 13–1. Diagram showing the different possibilities in twin placentation. (Reproduced with permission from: Smith, D. W., et al.: Monozygotic twinning and Duhamel anomalad [imperforate anus to sirenomelia]: A non-random association between two aberrations in morphogenesis. In Bergsma, D. [ed.]: *Cytogenetics, Environmental Malformation Syndromes.* New York: Alan R. Liss for the National Foundation-March of Dimes; BD:OAS XII [5], 1976.)

Another problem specific to twins is the twin-twin transfusion syndrome (or parabiotic syndrome), in which arteriovenous communication exists between placental blood vessels. The recipient twin may become plethoric and hyperviscous, whereas the donor twin may become anemic (Fig. 13–2). The recipient is frequently larger and the donor smaller, but both may develop hypoglycemia.

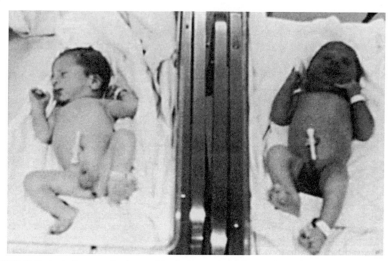

FIGURE 13–2. Twin-twin transfusion, with the anemic twin on the left and the "plethoric" twin on the right. The anemic twin was 20% smaller than the plethoric twin.

A summary of the problems of twins is provided in Table 13–1. In addition to the problems noted earlier, an unexplained observation of an increased prevalence of single umbilical artery was noted many years ago. However, in the absence of other findings, it is not clear that this condition is a marker for unsuspected congenital abnormalities. Another, more recent observation of an increased risk of group B streptococcal infection in twins is also difficult to explain, but because many twins are born with very low birth weight, mortality may be particularly high.

The second of twins born prematurely is generally considered to be at a greater risk of developing respiratory distress syndrome. Whether this is because a minimal amount of blood remains to be transfused from the placenta or

---

TABLE 13–1. PROBLEMS OF TWINS

Twin-twin transfusion
Anemia
Hyperviscosity
Hypoglycemia
High incidence of single umbilical artery
? Associated congenital anomalies
High incidence of GBS infection
High mortality of VLBW
More likely born preterm
Multiple problems (see Chapter 12)
RDS more likely in second twin

GBS = group B streptococcal; RDS = respiratory distress syndrome; VLBW = very low birth weight.

because of the greater likelihood of asphyxia (placental separation or breech delivery) is unclear. In any event, special preparations should be made in the delivery room whenever a multiple birth is anticipated. In addition to having enough equipment available (warmers, laryngoscopes, and so on), it is important to have enough people who can adequately perform resuscitation.

The follow-up of discordant twins has generally indicated that the smaller twin remains smaller and is usually intellectually inferior. However, notable exceptions have occurred, with remarkable capability of catch-up growth in some cases. Both environmental stimulation and good nutrition may be important in such catching up.

It has been suggested that the babies of multiple pregnancies (usually twins) be discharged at the same time, but it seems more important to make sure that the parents are comfortable with the planning arrangements for discharge. In particular, if one baby is significantly smaller than the other, it may be easier to get used to handling one (the larger) baby before coping with two.

The neonatal mortality of twins is primarily related to the increased incidence of low-birth-weight babies, as noted earlier. In a recent study, neonatal mortality for twins was 78 per 1000 live births, which was 6.6 times the rate for singletons. When weight-specific mortality for twins versus singletons was evaluated, they were similar. When one of a twin pair dies before delivery, the living twin may develop thrombocytopenia.

One observation about twins that has not been clearly documented in the intensive care nursery (but is certainly my impression) is that preterm twins frequently follow similar courses with regard to complications. For instance, if both babies have respiratory distress syndrome and one develops pneumothorax, it is very common for the other to have pneumothorax. If one develops pulmonary interstitial emphysema, the other usually follows suit. This phenomenon has been described with sudden infant death syndrome, with several twin pairs dying on the same day.

For commentary on grief response when one of a pair of twins dies, see p. 179.

BIBLIOGRAPHY

Buckler, J. N. H., and Robinson, A.: Matched development of a pair of monozygous twins of grossly different size at birth. *Arch. Dis. Child.* 1974, 49:472.

Editorial: Worldwide decline in dizygotic twinning. *B.M.J.* 1976, 1:1553.

Rothman, K. J.: Fetal loss, twinning and birth weight after oral contraceptive use. *N. Engl. J. Med.* 1977, 297:468.

Terasaki, P. I., Gjerton, D., Bernoco, D., et al.: Twins with two different fathers identified by HLA. *N. Engl. J. Med.* 1978, 299:590.

McCarthy, B. J., Sachs, B. P., Layde, P. M., et al.: Epidemiology of neonatal deaths in twins. *Am. J. Obstet. Gynecol.* 1981, 141:252–256.

Ron-El, R., Caspi, E., Schreyer, P., et al.: Triplet and quadruplet pregnancies and management. *Obstet. Gynecol.* 1981, 57:458–463.

Edwards, M. S., Jackson, C. V., and Baker, C. J.: Increased risk of group B streptococcal disease in twins. *J.A.M.A.* 1981, 245:2044–2046.

Altshuler, G.: Developmental aspects of twins, twinning and chimerism. *Perspect. Pediat. Pathol.* 1982, 7:121–136.

Galea, P., Scott, J. M., and Goel, K. M.: Feto-fetal transfusion syndrome. *Arch. Dis. Child.* 1982, 57:781–794.

Hecht, F., and Hecht, B. K.: Genetic and related biomedical effects of twinning. *Pediatr. Rev.* 1983, 5:179–183.

Robertson, E. G., and Neer, K. H.: Placental injection studies in twin gestation. *Am. J. Obstet. Gynecol.* 1983, 147:170–174.

Young, B. K., Suidan, J., Antoine, J., et al.: Differences in twins: The importance of birth order. *Am. J. Obstet. Gynecol.* 1985, 151:915–921.

Keet, M. P., Jaroszewicz, A. M., and Lombard, C. J.: Follow-up study of physical growth of monozygous twins with discordant within-pair birth weights. *Pediatrics* 1986, 77:336–344.

Annotation: Coping with three, four or more. *Lancet* 1990, 336:473.

Sassoon, D. A., Castro, L. C., Davis, J. L., and Hobel, C. J.: Perinatal outcome in triplet versus twin gestations. *Obstet. Gynecol.* 1990, 75:817–820.

Wolf, I. J., Vintzileos, A. M., Rosenkrantz, T. S., et al.: A comparison of predischarge survival and morbidity in singleton and twin very low birth weight infants. *Obstet. Gynecol.* 1992, 80:436–439.

Keith, L., Lopez-Zeus, J. A., and Luke, B.: Triplet and higher order pregnancies. *Contemp. Obstet. Gynecol.* 1993, June:36–50.

Collins, J. A.: Reproductive technology—The price of progress. *N. Engl. J. Med.* 1994, 331:270–271.

14

PARENT-INFANT INTERACTION

The realization that separating babies from their mothers and fathers for prolonged periods might be detrimental to establishing good parenting practices has resulted in some remarkable changes in delivery rooms and newborn nurseries in recent years. Fathers, who were once banished from delivery rooms, are now present to support the babies' mothers. Skin-skin contact immediately after delivery is encouraged, with mother and baby in a common recovery room. Not very long ago, the low-birth-weight newborn was placed in a premature nursery where the nurses looked after him. Parents were allowed to come to the window of the nursery and look at their baby through the window. Frequently, this view was from a considerable distance, but if the nursery was not too crowded, the incubator might be placed close to the window.

It is perhaps not surprising that some parents had great difficulty relating to their babies, and such attitudes almost certainly contributed to an increased incidence of child abuse in infants born with low birth weight. (Incidentally, other high-risk situations may be identifiable in the delivery room, when defenses are down.) In some centers, abuse and neglect continue to be problems, although in our own nursery population, these issues appear to be uncommon.

The importance of early and extended parent-infant interaction on subsequent development and behavior has been the subject of considerable debate in the past few years. The position that "all is lost" if contact is not made during a "critical period" is clearly not tenable. It seems safe to say that optimal parent-infant interaction is facilitated by early and frequent (subsequent) contact. However, some parents (because of anesthesia) or babies (because of immaturity) are unable to interact immediately after birth but later form attachment, which does not appear to be compromised and does not interfere with child rearing and development.

Current policies in intensive care nurseries usually permit unlimited visiting by both parents, who may not only see the baby at close quarters but may touch and even hold and participate in care when the baby's condition allows (Figs. 14–1 to 14–4). In addition, the complexity of modern neonatal intensive care is such that preparation of parents for what they will see and explanations of what procedure is being performed are almost always necessary. We have even allowed a mother to be present during an exchange transfusion (Fig. 14–5). The ability of parents to cope may be greatly helped by talking to somebody who is not directly involved in the care of the baby but who understands the difficulties they face. A medical social worker is invaluable in many nurseries.

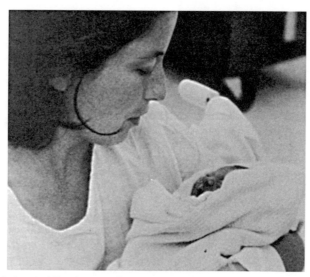

FIGURE 14–1. Mother holding her small premature infant shortly after delivery (note the wheelchair), demonstrating the classic en face position.

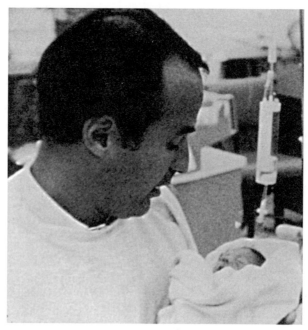

FIGURE 14–2. Fathers are also encouraged to participate in the care of their offspring.

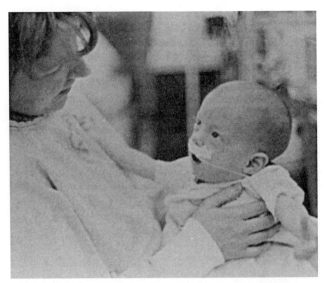

FIGURE 14–3. Even sick babies can benefit from parental contact. This baby being held by his mother has a nasal catheter that delivers low-flow oxygen for bronchopulmonary dysplasia.

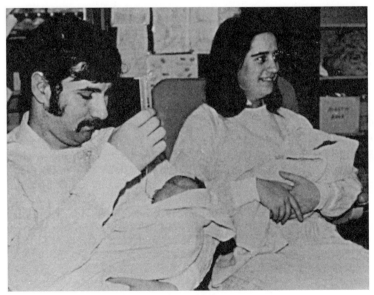

FIGURE 14–4. Parents of twins participating in the care of their babies. The father is gavage feeding one baby by use of gravity flow.

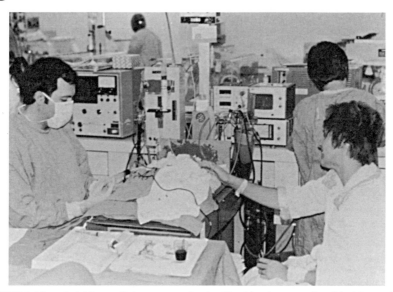

FIGURE 14–5. Liberal visiting policies are emphasized in this photograph, with this mother (a nurse) visiting her baby toward the end of an exchange transfusion.

One important contribution that mothers can make to the care of their premature infants is to provide breast milk. Even though it may not be possible to feed the tiny baby enterally for several days, mothers may be able to express milk from the breast either manually or by use of an electric breast pump. It can be very reassuring for some parents to know that provision of breast milk will help their baby. A feeling of helplessness is, to some extent, relieved by being involved.

It may be important to help parents understand that some babies may benefit from active intervention (e.g., massage), whereas others may be compromised by being disturbed (e.g., the labile baby with persistent pulmonary hypertension). Interventions may also need to be clustered, and an individualized approach (specific prescription) can be helpful.

From time to time, one is faced with difficult ethical decisions, particularly regarding continuation of assisted ventilation in babies with either brain damage or lethal congenital malformations. Parents need to be fully informed and involved to the greatest extent possible. This does not mean that parents have to make these decisions themselves, but that they are included in the decision-making process.

Another recent change in philosophy is largely the result of the work of Dr. T. Berry Brazelton. His major contribution has been to instill the idea that babies are not necessarily molded by their environment but that they have personalities that they impose on their caretakers. For example, there are fussy babies and placid babies. Parents need not feel guilty, if they have the former, believing that they have caused the fussiness. On the other hand, the placid baby is not necessarily easy to take care of because of the personal attributes of the parents but rather because of those of the baby.

In addition, the careful examination of newborns and young infants indicates a much greater ability to integrate and process information than they are commonly believed to possess.

Some workers have taken advantage of the demonstrable abilities of neonates to help parents of low-birth-weight infants better understand their infant's capabilities. This understanding seems to provide benefits for parents (usually mothers) and babies by improving interaction and appropriate stimulation.

Another concept that is worth mentioning is the idea that the things that we as physicians and nurses think are important are not necessarily what parents perceive as important. For instance, having a baby under phototherapy may be as disturbing for some parents as having a baby on a respirator. It is also common for two parents to receive quite different messages during a conversation about their baby. Some parents hear what they want to hear, whether that is an optimistic or a pessimistic outlook. Because parents of sick infants are frequently overwrought immediately after delivery, it may be necessary to relay information several times before it is well understood. On the other hand, we can do much to alleviate anxiety through careful explanation, but we must try not to engender anxiety by overdetailed (or pessimistic) explanations. Clearly, the more extended the hospital stay and the more complicated the hospital course, the greater the likelihood that parent-infant interaction will be disrupted. In addition, parent-parent interaction is more likely to be disrupted. Individual strengths and weaknesses are more likely to be revealed under such stress.

GRIEF RESPONSE

It is commonly appreciated that when a baby dies, the parents suffer a period of loss with associated grief. This process is fairly predictable and is little different for grief after the death of an infant than grief for any death. There are several stages, which can be summarized as follows: (1) denial, (2) anger, (3) bargaining, (4) depression, and (5) acceptance.

Feelings of guilt are particularly common and can be anticipated. Mothers in particular will pick some event during the pregnancy that they believe was responsible and may even focus on an event that could not remotely have been implicated. In many cases, such feelings can be relieved by sympathetic questioning and discussion.

Although it might seem that when one of a pair of twins dies the grief response might be attenuated (because parents can focus on the living child), this does not seem to be the case. As with other parents of babies who die, they should be given the opportunity to discuss the dead baby. Parents who have a stillborn baby also experience the same feelings and require the same understanding as parents of a liveborn baby who dies.

In the case of babies who die shortly after birth, it may be important to allow parents to see and hold the baby, if they so desire. Except for the most grotesquely deformed babies, this seems to be a wise policy in all cases, because the imagined is frequently much worse than the reality. When death occurs later, particularly after a protracted course, every effort should be made to let parents hold the baby before and after death, according to their wishes. This is sometimes the only opportunity they will ever have to feel that it is their baby. Depending on the hospital unit, they should be given as much privacy as possible at this time. As a result of this interaction, the grief response may be accelerated.

Follow-up visits or telephone calls to discuss how parents are coping and what their understanding is of the cause of death seem to be beneficial. It may also be important to explain that occasional depression may last as long as a year and that if this does happen, it is not abnormal.

Less commonly appreciated is the fact that when an infant with congenital abnormalities is born, the parents frequently go through a similar process in adjusting to the abnormal baby, presumably grieving for the "normal" baby that was anticipated. The sequence of behavior typically is (1) shock, (2) denial, (3) sadness and anger, (4) adaptation, and (5) reorganization.

Similarly, it is now apparent that parents of critically ill newborns may experience anticipatory grief. Most parents experience sadness, difficulty in sleeping, preoccupation, loss of appetite, and irritability. Less commonly, anger is experienced, and guilt seems to affect mothers more than fathers.

An appreciation of these feelings is important when dealing with parents of critically ill newborns. Tact and understanding are required in handling families who experience any of these grief-provoking circumstances. Whenever a major congenital abnormality is present (particularly the child with a chromosomal abnormality or ambiguous genitalia), it is important to offer immediate and long-term genetic counseling (see Chapter 8).

BIBLIOGRAPHY

Klaus, M. H., and Kennell, J. H.: *Parent-Infant Bonding*, 2nd ed. C. V. Mosby, St. Louis, 1982.

Parent-Infant Interaction

Widmayer, S. M., and Field, T. M.: Effects of Brazelton demonstration for mothers on the development of preterm infants. *Pediatrics* 1981, 67:711–714.
Chamberlin, R. W.: Bonding and screening: Myth and reality (Commentary). *Pediatr. Rev.* 1982, 3:203–204.
Charney, E.: Counseling of parents around the birth of a baby. *Pediatr. Rev.* 1982, 4:167–176.
Klaus, M., and Kennell, J.: Interventions in the premature nursery: Impact on development. *Pediatr. Clin. North Am.* 1982, 29:1263–1273.
Lamb, M. E., Campos, J. J., Hwang, C.-P., et al.: Joint reply to "maternal-infant bonding: A joint rebuttal." *Pediatrics* 1983, 72:574–576.
Lealman, G. T., Haigh, D., Phillips, J. M., et al.: Prediction and prevention of child abuse—an empty hope? *Lancet* 1983, i:1423–1424.
Minde, K., Whitelaw, A., Brown, J., and Fitzharding, P.: Effect of neonatal complications in premature infants on early parent-infant interactions. *Dev. Med. Child Neurol.* 1983, 25:763–777.
Schwab, F., Tolbert, B., Bagnato, S., and Maisels, M. J.: Sibling visiting in a neonatal intensive care unit. *Pediatrics* 1983, 71:835–838.
Brazelton, T. B.: Neonatal behavioral assessment scale. *Clin. Develop. Med.* No. 50, S.I.M.P. J. B. Lippincott, Philadelphia, 2nd ed., 1984.

Als, H., Lawhon, G., Brown, E., et al.: Individualized behavioral and environmental care for the very low birth weight preterm infant at high risk for bronchopulmonary dysplasia. *Pediatrics* 1986, 78:1123–1132.

Grief Response

Drotar, D., Baskiewiz, A., Irvin, N., et al.: The adaptation of parents to the birth of an infant with a congenital malformation: A hypothetical model. *Pediatrics* 1975, 56:710.
Benfield, D. G., Lieb, S. A., and Vollman, J. H.: Grief response of parents to neonatal death and parent participation in deciding care. *Pediatrics* 1978, 62:171.
Speck, W. T., and Kennell, J. H.: Management of perinatal death. *Pediatr. Rev.* 1980, 2:59–62.
Forrest, G. C., Claridge, R. S., and Baum, J. D.: Practical management of perinatal death. *B.M.J.* 1981, 282:31–32.
Wilson, A. L., Fenton, L. J., Stevens, D. C., and Soule, D. J.: The death of a newborn twin: An analysis of parental bereavement. *Pediatrics* 1982, 70:587–591.
Drell, M. J.: The call: Anticipatory guidance for the death of a family's newborn. *Pediatr. Rev.* 1987, 8:196–199.
Lewis, E., and Bryan, E. M.: Management of perinatal loss of a twin. *B.M.J.* 1988, 297:1321–1323.
Wessel, M. A.: Pediatrician's response to a stillborn or death of a neonate. *Pediatr. Rev.* 1990, 12:163–164.
Acolet, D., Modi, N., Giannakoulopoulos, X., et al.: Changes in plasma cortisol and catecholamine concentrations in response to massage in preterm infants. *Arch. Dis. Child.* 1993, 68:29–31.

15
NEONATAL INFECTION

BACTERIAL INFECTION

SEPSIS

Introduction

Despite considerable attention during the past 20 years, there is still no completely reliable way of making a rapid diagnosis of neonatal sepsis (septicemia). The major difficulty relates to the large number of predisposing risk factors and clinical manifestations of sepsis and meningitis. Because of this, many infants are investigated, but few prove to have sepsis or meningitis. In my studies in Vermont, and more recently in Maine, 8% of neonates investigated for infection in an intensive care nursery proved to have bacterial sepsis.

The incidence of sepsis varies from one center to another, but it ranges from 1 in 1000 to 4 in 1000 live births in most centers. In Houston, when early- and late-onset cases of both sepsis and meningitis were considered, the incidence varied between 4 in 1000 and 8 in 1000 live births between 1969 and 1978. There appears to be an increasing prevalence of sepsis with decreasing birth weight. Rates as high as 16% in infants between 1001 and 1500 g were reported 30 years ago, and similarly high rates have been reported recently from some intensive care units (admitting mostly low-birth-weight infants). With increased survival of infants with birth weights of less than 1000 g have come increased numbers of infants with late-onset infection.

Neonatal sepsis and meningitis remain important contributors to neonatal mortality. Very early onset of infection (within 24 hours of birth) in very-low-birth-weight infants is particularly lethal but seems to be decreasing in association with more liberal use by obstetricians of prenatal antibiotics when managing very preterm labor and preterm, premature rupture of the membranes. In some centers, the case fatality rate may be 20 to 25%, but the author's recent experience suggests that this rate can be lowered to 10 to 15%.

Etiology

The bacterial organisms accounting for neonatal sepsis have shown certain cyclic variations, and the organisms responsible for neonatal sepsis are usually quite different from those accounting for similar infections in older infants and children. Before the 1940s, the predominant pathogen appeared to be group A β-hemolytic streptococci. In the 1950s, *Staphylococcus aureus* assumed a relatively important role, and in the 1960s, gram-negative organisms, and particularly *Escherichia coli*, ruled supreme. The 1970s saw a virtually nationwide preponderance of group B streptococcal infection, although *E. coli* remained prominent. In the 1980s, group B streptococcal infection remained important, and coagulase-negative staphylococcal infection (usually *Staphylococcus epidermidis*) emerged as the most important late-onset infection, particularly in infants with birthweights of less than 1000 g. Both remain common problems for early- and late-onset infections, respectively, in the 1990s, although other organisms (*E. coli* and *S. aureus*) may be making a comeback. New serotypes of group B streptococci have recently been described, one of which (type V) has caused neonatal sepsis. Although anaerobic organisms can cause sepsis, they do not seem to play a prominent role at this time.

Certainly the most likely explanation for an individual baby developing neonatal sepsis relates to a defect in host defense mechanisms, and it is particularly noteworthy that there is an increased prevalence of neonatal infection in male infants (which is difficult to explain, although it has been suggested that male susceptibility relates to protection on the X chromosome). Other problems of host defense mechanisms implicate (1) a deficiency of opsonic activity, (2) an inability of polymorphonuclear leukocytes to migrate and phagocytose adequately, and (3) a deficiency of chemotactic factor. Complement factors (particularly C5) are functionally deficient. Evidence also suggests that deficient levels of fibronectin are present in neonates, and even lower levels are seen in neonates with sepsis. The ability to generate acute-phase proteins (which are also low in neonates) may also play an important role in survival. One other interesting observation is that many infants with galactosemia present with *E. coli* sepsis.

Transplacentally acquired antibodies fall into the immunoglobulin (IgG) class, and most antibodies to gram-negative organisms fall into the IgM class. This explanation of increased susceptibility to gram-negative organisms was offered (and accepted) for many years. The hypothesis is not proved, but preterm infants have enhanced susceptibility partly because the transfer of IgG increases with advancing gestational age, especially after 32 weeks. It now seems to be quite clear that susceptibility of an individual newborn to the group B streptococcus relates to the absence of type-specific antibody in the mother, so that protective IgG antibody cannot be transferred to the fetus and neonate.

Diagnosis

As noted earlier, many different clinical situations lead one to consider the diagnosis of sepsis. In view of the high mortality, the physician must maintain a high index of suspicion. Despite the fact that some authors have believed for many years that preterm labor and premature rupture of membranes (rupture before the onset of labor) might be precipitated by infected amniotic fluid, most authors have stressed the potential for acquiring infection after the rupture of membranes. The evidence is now clear that the former mechanism is quite common, and the latter is less likely to occur with conservative management (avoiding frequent vaginal examinations).

The following high-risk circumstances indicate the need to search for neonatal infection (sepsis, pneumonia, and meningitis):

1. Prolonged rupture of membranes (> 24 hours)
2. Premature (particularly preterm) rupture of membranes
3. Preterm labor without adequate explanation (e.g., in multiple pregnancy, abruptio placentae)
4. Meconium-stained amniotic fluid without adequate explanation (e.g., in a postterm or dysmature infant or with an infarcted placenta; unusual before 36 weeks' gestation—think of *Listeria*)
5. Maternal fever or other evidence of maternal infection
6. Fetal tachycardia
7. Foul-smelling amniotic fluid or malodorous baby

The clinical manifestations that may indicate sepsis are numerous, and some are more important at certain ages than others. Because the best hope for successful treatment is early diagnosis, the signs that present early are considered first:

1. Lethargy
2. Low Apgar scores (without other explanations)
3. Poor feeding
4. Abdominal distension
5. Temperature instability
6. Unexplained apnea
7. Unexplained cyanosis (dusky spells)
8. Unexplained jaundice
9. Respiratory distress (with pneumonia)
10. Irritability (with meningitis)
11. Hepatomegaly (and occasionally splenomegaly)
12. Diarrhea
13. Vomiting
14. Skin eruptions, such as pustules, bullae, necrotic lesions

Features that appear late and therefore suggest a bad prognosis are pallor or blotchiness (poor capillary filling), shock (hypotension), sclerema, petechiae and purpura, convulsions (seizures), and a bulging fontanel (with meningitis).

The only certain way of determining bacterial sepsis is having a positive blood culture. However, certain factors may strongly suggest that infection is present. In the immediate neonatal period, gastric aspirate may be obtained and sent to the laboratory for smear (with or without culture). Large numbers of gram-positive cocci on the gastric aspirate smear may be indicative of group B streptococcal infection. A large number of polymorphonuclear leukocytes (pus cells) suggests that the baby has been exposed to infection for some time. If the baby is premature and has low Apgar scores, this finding may be enough to initiate a full sepsis workup and administration of antibiotics. Further help may be obtained from a white blood count and differential. As a rule of thumb, in the immediate neonatal period, a white count greater than 30,000 or less than 5000/mm³ may be considered abnormal. Leukopenia (especially neutropenia less than 1000/mm³) seems to be more indicative of infection in the first week after birth, but after that time, elevated leukocyte counts ($> 20,000/mm^3$, particularly with neutrophilia) may be predictive. Although an increase in the absolute number of immature (band, myelocyte, and metamyelocyte) neutrophils may be helpful in term infants, the immature to total neutrophil ratio seems to be more reliable in predicting infection.

A search for an adequate laboratory investigation that might give reliable information about the presence or absence of infection has been undertaken by several authors. At present, no one test appears to be accepted as uniformly reliable.

Another approach is to use several different investigations, which by themselves may not be diagnostic but which in combination may support the diagnosis. The following tests have also been used to educe bacterial infection:

1. Mini–erythrocyte sedimentation rate determination
2. C-reactive protein determination
3. Haptoglobin determination
4. α_1-Acid glycoprotein (orosomucoid) determination
5. Nitroblue tetrazolium test
6. Examination of the buffy coat for ingested organisms
7. Degenerative changes in neutrophils (e.g., toxic granulation)

In the author's experience, any two (or more) of the following five findings strongly suggest infection:

1. Total white blood cell count of $< 5000/mm^3$ (or $> 20,000/mm^3$ after 5 days)
2. Immature to total neutrophils at least 0.2 (≥ 0.3 is even better)
3. Positive latex C-reactive protein
4. Mini–erythocyte sedimentation rate of at least 15 mm in the first hour
5. Positive latex haptoglobin

Although IgM level is sometimes elevated in gram-negative sepsis, this phenomenon seems to occur about 48 to 72 hours after the onset of infection. An elevated IgM level can be seen in about 70% of chronic intrauterine nonbacterial infections.

With the advent of techniques such as laser and rate nephelometry, it is now possible to obtain rapid quantitative determinations of acute phase proteins, such as C-reactive protein and α_1-acid glycoprotein. Evidence continues to accumulate to support the measurement of levels of these proteins (especially C-reactive protein) both to diagnose and to manage infections (but other inflammatory processes can produce increased levels to complicate interpretation). Semiquantitative measurements of C-reactive protein can be obtained with latex reagent by serial dilution of serum.

The search for the perfect rapid diagnostic test continues. Two additional tests that have shown some promise are elastase-α_1-proteinase inhibitor and interleukin-6. The latter seems to be the stimulus for C-reactive protein production and increases early in the course of infection. However, the test currently takes several hours to perform, which may not be useful in the clinical setting.

Management

Use of the tests noted earlier can make antibiotic therapy more rational. Certainly in the presence of an asymptomatic term baby and negative test results, it would seem reasonable if only a high-risk situation exists to defer antibiotic therapy. On the other hand, in the preterm baby or in the presence of clinical symptomatology that cannot be explained on other grounds (e.g., metabolic disorders), obtaining blood, urine, and cerebrospinal fluid cultures and initiating antibiotic treatment seems to be the safest course. The choice of antibiotics for treating bacterial sepsis is dictated by the most frequently encountered organisms, which means that coverage should be provided for both gram-negative and gram-positive organisms and in particular for *E. coli* and group B streptococcal infections. Local sensitivities may dictate which antibiotics are chosen, but a penicillin and aminoglycoside are the usual starting agents. Gentamicin in combination with ampicillin is usually effective therapy at this time. *Pseudomonas* sp. may require tobramycin and carbenicillin, and staphylococci may require methicillin, nafcillin, or (more frequently now) vancomycin. Some gram-negative enteric organisms may need third-generation cephalosporins (e.g., cefotaxime, ceftriaxone). In cases of sepsis, antibiotics are given by the intravenous route for 7 days to 2 weeks, depending on the organism and the clinical or C-reactive protein response (7 to 10 days for penicillin-susceptible organisms). If cultures are negative at 48 hours and no abnormality of white blood count, differential, and C-reactive protein is detected, antibiotics can be stopped.

With the increased use of prenatal antibiotics for preterm labor or preterm, premature rupture of the membranes, the incidence of neonates exposed to infection that have a negative blood culture has increased. Babies born under these circumstances should be investigated for infection (with some having positive blood cultures) and started on antibiotics. Based on the white blood count, differential, and C-reactive protein, antibiotic treatment can be limited to approximately 48 hours if the blood culture is negative and the test results are normal.

In addition to specific therapy, other supportive measures may be necessary. Attention to thermoregulation, correction of metabolic acidosis, and administration of oxygen may be required. The use of plasma or whole-blood transfusions, once considered nonspecific, may help to correct the defects in the complement system.

Clear evidence exists that plasma from different individuals contains differing amounts of antibody to group B streptococci. This finding seems to have affected survival when plasma, containing antibody, was transfused into neonates with group B streptococcal infection. Specific immunotherapy (intravenous immunoglobulin with specific antibody or monoclonal antibody) is desirable and may become available.

Numerous bacteria (but most frequently group B streptococci) may predispose to the development of persistent pulmonary hypertension (see p. 122). In a few infants with overwhelming sepsis, extreme measures, such as exchange transfusion or granulocyte transfusion, may be required. Profound neutropenia may also be responsive to granulocyte colony-stimulating factor.

Prophylaxis

Because of the high mortality from neonatal sepsis, particularly in response to experience with early-onset group B streptococcal sepsis, attempts to prevent infection have been made. These can be summarized as chemoprophylaxis and immunoprophylaxis. Chemoprophylaxis involves the administration of penicillin to neonates and penicillin or ampicillin to mothers. Although prenatal administration may prevent early-onset group B streptococcal infection, the evidence for postnatal antibiotics is somewhat conflicting. It may be useful in term infants but is unlikely to be beneficial in preterm infants. Prenatal immunoprophylaxis is the selective immunization of mothers against specific organisms likely to cause neonatal sepsis. This approach may work, but maternal response to vaccine is variable and cost/benefit analysis has not been completed. Postnatal immunoprophylaxis involves administration of intravenous immunoglobulin to very-low-birth-weight infants every 1 to 2 weeks after delivery. In the two largest studies published so far, the results were contradictory, with a decrease in nosocomial infection in the earlier study (Baker, 1992) and no decrease in the later study (Fanaroff, 1994).

MENINGITIS (BACTERIAL)

Introduction

It is difficult to separate meningitis from sepsis in most cases because many of the signs are common to both disorders. It has been estimated that one quarter to one third of all cases of sepsis have concomitant meningitis, but more recently, this figure may be down to one tenth. Despite antibiotic use, the case fatality from neonatal meningitis remains depressingly high. Approximately 25 to 30% of babies with neonatal meningitis die, and many others have neurologic sequelae.

Etiology

The organisms responsible for neonatal meningitis do not differ to any significant extent from those resulting in sepsis. Both *E. coli* and group B streptococcal bacteria are the most likely organisms to be isolated, *E. coli* being more common in the first few days of life and group B streptococcal meningitis occurring more frequently toward the end of the first week to 10 days of age. It has been suggested that the type of *E. coli* responsible for meningitis is different from types producing other kinds of pathogenicity. The variance appears to rest in the type K1 polysaccharide capsular antigen. Another organism that should be considered when meningitis is suspected is *Listeria monocytogenes*. In the older neonate, salmonella meningitis becomes more likely, but a wide variety of organisms have been implicated. Of note is *Citrobacter diversus*, which is frequently associated with brain abscess.

Diagnosis

As noted in the list of clinical manifestations for sepsis, irritability may be striking, as may a bulging anterior fontanel. Frequently, metabolic acidosis is a prominent feature. The diagnosis may be confirmed on examination of cerebrospinal fluid obtained by lumbar puncture. A white blood count higher than 30/mm³, particularly with an increased number of polymorphonuclear leukocytes, would suggest bacterial meningitis. However, frequently, fewer than 25 cells are initially present in the cerebrospinal fluid (CSF) from which bacteria are subsequently cultured. In one study, only 12 of 21 CSF samples in infants with bacterial meningitis had more than 25 cells/mm³. In gram-negative meningitis, eradication of bacteria from CSF takes about 3 days after initiation of antibiotic therapy. The protein level in CSF is usually significantly elevated but may be difficult to distinguish in the neonatal period because protein levels are frequently elevated in the neonate, particularly the premature infant. Such levels may be as high as 200 mg/dl in the first days of life, falling to closer to 100 mg/dl in the second week of life. To interpret the CSF glucose level, it is important to at least check the peripheral blood with test strips and preferably to perform a blood sugar determination at the same time as the lumbar puncture is performed. If the CSF glucose level is less than 50% of the blood glucose level, this would help to confirm bacterial meningitis.

Management

Supportive management includes intravenous (or intraarterial) fluids and occasionally alkali (sodium bicarbonate) for metabolic acidosis. Incubator observation is important because convulsions are a common complication of neonatal meningitis. Appropriate anticonvulsant therapy may be required. Intracranial pressure monitoring may be of some assistance, but it is not clear that pharmacologic agents (e.g., mannitol, glycerol, and dexamethasone) have sustained beneficial effects. Hyperventilation, with assisted ventilation, may be the most reliable way of decreasing intracranial pressure.

The definitive treatment includes initiation of antibiotic treatment with a penicillin and an aminoglycoside. Ampicillin is usually effective in treating both *E. coli* and group B streptococcal meningitis. However, if the *E. coli* is ampicillin resistant, alternative therapy may be necessary because the aminoglycosides (e.g., gentamicin) enter CSF poorly. Under such circumstances, it may be necessary to use chloramphenicol, which penetrates into CSF much more readily. Intraventricular gentamicin in gram-negative bacillary meningitis was found to have a higher case fatality rate in one study. Thus, intraventricular gentamicin should not be used in routine management. If chloramphenicol is used, chloramphenicol levels must be measured at intervals, to avoid the potential toxicity of the gray baby syndrome and to know that adequate dosages are being given. In addition, experience with third-generation cephalosporins has been encouraging, and further trials are in progress. Imipenem-cilastatin has been used successfully to treat *C. diversus* meningitis. Daily head circumference measurements are probably needed to detect any rapid increase that may reflect developing hydrocephalus, but this may be a relatively crude estimate of the development of this complication. Cephalic ultrasound is an adjunct that can be employed to detect early ventriculomegaly and thalamic echodensities. Neurosurgical consultation will then dictate what form of therapy is to be employed. Antibiotic therapy is usually continued for 2 or 3 weeks by the intravenous route, depending on the causative organism. Measurement of C-reactive protein level may be helpful in deciding duration of antibiotic therapy. It is unwise to stop therapy until the serum C-reactive protein level is normal. Failure to eliminate an organism from CSF should suggest the possibility of ventriculitis. This too may be detectable with ultrasound in some cases. Despite apparently adequate therapy, there may be long-term sequelae in the form of profound mental retardation, soft neurologic signs, and/or deafness, in as many as 50% of cases.

Dexamethasone has been shown to decrease the incidence of neurologic sequelae of meningitis in children beyond the neonatal period, apparently by inhibiting inflammatory mediators (cytokines). It is not clear whether a similar benefit occurs in the neonate.

Summary

Neonatal meningitis is relatively uncommon, but despite appropriate antibiotic therapy, it still carries a rather high mortality and morbidity. *E. coli* and group B streptococci are the most frequently isolated organisms. Irritability and a bulging fontanel may be important clinical signs in addition to those normally associated with neonatal sepsis. Intravenous antibiotic therapy for 2 or 3 weeks and other supportive measures are usually successful in avoiding complications, but both short- and long-term sequelae may be observed.

OTHER BACTERIAL INFECTIONS

PNEUMONIA

This subject has been discussed earlier (see Chapter 9).

OMPHALITIS

Redness and induration of the umbilical region are most likely the result of infection caused by *S. aureus* (coagulase positive). The portal of entry is the cut surface of the umbilical cord. It is perhaps more likely to be seen if a catheter has been inserted into an umbilical vessel. Using various prophylactic measures (e.g., triple dye, bacitracin, povidone-iodine—see Chapter 4), this type of infection is now relatively uncommon. Should *S. aureus* (coagulase positive) again become a serious problem in nurseries, undoubtedly this kind of manifestation will be seen more frequently. Omphalitis is a potentially serious illness. It needs to be treated with appropriate intravenous antibiotics to prevent necrotizing fasciitis, which may require surgical consultation and intervention (debridement).

CONJUNCTIVITIS

Inflammation and drainage from the conjunctiva are most likely the result of chemical conjunctivitis secondary to instillation of silver nitrate, but this phenomenon is less common since the introduction of erythromycin and tetracycline for topical prophylaxis.

On the second day of life and thereafter, particularly if adequate eye prophylaxis has not been carried out, the diagnosis of gonococcal ophthalmia should be considered. From approximately 4 or 5 days of age onward, staphylococcal infection should be considered the most likely cause of the problem (Fig. 15–1). Chlamydial infection may be an important cause of ophthalmia neonatorum. This is sometimes referred to as inclusion conjunctivitis and requires examination of conjunctival scrapings. Erythromycin ointment may be valuable for prophylaxis against chlamydial conjunctivitis (but not against chlamydial pneumonia), although it is not apparently superior to silver nitrate.

URINARY TRACT INFECTION

In all cases in which sepsis is suspected, it is important to rule out urinary tract infection, just as it is important to rule out meningitis. This is usually accomplished by examination and culture of urine obtained by suprapubic bladder aspiration, although culture may be unrewarding in the first few days after birth. Examination of urine obtained by bag specimens is notoriously unreliable, particularly with respect to culture. Vomiting may be a more common accompaniment of this type of infection than of generalized sepsis. When jaundice is observed, the direct (conjugated) bilirubin is frequently more elevated than anticipated. *E. coli* is the most frequently encountered organism. A search for an underlying congenital urinary tract abnormality should be carried out in

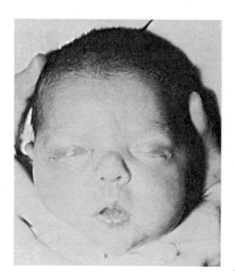

FIGURE 15–1. Purulent conjunctivitis, exhibiting drainage from both eyes (more obvious from the right eye).

all cases in which urinary tract infection is detected. Vesicoureteric reflux is especially important in this regard. Abnormalities of the urinary system were found in 45% of the girls in one study.

ENTERITIS

Whenever more than two infants in the nursery have diarrhea (frequent, loose, watery stools), an epidemic should be suspected. This is most frequently the result of viral infection with different agents but in the past has been associated with infection with various strains of E. coli, referred to as enteropathogenic strains. With the passage of time, other strains not formerly considered pathogenic have been associated with epidemics. Consequently, it is difficult to test for pathogenic strains unless an epidemic occurs. Occasionally other causative organisms are found, such as S. aureus, Shigella, and Salmonella. Blood in the stool usually indicates one of the more serious infections, but attention has been drawn to the possibility of infection with Campylobacter fetus, causing a mild illness with bloody diarrhea. After some initial enthusiasm regarding the role of Clostridium difficile in diarrhea, considerable caution in interpretation needs to be exercised when this organism is found in diarrheal stools of the neonate. Whenever diarrhea is encountered, the stools should be cultured and increased attention paid to isolation technique, which may necessitate wearing gloves and carefully disposing of all materials coming out of the incubator (see also Diarrhea section on p. 311).

OSTEOMYELITIS

There is a wide spectrum of involvement of bones by infection, from the relatively benign to the severe. S. aureus remains the most likely causative organism, but more recently, group B streptococci have been implicated. Any bone can be involved, but a long bone is most likely, although facial bones are also frequently involved. Swelling over the affected bone may be the only obvious sign, but other manifestations of more generalized infection (sepsis) may be present. Sometimes, movement of a limb seems to cause pain. Prolonged (≥ 4 weeks) antibiotic therapy is usually required in addition to other supportive measures. It may be difficult to distinguish septic arthritis from osteomyelitis.

PERITONITIS

Peritonitis is an uncommon form of neonatal infection. Most commonly, it occurs secondary to intestinal perforation, but primary peritonitis can also occur. A shiny, erythematous appearance of the abdomen may suggest the diagnosis.

OTITIS MEDIA

Otitis media is not frequently suspected in the neonatal period. However, it has been associated with prolonged nasotracheal intubation. It may give rise to facial palsy (as indicated by a series of one).

TETANUS

In certain parts of the world (partly on the basis of religious custom), tetanus is a common neonatal problem. Although rare, it can occur in the United States. Clinical features include poor suck, hypertonicity, and generalized spasms starting toward the end of the first week. The spasms may be confused with seizures. If infants can be helped through the acute illness with neuromuscular blockade and assisted ventilation, the long-term outlook seems to be good.

TUBERCULOSIS

Another problem that is encountered more frequently in underdeveloped countries than in developed nations is congenital tuberculosis. As a result of increased immigration from some of these underdeveloped countries, cases have also been encountered in the United States. Hepatomegaly is common, whereas failure to thrive, jaundice, and central nervous system involvement are unusual. Beyond the immediate neonatal period, cough and tachypnea are seen frequently. Useful diagnostic procedures seem to be liver biopsy, biopsy of skin lesions when present, and cultures of gastric aspirates. Treatment with isoniazid alone may be sufficient.

NONBACTERIAL INFECTIONS

THE TORCH SYNDROME

Introduction and Etiology

The commonly used acronym TORCH is derived from T for toxoplasmosis, O for other (includes other viruses and congenital syphilis), R for rubella (expanded rubella syndrome), C for cytomegalovirus, and H for herpes simplex. These infections have been grouped together because of their common clinical manifestations (Figs. 15–2 to 15–5), which range from asymptomatic infection to overwhelming infection (and death). It is usually the case that infection is acquired quite early in intrauterine life, giving rise to chronic intrauterine infection. Those infants who appear normal at birth may have acquired infection (e.g., herpes) late in pregnancy or at the time of delivery. A few years ago, it looked as if congenital rubella syndrome had been eliminated, but a resurgence was noted recently.

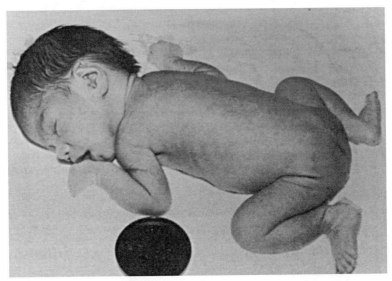

FIGURE 15–2. This baby had marked intrauterine growth retardation. The posture was that of a term baby, but the weight was approximately 1200 g (the lens cover from the camera provides a contrast). This baby had had chronic intrauterine infection with rubella.

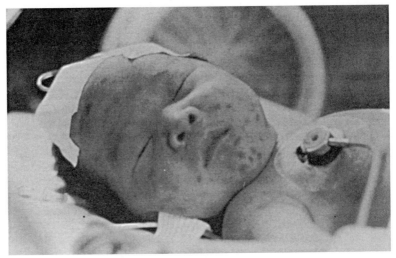

FIGURE 15–3. Purpuric spots on the face of a baby who had congenital toxoplasmosis.

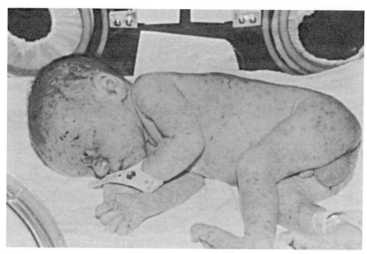

FIGURE 15–4. The generalized purpura and petechiae, giving rise to the name "blueberry muffin baby," associated with congenital rubella are shown here. This baby had cytomegalovirus infection.

Diagnosis

Apart from a few specific points that enable a more enlightened appraisal (see Table 15–1), one is generally unable to distinguish between the members of this group based on the most frequently encountered features. Such features are (1) small size for gestational age, (2) petechiae and purpura, (3) hepatospleno-megaly, (4) jaundice, (5) chorioretinitis, (6) anemia and thrombocytopenia, and (7) bone lesions.

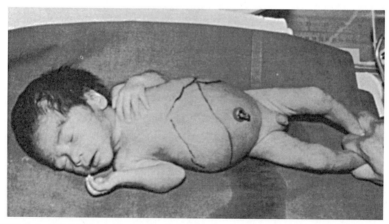

FIGURE 15–5. Another baby with congenital toxoplasmosis, showing intrauterine growth retardation, hepatosplenomegaly (especially the spleen), and dilated veins over the upper abdomen.

TABLE 15–1. SOME HELPFUL FEATURES IN DISTINGUISHING BETWEEN THE COMMON AGENTS IN THE TORCH SYNDROME

Toxoplasmosis	Rubella	CMV	Herpes	Congenital Syphilis
Intracranial calcification	Cataract	Intracranial calcification	Vesicles (especially over scalp)	Snuffles
Microcephaly	Congenital heart defects	Microcephaly	Meningoencephalitis	Peeling hands and feet
Hydrocephaly	Rubella virus recoverable	Inguinal hernia (males)	Maternal herpetic vulvovaginitis	Positive serologic test for syphilis
Splenomegaly more prominent than hepatomegaly	Deafness (detected later)	Cytomegalovirus recoverable	Herpesvirus recoverable (especially from vesicles)	
Positive dye test (Sabin-Feldman)		Deafness (detected later)		

CMV = cytomegalovirus; TORCH = toxoplasmosis, other, rubella, cytomegalovirus, herpes simplex.

Table 15–1 lists features that, if seen, allow more certainty about diagnosis. Absence of these features does not exclude a specific diagnosis. More recently, chronic lung disease of prematurity has been associated with postnatal acquisition of cytomegalovirus.

Management

Unfortunately, effective therapy is not available for most viral infections. Improvement in herpes simplex meningoencephalitis was first noted with adenine arabinoside (Ara-A) and more recently with acyclovir, but the treatment is not always beneficial. The prognosis in cases involving herpes simplex virus is largely dependent on the classification of illness. When infection is localized, survival is to be expected. However, case fatality with encephalitis is approximately 15% and with disseminated infection is over 50%. Congenital syphilis may be treated with penicillin, and prevention of progression of toxoplasmosis may result from sulfadiazine and pyrimethamine (or spiramycin) therapy.

Initially, some confirmation of diagnosis may be obtained by using serum IgM determination (a rapid determination may be obtained when laser nephelometry is available). If IgM level is elevated, serum for acute titers and specimens for viral culture should be analyzed. It is always better to try to make a specific diagnosis by sending specimens for viral culture than by blindly asking for TORCH titers. Although the latter may occasionally be helpful, especially when convalescent serum can be obtained in survivors, the yield from TORCH titers has been low. Differentiation from bacterial sepsis is frequently not possible, so that a sepsis workup followed by antibiotic therapy is frequently instituted.

Summary

Toxoplasmosis, rubella, cytomegalovirus, herpes, and other viral infection (plus syphilis) constitute the disorders classified as the TORCH syndrome. Common clinical manifestations are smallness for gestational age, jaundice, hepatosplenomegaly, petechiae, and purpura. Special features occasionally allow the specific disorder to be rapidly identified. Cultures for specific viruses or determination of specific IgM level seem to be more valuable than a TORCH screen. Apart from the agents used to treat herpes and syphilis, little specific therapy is available.

HERPES SIMPLEX

Transmission of Virus

Frequently, one is asked if personnel with herpes simplex lesions should be allowed to work in nurseries and whether or not a mother may infect her baby. The highest risk before delivery occurs with primary genital infection. Delivery by cesarean section within 4 hours of membrane rupture seems to protect the baby. It is not clear that postpartum transmission of virus from genital lesions has occurred. Because the potential exists for life-threatening illness (a high percentage of deaths have occurred in reported cases), it seems wise to adhere to the following recommendations:

1. Any infant with herpes simplex virus should be isolated from other infants.

2. Nursery personnel and other adults with lesions caused by the herpes simplex virus should be excluded from contact with newborn infants.

3. Mothers with active oral lesions caused by herpes simplex virus should probably be temporarily separated from their infants.

ACQUIRED IMMUNODEFICIENCY SYNDROME

The acquired immunodeficiency syndrome (AIDS) is caused by the human immunodeficiency virus (HIV). Although HIV is already of great concern to many neonatal centers, it is likely to be encountered by all clinicians in the years ahead. Evans (1994) observed: "A catastrophic phenomenon rather than a disease would be a more accurate characterization of AIDS. Lethal, increasing in its global scope, infecting ever-larger numbers of people, frustratingly difficult to treat effectively, it casts a long, ominous shadow."

A full discussion of this subject is beyond the scope of this book, but it is important to have some understanding of perinatal transmission of HIV. At this time, it is not possible to accurately diagnose AIDS in the neonatal period.

HIV is transmitted from mother to fetus in 20 (Europe) to 40% (Africa) of cases. Breast feeding by HIV-infected women is a risk factor for transmission of HIV. In cases of transmission of maternal antibody, it may not be possible to determine whether or not a neonate is infected until many months have passed.

Protection against other illnesses (e.g., measles) may be compromised because of depleted maternal antibody.

Attempts to prevent transmission, either by the use of pharmaceutical agents or by vaccines, have been initiated, but is not yet clear how effective they will be. Early results suggest that zidovudine may decrease perinatal transmission.

OTHER VIRAL INFECTIONS

VARICELLA-ZOSTER VIRUS

Although they are infrequently encountered, a pattern of fetal malformations may be associated with this virus. This pattern may include skin scarring, hypotrophic muscles, and eye changes. More typically, a neonate has the usual vesicular eruption of chickenpox in the neonatal period, the mother having displayed the same shortly before delivery. The postnatal appearance of the rash has important prognostic significance. If the rash in the mother appears within 4 days of delivery, there is high neonatal mortality. If the rash appears in the neonate in the first 4 days, the baby almost always does well, but if it appears within 5 to 10 days, the mortality is high. Varicella-zoster immune globulin in a dose of 1.25 ml is now available (but expensive) for high-risk cases.

HEPATITIS B

Although hepatitis caused by hepatitis B virus in the early neonatal period is unusual, a mother who is a carrier, who is hepatitis B surface antigen (HB$_s$-Ag) positive is not unusual. Although the rate is comparatively low in the United States, it is extremely common in Asian and African women. In these populations, a high percentage of neonates acquire hepatitis, which appears to be perinatally transmitted, which may later contribute to a very high incidence of hepatic carcinoma. Transmission seems to be greatest in infants born to HB$_s$-Ag- and HB$_e$-Ag-positive mothers. Several carefully controlled studies conducted in Taiwan and Senegal documented the efficacy of hepatitis B immune globulin and hepatitis B vaccine. Best results are achieved with a combination of these products.

It seems wise to administer hepatitis B immune globulin regardless of maternal e-antigen status because occasional cases of fulminant hepatitis can occur up to 3 months after birth. The dosage of hepatitis B immune globulin is 0.5 ml, to be given shortly after birth, with two additional doses given in the first year (e.g., 3 and 6 months) if vaccine is not given. Universal administration of hepatitis B vaccine is now recommended, but if used selectively, it should always be given in high-risk situations. It should be administered as early as possible. When vaccine is given within 7 days, it should be repeated at 1 and 6 months.

COXSACKIE B VIRUSES

This group occasionally presents a picture that is indistinguishable from herpes simplex infection (and hence others in the TORCH group), but more classically, an encephalitis-myocarditis syndrome is seen. These viruses have also been implicated as the cause of some cases of congenital heart disease.

OTHER ENTEROVIRUSES

The range of clinical manifestations may be enormous. Overwhelming infection resulting in death (with hemorrhage and hepatic necrosis as prominent features) has been reported with echovirus 19 (Fig. 15–6) and echovirus 11.

PARVOVIRUS B19

In 1983, human parvovirus B19 was shown to be the organism responsible for fifth disease (erythema infectiosum, characterized by the "slapped cheek" appearance). Shortly after this discovery, the virus was associated with fetal hydrops, occurring in association with severe anemia. However, prospective studies showed the fetus is affected relatively rarely when the virus is acquired during pregnancy.

Although correction of anemia with intrauterine transfusion may occasionally be needed, spontaneous resolution has also been reported. Parvovirus B19 has not been associated with specific teratogenesis.

RESPIRATORY SYNCYTIAL VIRUS

Although infection with respiratory syncytial virus in the immediate neonatal period is unusual, certain groups are more susceptible to the virus. These

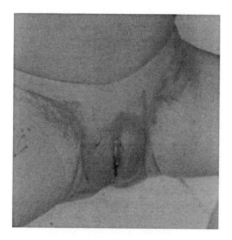

FIGURE 15–6. Petechiae and ecchymotic areas in both groins of this baby who had overwhelming infection with echovirus type 19.

groups include infants with bronchopulmonary dysplasia and those with complicated congenital heart disease. Therapy with ribavirin was strongly endorsed by the American Academy of Pediatrics Committee on Infectious Diseases, especially when infants require assisted ventilaton, but the need for and efficacy of ribavirin continues to be debated.

INFLUENZA VIRUS

Influenza virus has been linked to congenital malformations, especially neural tube defects.

MEASLES VIRUS

Measles virus is another virus that has been linked with fetal defects.

MUMPS VIRUS

Mumps virus is linked to endocardial fibroelastosis, but this association has not been proved. This virus has also been associated with perinatal infection, including pneumonia.

CANDIDA

Infection with the yeast-like organism *Candida albicans* is called monilial infection. It is more likely to occur after use of broad-spectrum antibiotics and in premature infants. Occasionally, a systemic (generalized) infection occurs, which seems to be more likely associated with central venous catheters (used for total parenteral nutrition). When this infection involves the mouth, it is called thrush and results in white plaques distributed on the buccal mucosa, tongue, gums, and even lips (Fig. 15–7). Involvement of skin in the diaper area produces a bright red, well-demarcated eruption. Treatment is with nystatin, orally for thrush and topically for skin involvement. When thrush is resistant to nystatin, gentian violet may be worth trying. Systemic infection may be responsive to 5-fluorocytosine and amphotericin B. Although miconazole was proposed as a useful alternative, it does not seem to be the drug of first choice.

CONGENITAL MALARIA

Parasitized erythrocytes may cross the placenta and cause malaria within weeks of birth, even in nonendemic areas (e.g., Canada).

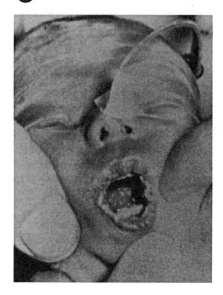

FIGURE 15-7. Thrush *(Monilia)* in the mouth of a small premature infant.

BIBLIOGRAPHY

Remington, J. S., and Klein, J. O.: *Infectious Disease of the Fetus and Newborn Infant*, 3rd ed. W. B. Saunders, Philadelphia, 1900.

Sepsis

Levy, H. L., Sepe, S. J., Shih, V. E., et al.: Sepsis due to *Escherichia coli* in neonates with galactosemia. *N. Engl. J. Med.* 1977, 297:823–825.
Miller, M. E.: Host defenses in the human neonate. *Pediatr. Clin. North Am.* 1977, 24:413.
Sabel, K. G., and Wadsworth, C.: C-reactive protein (CRP) in early diagnosis of neonatal septicemia. *Acta Paediatr.* 1979, 68:825–831.
Visser, V. E., and Hall, R. T.: Urine culture in the evaluation of suspected neonatal sepsis. *J. Pediatr.* 1979, 94:635–638.
Eriksson, M.: Neonatal septicemia. *Acta Paediatr.* 1983, 72:1–8.
Interview with Carol J. Baker, M. D.: Prevention of neonatal group B streptococcal disease. *Pediatr. Infect. Dis.* 1983, 2:1–5.
Klein, J. O., Dashefsky, B., Norton, E. R., and Mayer, J.: Selection of antimicrobial agents for treatment of neonatal sepsis. *Rev. Infect. Dis.* 1983, 5(Suppl):S55–S62.
Placzek, M. M., and Whitelaw, A.: Early and late neonatal septicemia. *Arch. Dis. Child.* 1983, 58:728–731.
Pyati, S. P., Pildes, R. S., Jacobs, N. M., et al.: Penicillin in infants weighing two kilograms or less with early-onset group B streptococcal disease. *N. Engl. J. Med.* 1983, 308:1383–1388.
Philip, A. G. S.: Acute phase proteins in neonatal infection. *J. Pediatr.* 1984, 105:940–942.
Philip, A. G. S.: *Neonatal Sepsis and Meningitis.* G. K. Hall Medical Publishers, Boston, 1985.
Wilson, C. B.: Immunologic basis for increased susceptibility of the neonate to infection. *J. Pediatr.* 1986, 108:1–12.
Hill, H. R.: Granulocyte transfusions in neonates. *Pediatr. Rev.* 1991, 12:298–302.
Baker, C. J., Mellish, M. E., Hall, R. T., et al.: Intravenous immune globulin for the prevention of nosocomial infection in low-birthweight neonates. *N. Engl. J. Med.* 1992, 327:213–219.

Rench, M. A., and Baker, C. J.: Neonatal sepsis caused by a new group B streptococcal serotype. *J. Pediatr.* 1993, 122:638–640.

Buck, C., Bundschu, J., Gallati, H., et al.: Interleukin-6: A sensitive parameter for the early diagnosis of neonatal bacterial infection. *Pediatrics* 1994, 93:54–58.

Fanaroff, A. A., Korones, S. B., Wright, L. L., et al.: A controlled trial of intravenous immune globulin to reduce nosocomial infections in very-low-birth-weight infants. *N. Engl. J. Med.* 1994, 330:1107–1113.

Philip, A. G. S., Tito, A. M., Gafeller, O., and Speer, C. P.: Neutrophil elastase in the diagnosis of neonatal infection. *Pediatr. Infect. Dis. J.* 1994, 13:323–326.

Philip, A. G. S.: The changing face of neonatal infection: Experience at a regional medical center. *Pediatr. Infect. Dis. J.* 1994, 13:1098–1102.

Meningitis

Visser, V. E., and Hall, R. T.: Lumbar puncture in the evaluation of suspected neonatal sepsis. *J. Pediatr.* 1980, 96:1063–1067.

Hill, A., Shackelford, G. D., and Volpe, J. J.: Ventriculitis with neonatal bacterial meningitis: Identification of real-time ultrasound. *J. Pediatr.* 1981, 99:133–136.

Fulginiti, V. A.: Treatment of meningitis in the very young infant (Editorial). *Am. J. Dis. Child.* 1983, 137:1043.

Barza, M.: Listeriosis and milk (Editorial). *N. Engl. J. Med.* 1985, 132:438–440.

Bortolussi, R.: Neonatal listeriosis: Where do we go from here? *Pediatr. Infect. Dis.* 1985, 4:228–229.

De Louvois, J., Blackbourn, J., Hurley, R., and Harvey, D.: Infantile meningitis in England and Wales: A two year study. *Arch. Dis. Child.* 1991, 66:603–607.

Franco, S. M., Cornelius, V. E., and Andrews, B. F.: Long-term outcome of neonatal meningitis. *Am. J. Dis. Child.* 1992, 146:567–571.

Perlman, J. M., Rollins, N., and Sanchez, P. J.: Late-onset meningitis in sick, very-low-birth-weight infants: Clinical and sonographic observations. *Am. J. Dis. Child.* 1992, 146:1297–1301.

Unhanand, M., Mustafa, M. M., McCracken, G. H., Jr., and Nelson, J. D.: Gram-negative enteric bacillary meningitis: A twenty-one year experience. *J. Pediatr.* 1993, 122:15–21.

Hristeva, L., Booy, R., Bowler, I., and Wilkinson, A. R.: Prospective surveillance of neonatal meningitis. *Arch. Dis. Child.* 1993, 69:14–18.

Haimi-Cohen, Y., Amir, J., Weinstock, A., and Varsano, I.: The use of imipenem-cilastatin in neonatal meningitis caused by *Citrobacter diversus. Acta Paediatr. Int. J. Paediatr.* 1993, 82:530–532.

Other Bacterial Infections

Gangarosa, E. J., and Merson, M. H.: Epidemiologic assessment of the relevance of the so-called enteropathogenic serogroups of *Escherichia coli* in diarrhea. *N. Engl. J. Med.* 1977, 296:1210.

Brill, P. W., Winchester, P., Krauss, A. N., and Symchych, P.: Osteomyelitis in a neonatal intensive care unit. *Radiology* 1979, 131:83.

Bell, M. J., Ternberg, J. L., and Bower, R. J.: The microbial flora and antimicrobial therapy of neonatal peritonitis. *J. Pediatr. Surg.* 1980, 15:569–573.

Philip, A. G. S.: Otitis media and facial palsy in a neonate. *Hosp. Pract.* 1980, 15:21–24.

Anders, B. J., Lauer, B. A., and Paisley, J. W.: *Campylobacter* gastroenteritis in neonates. *Am. J. Dis. Child.* 1981, 135:900–902.

Ginsburg, C. M., and McCracken, G. H., Jr.: Urinary tract infection in young infants. *Pediatrics* 1982, 69:409–412.

Welch, D. F., and Marks, M. I.: Is *Clostridium difficile* pathogenic in infants? *J. Pediatr.* 1982, 100:393–395.

DeSa, D. J.: Mucosal metaplasia and chronic inflammation in the middle ear of infants receiving intensive care in the neonatal period. *Arch. Dis. Child.* 1983, 58:24–28.

Teknetzi, P., Manios, S., and Katsouyanopoulos, V.: Neonatal tetanus: Long-term residual handicaps. *Arch. Dis. Child.* 1983, 58:68–69.

Sandstrom, K. I., Bell, T. A., Chandler, J. W., et al.: Microbial causes of neonatal conjunctivitis. *J. Pediatr.* 1984, 105:706–711.
Editorial: Ophthalmia neonatorum today. *Lancet* 1984, ii:1375–1376.
Galaska, A., and Cook, R.: Preventing neonatal tetanus: Failure of the possible. *Lancet* 1984, i:789–790.
Editorial: Epidemic pyelonephritis in babies? *Lancet* 1985, i:87.
Cushing, A. H.: Omphalitis: A review. *Pediatr. Infect. Dis.* 1985, 4:282–285.
Hammerschlag, M. R., Cummings, C., Roblin, P. M., et al: Efficacy of neonatal ocular prophylaxis for the prevention of chlamydial and gonococcal conjunctivitis. *N. Engl. J. Med.* 1989, 320:769–772.
Crain, E. F., and Gershel, J. C.: Urinary tract infections in febrile infants younger than 8 weeks of age. *Pediatrics* 1990, 86:363–367.
Williamson, J. B., Galasko, C. S. B., and Robinson, M. J.: Outcome after acute osteomyelitis in preterm infants. *Arch. Dis. Child.* 1990, 65:1060–1062.
Frederiksen, B., Christiansen, P., and Knudsen, F. U.: Acute osteomyelitis and septic arthritis in the neonate: Risk factors and outcome. *Eur. J. Pediatr.* 1993, 152:577–580.
Schaaf, H. S., Gie, R. P., Beyers, N., et al.: Tuberculosis in infants less than 3 months of age. *Arch. Dis. Child.* 1993, 69:371–374.
Cantwell, M. F., Shehab, Z. M., Costello, A. M., et al.: Brief report: Congenital tuberculosis. *N. Engl. J. Med.* 1994, 330:1051–1054.

The TORCH Syndrome

Nahmias, A. J.: The TORCH complex. *Hosp. Pract.* 1974, 9:65.
Ballard, R. A., Drew, W. L., Hufnagle, K. G., and Riedel, P. A.: Acquired cytomegalovirus infection in preterm infants. *Am. J. Dis. Child.* 1979, 133:482.
Andreasson, B., Svenningsen, N. W., and Nordenfelt, E.: Screening for viral infections in infants with poor intra-uterine growth. *Acta Paediatr.* 1981, 70:673–676.
Bambirra, E. A., Pittella, J. E. H., and Rezenda, M.: Toxoplasmosis and hydranencephaly. *N. Engl. J. Med.* 1982, 306:1112–1113.
Griffiths, P. D., Stagno, S., and Pass, R. F.: Congenital cytomegalovirus infection: Diagnostic and prognostic significance of the detection of specific immunoglobulin M antibodies in cord serum. *Pediatrics* 1982, 69:544–549.
Saigal, S., Lunyk, O., Larke, R. P. B., and Chernesky, M. A.: The outcome in children with congenital cytomegalovirus infection: A longitudinal follow-up study. *Am. J. Dis. Child.* 1982, 136:896–901.
Editorial: Congenital cytomegalovirus infection. *Lancet* 1983, i:801–802.
Leland, D., French, M. L. V., Kleiman, M. B., and Schreiner, R. L.: The use of TORCH titers. *Pediatrics* 1983, 72:41–43.
Sander, J., and Niehaus, C.: Screening for rubella IgG and IgM using an ELISA test applied to dried blood on filter paper. *J. Pediatr.* 1985, 106:457–461.
Desmonts, G., Daffos, F., Forestier, F., et al.: Prenatal diagnosis of congenital toxoplasmosis. *Lancet* 1985, i:500–504.
Sanchez, P. J., Wendel, G. D., and Norgard, M. V.: IgM antibody to *Treponema pallidum* in cerebrospinal fluid of infants with congenital syphilis. *Am. J. Dis. Child.* 1992, 146:1171–1175.
Lee, S. H., Ewert, D. P., Frederick, P. D., and Mascola, L.: Resurgence of congenital rubella syndrome in the 1990s: Report on missed opportunities and failed prevention policies among women of child bearing age. *J.A.M.A.* 1992, 267:2616–2620.
Guerina, N. G., Hsu, H-W, Meissner, H. C., et al.: Neonatal serologic screening and early treatment for congenital *Toxoplasma gondii* infection. *N. Engl. J. Med.* 1994, 330:1858–1863.
Evans, H. E., and Frenkel, L. D.: Congenital syphilis. *Clin. Perinatol.* 1994, 21:149–162.

Herpes Simplex

Kleiman, M. B., Schreiner, R. L., Eitzen, H., et al.: Oral herpes virus infection in nursery personnel: Infection control policy. *Pediatrics* 1982, 70:609–612.

Whitley, R. J., and Hutto, C.: Neonatal herpes simplex virus infections. *Pediatr. Rev.* 1985, 7:119–126.

Englund, J. A., Fletcher, C. V., and Balfour, H. H., Jr.: Acyclovir therapy in neonates. *J. Pediatr.* 1991, 119:129–135.

Whitley, R., Arvin, A., Prober, C., et al.: Predictors of morbidity and mortality in neonates with herpes simplex virus infections. *N. Engl. J. Med.* 1991, 324:450–454.

Acquired Immunodeficiency Syndrome

De Moraes-Pinto, M. I., Farhat, C. K., Carbonare, S. B., et al.: Maternally acquired immunity in newborns from women infected by the human immunodeficiency virus. *Acta Paediatr. Int. J. Paediatr.* 1993, 82:1034–1038.

Evans, H. E. (ed.): Perinatal AIDS. *Clin. Perinatol.* 1994, 21:1–204.

Connor, E. M., Sperling, R. S., Gelber, R., et al.: Reduction of maternal-infant transmission of human immunodeficiency virus type I with zidovudine treatment. *N. Engl. J. Med.* 1994, 331:1173–1180.

Other Viral Infections

Hanshaw, J. B., and Dudgeon, J. A.: *Viral Diseases of the Fetus and Newborn.* W. B. Saunders, Philadelphia, 1978.

Gear, J. H. S., and Measroch, V.: Coxsackie virus infections in the newborn. *Prog. Med. Virol.* 1973, 15:42.

Mackenzie, J. S., and Houghton, M.: Influenza infections during pregnancy: Association with congenital malformations and with subsequent neoplasms in children and potential hazards of live virus vaccines. *Bact. Rev.* 1974, 38:356.

Jespersen, C. S., Littaner, J., and Sagild, U.: Measles as a cause of fetal defects: A retrospective study of ten measles epidemics in Greenland. *Acta Paediatr.* 1977, 66:367.

Murphy, A. M., Albrey, M., and Crewe, E.: Rotavirus infections of neonates. *Lancet* 1977, ii:1149.

Jones, J. F., Ray, C. G., and Fulginiti, V. A.: Perinatal mumps infection. *J. Pediatr.* 1980, 96:912–914.

Modlin, J. F.: Fatal echovirus 11 disease in premature neonates. *Pediatrics* 1980, 66:775–780.

Editorial: Prevention of perinatally transmitted hepatitis B infection. *Lancet* 1984, i:939–941.

Isaacs, D., Dobson, S. R. M., Wilkinson, A. R., et al.: Conservative management of an echovirus 11 outbreak in a neonatal unit. *Lancet* 1989, i:543–545.

Lipton, S. V., and Brunell, P. A.: Management of varicella exposure in a neonatal intensive care unit. *J.A.M.A.* 1989, 261:1782–1784.

Humphrey, W., Magoon, M., and O'Shaughnessy, R.: Severe nonimmune hydrops secondary to parvovirus B-19 infection: Spontaneous reversal in utero and survival of a term infant. *Obstet. Gynecol.* 1991, 78:900–902.

Kumar, M. L.: Human parvovirus B19 and its associated diseases. *Clin. Perinatol.* 1991, 18:209–225.

Freed, G. L., Bordley, W. C., Clark, S. J., and Konrad, T. R.: Universal hepatitis B immunization of infants: Reactions of pediatricians and family physicians over time. *Pediatrics* 1994, 93:747–751.

Pastuszak, A. L., Levy, M., Schick, B., et al.: Outcome after maternal varicella infection in the first 20 weeks of pregnancy. *N. Engl. J. Med.* 1994, 330:901–905.

Wald, E. R., and Dashefsky, B.: Ribavirin: Red book committee recommendations questioned. *Pediatrics* 1994, 93:672–673.

Candida

Jennison, R. F.: Thrush in infancy. *Arch. Dis. Child.* 1977, 52:747.

Johnson, D. E., Thompson, T. R., Green, T. P., and Ferrieri, P.: Systemic candidiasis in very low-birth-weight infants (<1,500 g). *Pediatrics* 1984, 73:138–143.

Baley, J. E.: Neonatal candidiasis: The current challenge. *Clin. Perinatol.* 1991, 18:263–280.

Congenital Malaria

Davies, H. D., Kaystone, J., Lester, M. L., and Gold, R.: Congenital malaria in infants of asymptomatic women. *Can. Med. Assoc. J.* 1992, 146:1755–1756.

16
DISORDERED GROWTH

INFANTS OF DIABETIC MOTHERS

INTRODUCTION

Before the introduction of insulin, it was uncommon to have to deal with pregnancy in women with diabetes mellitus. However, many women with diabetes have delivered babies since insulin was introduced. In 1959, Dr. James Farquhar wrote the following delightful description:

> These infants are remarkable not only because like foetal versions of Shadrach, Meshach and Abednego, they emerge at least alive from within the fiery metabolic furnace of diabetes mellitus, but because they resemble one another so closely that they might well be related. They are plump, sleek, liberally coated with vernix caseosa, full-faced and plethoric. The umbilical cord and the placenta share in the gigantism. During their first 24 or more extrauterine hours they lie on their backs, bloated and flushed, their legs flexed and abducted, their lightly closed hands on each side of the head, the abdomen prominent and their respiration sighing. They convey a distinct impression of having had such a surfeit of both food and fluid pressed upon them by an insistent hostess that they desire only peace so that they may recover from their excesses. And on the second day their resentment of the slightest noise improves the analogy, while their trembling anxiety seems to speak of intrauterine indiscretions of which we know nothing.

PATHOPHYSIOLOGY

Although the subject of diabetes mellitus is not a simple one and some newer facts confuse and complicate the issue, some oversimplification seems justified. For all practical purposes, the main problem relates to elevated levels of blood glucose in the diabetic mother. There is normally a gradient of blood glucose from mother to fetus of about 75%. Because most diabetic mothers have hyperglycemic levels, relative hyperglycemia exists in the fetus. This condition results in stimulation of the fetal pancreas and accounts for the marked hypertrophy of the beta cells of the islets of Langerhans observed in infants of diabetic mothers (IDMs) who die. The increased output of insulin combined with the availability of glucose substrate results in accelerated growth rates (with macrosomia) and deposition of fat. This situation is most marked in infants born to mothers who are insulin dependent, and for obstetric reasons (e.g., higher stillbirth rate, cephalopelvic disproportion), delivery at 36 or 37 weeks gestation was frequently accomplished in these mothers. With tighter control of diabetes, delivery closer to term is now more usual. Some mothers demonstrate an abnormality of glucose tolerance only during pregnancy and are said to have gestational diabetes. The same problems as those seen in insulin-dependent diabetes are likely to be seen in gestational diabetes, but to a lesser extent. By careful dietary regulation, the tendency to macrosomia can be decreased, with delivery occurring at or close to term.

Diabetes mellitus in the mother is usually subdivided according to the classification of White:

Group A	Abnormal glucose tolerance test results only (chemical diabetes)
Group B	Onset after age 20, duration less than 10 years
Group C	Onset ages 10 to 19, duration 10 to 19 years
Group D	Onset before age 10, or duration 20 years or more; vascular disease in legs; retinal changes or fundoscopic change
Group E	Same as D, with pelvic arteriosclerosis
Group F	Kidney involvement
Group R	Active retinitis proliferans

In some cases of diabetes, intrauterine growth retardation (IUGR) may occur, which has usually been associated with the more severe grades of diabetes and is presumably secondary to vascular problems. However, in some cases, it may occur very early in pregnancy. Another interesting clinical association is that diabetic women whose glucose levels are poorly controlled around the time of conception may have a higher incidence of infants with congenital abnormalities. These malformations seem to be related to increased amounts of glycosalated hemoglobins (particularly HbA_{1c}) and may be decreased by tight glucose control in the periconceptional period.

It has been reported that macrosomia correlates with the amount of animal insulin found in cord serum and that increased amounts of animal insulin are transferred when large amounts of insulin antibody are found in the mother. Transfer of insulin takes place as an insulin-antibody complex. This does not seem to be a problem with recombinant human insulin.

DIAGNOSIS AND CLINICAL COURSE

The classic IDM, as described by Dr. Farquhar, resembles other babies who are IDM so closely that there is usually no doubt about the diagnosis (Fig. 16–1). Because of their increased intrauterine growth, they are frequently very large for gestational age. For the uninitiated, such increase in size can lead to the false assumption that a baby born prematurely is at term. Convincing evidence now exists to corroborate the long-held opinion that IDMs may behave in a less mature way at a given gestational age, at least as far as pulmonary function is concerned (resulting in a higher frequency of respiratory distress syndrome).

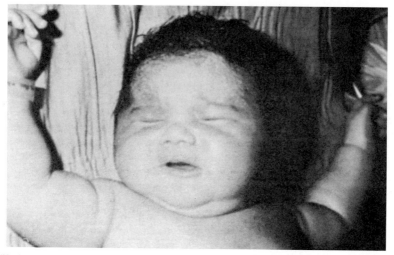

FIGURE 16–1. Typical features of the infant of a diabetic mother, showing the "tomato-face" and ". . . lightly closed hands on either side of the face . . . ."

This condition seems to be the result of fetal hypersecretion of insulin, blocking the enzyme-inductive capability of cortisol in the lung.

The neonatal problems likely to be encountered in IDMs are as follows:

1. Hypoglycemia secondary to hyperinsulinemia (see previous discussion)
2. Respiratory distress syndrome (see previous discussion)
3. Hypocalcemia
4. Hyperbilirubinemia
5. Hypertrophic cardiomyopathy
6. Congenital abnormalities
7. Renal vein thrombosis

The first four problems are discussed in other sections. Hypertrophic cardiomyopathy is important because using digoxin may be deleterious with this problem. It appears to be a benign disorder that resolves spontaneously, but propranolol may be needed. The incidence and type of congenital abnormalities has varied in different series of IDMs. In Boston, congenital heart disease is prominent; in Copenhagen, neural tube or osseous defects predominate; and in Edinburgh, there was no statistically significant difference in the incidence of defects compared with the non-diabetic population. Another unusual abnormality is the small left colon syndrome. There does seem to have been some decrease in the number of abnormalities as a result of good control of maternal diabetes. Renal vein thrombosis has been reported to be a problem that occurs with markedly increased frequency in IDMs when compared with other infants. With present management, it is rarely encountered.

MANAGEMENT

Infants born to insulin-dependent mothers and those of gestational diabetics who look like IDMs should be cared for in a special care nursery. It seems wise to replace the constant infusion of glucose via the placenta with an extrauterine infusion of glucose to prevent the rapid development of hypoglycemia, although the evidence showing that low levels of glucose in IDMs cause long-term sequelae is far from conclusive. This infusion is usually given by the intravenous route, but in the very obese baby, finding a vein may be difficult. Under such circumstances, we frequently elect to use an umbilical artery catheter until feeding is established.

Because of the frequency of respiratory difficulty and the tendency of IDMs to vomit on the first day, oral feedings are usually deferred for 12 to 24 hours.

Measurement of blood glucose using a test strip (see p. 36) seems particularly valuable for detecting hypoglycemia and may be performed on a drop of blood obtained from a warmed heel stick. Hourly determinations for the first 4 to 6 hours, followed by determinations at 4-hour intervals, are usually performed. If an infusion has not been started, some people prefer to use glucagon to treat hypoglycemia. It seems easier to anticipate hypoglycemia and begin a glucose infusion before it occurs. If low blood glucose level occurs despite 10% dextrose infusion, it may be necessary to give a 15% solution or to resort (in refractory cases) to corticosteroids. Subsequent intellectual impairment has been described in some IDMs but does not seem to be the result of hypoglycemia.

After oral feeding is begun, the glucose solution by infusion should be gradually decreased or changed to 5% to prevent reactive hypoglycemia. This change usually occurs at 24 hours and is discontinued at 48 hours of age.

Treatment of the respiratory distress syndrome in IDMs differs little from that in other babies (see Chapter 9). Hypocalcemia may be corrected if necessary with calcium gluconate, and hyperbilirubinemia may be controlled with phototherapy in most instances. Conservative management is usually employed in the rare cases of renal vein thrombosis.

Some babies appear to lose a lot of weight, but if on calculation this loss does not exceed 10% of birth weight, it can probably be accepted as being within normal limits. In other words, the absolute weight loss (e.g., 400 g) may be unremarkable when the baby's birth weight is also very high (e.g., $\geq$ 4.5 kg, which is not an unusual birth weight for an IDM).

SUMMARY

The typical IDM may be seen less frequently now and in the future, thanks to tighter control of the glucose level in the mother. However, it is still common to see infants of insulin-dependent diabetic mothers who are large for gestational age as a result of macrosomia (presumably secondary to increased endogenous insulin production). Neonatal management is primarily concerned with (1) prevention and treatment of hypoglycemia, and (2) treatment of the respiratory distress syndrome. These babies require special care nursing, as may infants born to mothers with gestational diabetes.

INTRAUTERINE GROWTH RETARDATION

INTRODUCTION AND INCIDENCE

The designation IUGR describes a problem more than a specific diagnosis because this is a very heterogeneous group of babies. The topic is discussed more or less as a single entity because a uniform approach is required and management is likely to be similar, regardless of cause.

A large number of terms have been used synonymously with IUGR and may or may not prove superior or more popular. The reader may choose from the following: small for gestational age (SGA), small for date, light for date, dysmature, fetal malnutrition (undernutrition), placental insufficiency syndrome, runting syndrome, and fetal growth retardation.

Approximately one quarter to one third of all infants of low birth weight (< 2500 g) have been considered to fall into this category of IUGR. It is generally agreed that all babies falling below the 10th percentile are SGA, but some who fall above may also represent IUGR. Such babies usually appear scrawny.

ETIOLOGY AND PATHOPHYSIOLOGY

The factors associated with growth are multiple, and it is not always possible to determine which of several factors produced an effect in a particular pregnancy. Genetic and chromosomal factors obviously play a part. If both parents are of short stature it is likely that a small baby will result from their union. Prepregnancy (preconceptional) weight may be as important as weight gain during pregnancy in determining fetal weight. It seems clear that women whose preconceptional weight is less than 50kg (110 pounds) and/or whose height is below 153 cm (60 inches) are more likely to have infants whose birth weight is below the 10th percentile.

These factors are likely to exert an effect throughout pregnancy and may be classified as producing chronic IUGR. When the influence of a factor is felt only in the last weeks of pregnancy (e.g., infarction of a large portion of the placenta, acute maternal cardiopulmonary insufficiency), the resultant IUGR may be considered acute. Such a concept may have an important bearing on the approach to the baby. Chronic IUGR has been considered to result in a decrease in cell number, whereas acute IUGR was thought likely to produce a decrease in cell size. These concepts have been questioned, and it seems probable that both cell number and cell size can be affected, either by chronic or acute insults. In addition, mixed patterns may exist, with acute, chronic, or subacute forms. Perhaps the simplest way of approaching the etiology of IUGR is that anything that compromises nutrition or oxygenation is likely to produce IUGR. Using this basic premise, the causes of IUGR may be divided into three basic groups: (1) maternal, (2) placental, and (3) fetal (Table 16–1).

TABLE 16–1. CONDITIONS CONTRIBUTING TO IUGR

Maternal	Placental
Small stature	Poor implantation site
<50 kg/<153 cm	Infarction
Under nutrition or	Structural abnormality
malnutrition	Functional abnormality
Hypoxia	
High altitude	Fetal
Cardiac disease	Chromosomal abnormality
Pulmonary disease	Trisomy 18
Anemia	Other
Vascular compromise	Genetic (hereditary)
Stressful life events	Chronic infection
Toxemia	TORCH syndrome
Essential hypertension	Twinning
Renal disease	Single umbilical artery
Diabetes, groups D–F	Congenital abnormalities
Heavy smoking	Cardiac
Drug ingestion	Renal
including alcohol	Other

TORCH = toxoplasmosis, other, rubella, cytomegalovirus, and herpes simplex.

DIAGNOSIS AND PROBLEMS

The diagnosis may be suspected by the obstetrician before delivery on the basis of decreased uterine growth and ultrasonography. Unless a reasonably accurate assessment of gestational age is available, it is difficult to clinically diagnose infants who have chronic IUGR because the degree of involvement of different organ systems may be relatively equal. Improved techniques, using femur length, abdominal circumference, and total intrauterine volume, have increased the accuracy of assessment (see Chapter 1). Clinical evaluation (via the Dubowitz score, and so on) is usually sufficiently accurate to make a firm statement that a baby is definitely IUGR or SGA. Frequently, one has to modify such a statement to borderline IUGR if the weight for gestational age is close to the 10th percentile.

In infants with subacute IUGR, discrepancies in the body measurements are more likely than in those with chronic IUGR so that head circumference appears disproportionately large. When head circumference is plotted against gestational age, it may be found to be the only normal measurement or it may be below the mean. This is sometimes referred to as the brain-sparing effect. Such infants will appear scrawny if they are close to normal length. The baby who is wasted will have a decreased ponderal index* (weight to length ratio), but this finding does not always indicate that the insult to growth has been of short duration. The author has found that babies with a low ponderal index were lighter than those with a normal ponderal index and had a greater decrease in ossification.

---

*Ponderal index $= \dfrac{\text{weight (g)} \times 100}{\text{length (cm)}^3}$.

Although the Dubowitz score is helpful, gestational age may, if anything, be underestimated in term infants because of three specific physical findings: (1) soft ear cartilage, (2) absence of breast tissue, and (3) lack of subcutaneous fat, making small blood vessels more readily visible.

These findings may alter the score by 4 or 5 points and decrease the assessed gestational age by 1 to 1½ weeks. However, a compensatory increase frequently occurs in neurologic maturation (see figures and discussion, Chapter 6).

The following problems are likely to be encountered in babies with IUGR.

FETAL DISTRESS AND NEONATAL ASPHYXIA. These conditions occur (with or without meconium aspiration) as a result of the increased likelihood of hypoxia as labor progresses if the placenta is insufficient to meet the demands.

HYPOGLYCEMIA. This condition presents as a result of minimal reserves of both liver glycogen and fat (white and brown).

TEMPERATURE INSTABILITY. This instability is primarily hypothermia, because of decreased subcutaneous fat (i.e., lack of insulation), increased surface area to body weight ratio, and lack of brown adipose tissue to respond to cold stress.

HYPOCALCEMIA. This condition is known to occur in infants with IUGR with increased frequency only when it is preceded by asphyxia, and it appears to be the result of transient hypoparathyroidism.

HIGH HEMATOCRIT SYNDROME (HYPERVISCOSITY). This condition is probably the result of two factors: (1) a response to chronic intrauterine hypoxia and (2) the relatively high red cell volume. The latter may be explained in an oversimplified way: relative blood volume is increased, whereas absolute blood volume is decreased.

In a 3-kg baby, the blood volume is approximately 80 ml/kg or 240 ml, and if the hematocrit value is 50%, the red cell volume is 120 ml.

In a 2-kg IUGR baby, blood volume is approximately 100 ml/kg or 200 ml, and to accommodate 120 ml of red cells, the hematocrit value would have to be 60%.

NECROTIZING ENTEROCOLITIS. This condition seems to be directly related to hyperviscosity, resulting in decreased mesenteric blood flow and ischemia.

PULMONARY HEMORRHAGE. This condition is infrequently encountered but may be secondary to intrauterine or neonatal asphyxia (or hypothermia).

HYPERGLYCEMIA. This condition is sometimes seen as a baby with hypoglycemia is being treated with a glucose infusion, and it is sometimes seen in the rare syndrome of transient diabetes mellitus of the newborn.

INCREASED NUCLEATED RED BLOOD CELLS. The response to chronic intrauterine hypoxia may not always result in a high hematocrit value, but may be associated with increased numbers of immature (nucleated) red blood cells (erythroblasts), especially in very-low-birth-weight infants. This phenomenon may be accompanied by a decrease in platelet or neutrophil counts, as the pluripotent stem cell is selectively directed toward the erythroid cells.

In contrast to these problems, infants with IUGR rarely develop the respiratory distress syndrome (unless they are very premature as well) or develop significant jaundice (except with the TORCH complex of infection). On the other hand, behavior may be altered on the Brazelton evaluation (see p. 30), which may result in parental anxiety.

One other abnormality may be encountered in IUGR that may give rise to confusion: decreased ossification of both membranous and enchondral bone. The observed abnormalities are a markedly enlarged anterior fontanel of the skull and decreased epiphyseal ossification at the knee. The latter observation makes radiologic confirmation of maturity of little value because absence of epiphyseal ossification does not exclude a baby born at term. (However, the presence of epiphyseal ossification at the knee could confirm a term birth.)

MANAGEMENT AND PROGNOSIS

Problems in the delivery room may be anticipated and appropriate resuscitation provided, particularly to prevent meconium aspiration syndrome. Whenever a baby who appears to be SGA is admitted to the nursery, a clinical estimate of gestational age should be performed. If the baby is confirmed as being SGA, then the neonatal examination should be directed toward a search for clinically apparent causes. These are: (1) chromosomal abnormalities, (2) other congenital abnormalities, and (3) chronic intrauterine infection (TORCH complex).

Whenever the IUGR is more than borderline, a glucose infusion should be started to prevent hypoglycemia, and blood glucose estimations should be made with a test strip on an hourly basis for the first few hours. Early oral feeding (4 to 6 hours of age) may be started if the baby is having no apparent difficulties. The amount of feeding taken may need to be quite large on a per-kilogram basis, especially if the head circumference is normal. In other words, calculation may need to be based on what the weight should have been, rather than on what it is. If asphyxia occurred at delivery, hypocalcemia should be looked for. A hematocrit determination is always in order, and if increased numbers of nucleated red blood cells are found, thrombocytopenia and neutropenia may be anticipated. It seems sound to determine the immunoglobulin M level as a screen for chronic intrauterine infection. Although not always elevated with such infection, a greatly elevated IgM level (> 30 mg/dl) should lead to further investigation with viral cultures, and so on.

The follow-up of babies born SGA has shown both physical and intellectual retardation based on the management provided in the 1960s. More recent results suggest a more optimistic outlook, particularly if adequate nutrition and appropriate stimulation are provided during the first month of life. Great variability undoubtedly exists in subsequent growth, but considerable catch-up growth is possible in some infants with IUGR. Almost invariably, this catching up is in the group with acute or subacute growth retardation. In one long-term follow-up study, the ability to catch up seemed to be limited to those who displayed late-onset IUGR as determined by serial ultrasound studies. Those displaying early and chronic IUGR (the low profile on sequential ultrasound) failed to achieve normal stature.

SUMMARY

Infants with IUGR comprise a very heterogeneous group. Depending on the duration of effect of various causal agents, chronic or acute IUGR may be produced. A reduction in cell number, or cell size, or both, may occur. Careful gestational age assessment is important in diagnosis. The major problems are fetal and neonatal asphyxia, hypoglycemia, and high hematocrit (hyperviscosity) syndrome. A search for congenital abnormalities and chronic intrauterine infection, followed by careful observation and glucose infusion, provide the essentials of management. Prognosis in many cases (without congenital abnormalities) may be more optimistic than was formerly thought.

BIBLIOGRAPHY

Infants of Diabetic Mothers

Farquhar, J. W.: The child of the diabetic woman. *Arch. Dis. Child.* 1959, 34:76.

Farquhar, J. W.: The infant of the diabetic mother. *Clin. Endocrinol. Metab.* 1976, 5:237.

North, A. F., Jr., Mazumdar, S., and Logrillo, V. M.: Birth weight, gestational age, and perinatal deaths in 5,471 infants of diabetic mothers. *J. Pediatr.* 1977, 90:444.

Halliday, H. L.: Hypertrophic cardiomyopathy in infants of poorly-controlled diabetic mothers. *Arch. Dis. Child.* 1981, 56:258–263.

Cowett, R. M., and Schwartz, R.: The infant of the diabetic mother. *Pediatr. Clin. North Am.* 1982, 29:1213–1231.

Pedersen, J. F., and Pedersen, L. M.: Early growth delay predisposes the fetus in diabetic pregnancy to congenital malformation. *Lancet* 1982, i:737.

Cowett, R. M., Susa, J. B., Giletti, B., et al.: Glucose kinetics in infants of diabetic mothers. *Am. J. Obstet. Gynecol.* 1983, 146:781–786.

Neave, C.: Congenital malformation in offspring of diabetics. *Perspect. Pediatr. Pathol.* 1984, 8:213–222.

Morriss, F. H., Jr.: Infants of diabetic mothers: Fetal and neonatal pathophysiology. *Perspect. Pediatr. Pathol.* 1984, 8:223–234.

Menon, R. K., Cohen, R. M., Sperling, M. A., et al.: Transplacental passage of insulin in pregnant women with insulin-dependent diabetes mellitus: Its role in fetal macrosomia. *N. Engl. J. Med.* 1990, 323:309–315.

Becerra, J. E., Khoury, M. J., Cordero, J. F., and Erickson, J. D.: Diabetes mellitus during pregnancy and the risks for specific birth defects: A population-based case-control study. *Pediatrics* 1990, 85:1–9.

Kitzmiller, J. L., Gavin, L. A., Gin, G. D., et al.: Preconception care of diabetes: Glycemic control prevent congenital anomalies. *J.A.M.A.* 1991, 265:731–736.

Jovanovic-Peterson, L., Kitzmiller, J. L., and Peterson, C. M.: Randomized trial of human versus animal species insulin in diabetic pregnant women: Improved glycemic control, not fewer antibodies to insulin, influences birth weight. *Am. J. Obstet. Gynecol.* 1992, 167:1325–1330.

Ballard, J. L., Rosenn, B., Khoury, J. C., and Miodovnik, M.: Diabetic fetal macrosomia: Significance of disproportionate growth. *J. Pediatr.* 1993, 122:115–119.

Piper, J. M., and Langer, O.: Does maternal diabetes delay fetal pulmonary maturity? *Am. J. Obstet. Gynecol.* 1993, 168:783–786.

Landon, M. B. (ed.): Diabetes in pregnancy. *Clin. Perinatol.* 1993, 20:507–667.

Intrauterine Growth Retardation

Warkany, J., Monroe, B. B., and Sutherland, B. S.: Intrauterine growth retardation. *Am. J. Dis. Child.* 1961, 102:249.

Ounsted, M., and Ounsted, C.: On fetal growth rate. *Clin. Dev. Med.* 46, S.I.M.P., J. B. Lippincott, Philadelphia, 1973.

Size at Birth. Ciba Foundation Symposium 27 (new series). Associated Scientific Publishers, Amsterdam, 1974.

Philip, A. G. S.: Fetal growth retardation: Femurs, fontanels and follow-up. *Pediatrics* 1978, 62:446.

Redmond, G. P.: Effect of drugs on intrauterine growth. *Clin. Perinatol.* 1979, 6:5.

Sands, J., Dobbing, J., and Gratrix, C.: Cell number and cell size: Organ growth and development and the control of catch-up growth in rats. *Lancet* 1979, ii:503.

Miller, H. C.: Intrauterine growth retardation: An unmet challenge. *Am. J. Dis. Child.* 1981, 135:944–948.

Sly, P. D., and Drew, J. H.: Massive pulmonary hemorrhage: A cause of sudden unexpected deaths in severely growth retarded infants. *Aust. Paediatr. J.* 1981, 17:32–34.

Walter, F. J., and Ramaerkers, L. H. J.: Neonatal morbidity of SGA infants in relation to their nutritional status at birth. *Acta Paediatr.* 1982, 71:437–440.

Westwood, M., Kramer, M. S., Munz, D., et al.: Growth and development of full-term non-asphyxiated small-for-gestational age newborns: Follow-up through adolescence. *Pediatrics* 1983, 71:376–382.

Briend, A.: Do maternal energy reserves limit fetal growth? *Lancet* 1985, i:38–40.

Warshaw, J. B.: Intra-uterine growth retardation. *Pediatr. Rev.* 1986, 8:107–114.

Philip, A. G. S., and Tito, A. M.: Increased nucleated red blood cell counts in small for gestational age infants with very low birth weight. *Am. J. Dis. Child.* 1989, 143:164–169.

Bakketeig, L. S., Jacobsen, G., Hoffman, H. J., et al.: Pre-pregnancy risk factors of small-for-gestational age births among parous women in Scandinavia. *Acta Obstet. Gynecol. Scand.* 1993, 72:273–279.

Hawdon, J. M., and Ward-Platt, M. P.: Metabolic adaptation in small for gestational age infants. *Arch. Dis. Child.* 1993, 68:262–268.

Snijders, R. J. M., Sherrod, C., Gosden, C. M., and Nicolaides, K. H.: Fetal growth retardation: Associated malformations and chromosomal abnormalities. *Am. J. Obstet. Gynecol.* 1993, 168:547–555.

Sung, I-K., Vohr, B., and Oh, W.: Growth and neurodevelopmental outcome of very low birth weight infants with intra-uterine growth retardation. *J. Pediatr.* 1993, 123:618–624.

17
METABOLIC DISORDERS

HYPOGLYCEMIA

INTRODUCTION

Low levels of blood glucose are found in a considerable number of babies when looked for in a routine (or screening) manner. However, the number of babies who present with specific symptoms relating to low levels of blood glucose is relatively small. The incidence therefore is not well established for different populations. The question of what dangers are inherent in allowing a baby to remain hypoglycemic are not yet completely answered, because it is quite possible that many infants with hypoglycemia go undetected and may have no subsequent abnormality. There is *some* evidence (pathologically) to suggest that hypoglycemia by itself may produce specific changes in the brain. This is in contrast to pure "metabolic" hypocalcemia, in which the evidence supports the view (with clinical and electroencephalographic support) that no permanent damage ensues, even in the face of frank convulsions.

There is continued debate about what constitutes significant hypoglycemia, and currently no definition exists on which clinicians agree. Evidence has been presented that suggests that glucose levels that are persistently below 45 mg/dl (2.5 mmol/L) may impair neurodevelopmental outcome. Most clinicians would agree that glucose levels less than 25 mg/dl (1.4 mmol/L) should be treated with parenteral (intravenous or intraarterial) glucose. Although glucose levels that are low for brief periods may not be harmful, it seems reasonable (especially in a symptomatic infant) to correct, or adjust, the level toward normal.

ETIOLOGY

There are probably five main categories of infants who develop hypoglycemia:

1. The truly immature infant
2. The dysmature or small-for-date infant
3. The infant of a diabetic mother
4. The infant with brain damage
5. The infant with sepsis or meningitis

In the first two categories, liver glycogen is usually deficient although hyperinsulinemia may also be present; in the third, hyperinsulinemia is present; and central mechanisms are implicated in the fourth. With sepsis, it is not clear what the mechanism is, but increased glucose utilization is well documented. Hyperinsulinism is not present, and a hypermetabolic state is unlikely (because fever is unusual).

In the first three categories, specific symptoms should be looked for, and in the fourth, a combination of metabolic problems may give a clue to the underlying problem (e.g., when hypoglycemia and hypocalcemia coexist). Sepsis is discussed in Chapter 15. Hypoglycemia has also been encountered in severe cases of erythroblastosis fetalis, apparently because of hyperinsulinemia, and is rarely the result of an insulin-secreting pancreatic tumor (nesidioblastoma). It may also accompany neonatal cold injury, when glycogen stores are depleted.

DIAGNOSIS

Certain symptoms and signs of hypoglycemia are better known than others, and several (if not all) tend to overlap with the manifestations of other disorders. They are (1) irritability, manifested by jitteriness or tremulousness, eye rolling, and convulsions; (2) cyanosis and apneic episodes; (3) listlessness (apathy) and poor feeding; (4) hypothermia; and (5) hypotonia. In addition, hypoglycemia may produce cardiomegaly.

Although test strips (Dextrostix and Chemstrip) are frequently used, their reliability has been questioned. Confirmation of abnormal values is needed, using laboratory determinations.

MANAGEMENT

It is probably wise to try to prevent hypoglycemia, and many infants in the at-risk group are treated by use of parenteral fluids (usually intravenous 10% dextrose). This should always be used if test strip levels are below 25 mg/dl. The best method is to give a bolus of 2 ml/kg of 10% dextrose, followed by a constant infusion of glucose to provide 8 mg/kg/min. In some cases, it may be necessary to use up to 12 mg/kg/min. Glucagon has also been recommended for emergency treatment in the infant of a diabetic mother. The oral route (gavage feeding) has been used for early feedings in some centers to prevent hypoglycemia in small babies, and bottle feeding may be well tolerated in the more mature infant. Early feeding is appropriate if test strip glucose levels fall to 25 to 45 mg/dl. Occasionally, a refractory case of hypoglycemia requires corticosteroid therapy.

SUMMARY

With modern neonatal intensive care, hypoglycemia is anticipated in small-for-gestational-age babies, very premature babies, and infants of diabetic mothers, and it is now rarely seen with the use of early parenteral or oral feeding. Clinical manifestations range from jitteriness and convulsions to poor feeding, hypotonia, and apneic episodes. Screening with glucose test strips can be very useful, but their reliability is questioned. Evaluation of the long-term effects of hypoglycemia is complicated by other problems associated with babies who are at greatest risk.

HYPERGLYCEMIA

Although not as common as hypoglycemia, hyperglycemia is being seen with increasing frequency as a result of the aggressive management and improved survival of very-low-birth-weight infants (< 1500 g, and particularly < 1000 g). Hyperglycemia may produce glycosuria, which may result in an osmotic diuresis if the amount of glucose is large. The small-for-gestational-age baby (or the smaller of discordant twins) may also have difficulty handling glucose when treated for hypoglycemia. In extreme cases, this problem manifests itself as transient diabetes mellitus of the newborn. This condition may last for a variable length of time but usually requires insulin therapy (the dose is usually 0.01 to 0.1 U/kg/hr). Although uncommon, hyperglycemia may also be seen with sepsis (see Chapter 15).

Part of the problem with very-low-birth-weight infants is their increased fluid requirement. It is therefore important to calculate the rate of glucose infusion and to modify the concentration of glucose accordingly. Most babies tolerate 6 mg of glucose/kg/min, and some tolerate more.

HYPOCALCEMIA

INTRODUCTION

The easiest way to approach hypocalcemia is to take the at-risk groups for hypoglycemia and their clinical manifestations and say, "anything hypoglycemia can do, hypocalcemia can do better." There appears to be one further refinement, namely, differentiation into early and late hypocalcemia.

ETIOLOGY

Early hypocalcemia, seen in the first 2 days, has been observed in (1) very premature infants (immature), (2) small-for-gestational-age infants who have suffered asphyxia at birth, (3) infants of diabetic mothers, (4) infants with brain damage, (5) infants whose mothers had hypercalcemia (as a result of hyperparathyroidism), and (6) after exchange transfusion.

The work of Tsang and his coworkers (1976) has demonstrated a common cause: transient hypoparathyroidism. Because of responsiveness to exogenous parathormone, end-organ (kidney) unresponsiveness seems to be largely eliminated. Late hypocalcemia occurs at approximately 5 to 7 days of age and seems to be the result of accumulation of phosphate, either as a result of too great a phosphate load (relative to calcium) in the milk or inability of the kidney to excrete phosphate satisfactorily.

DIAGNOSIS

The clinical manifestations of hypocalcemia are outlined under hypoglycemia. One other feature is occasionally present if hypocalcemia remains uncorrected. This is a conduction defect in the heart (which may produce a 2:1 heart block). A fairly rapid means of detection is to measure the Q_oT_c interval on the electrocardiograph. This calculation correlates reasonably well with serum calcium levels and is derived from the following formula:

$$Q_oT_c = \frac{Q - {}_oT}{\sqrt{R - R}}$$

where ${}_oT$ = origin of the T wave and $R - R$ = interval between successive R waves. Levels above 0.2 (sec) are considered abnormal. In the sick preterm infant, the correlation of Q_oT_c with calcium levels may not be reliable.

Although one is most interested in the ionized calcium, many laboratories perform only total calcium level determinations. Total calcium levels below 8 mg/dl on the first day and subsequently below 7 mg/dl are generally regarded as abnormal. Fetal serum calcium levels are usually somewhat higher than maternal levels. Reliable measurements of ionized calcium are now available and will probably be used increasingly.

MANAGEMENT

Although it is unlikely that any permanent sequelae result from hypocalcemia that is metabolic in origin, it seems sensible to maintain the calcium level above 7 mg/dl. Prevention has been achieved by giving oral calcium supplements every 6 hours between 12 and 72 hours (dosage, 75 mg/kg/day) to infants at risk. Immediate treatment can be given with a SLOW infusion (no faster than 1 ml/min) of 100 to 200 mg/kg of 10% calcium gluconate. This needs to be followed either by further increments (100 to 200 mg/kg) at intervals (6 to 8 hours) or the same dosage given continuously by intravenous (or intraarterial) infusion (i.e., approximately 400 mg/kg/day). Care should be taken to ensure that sodium bicarbonate is not in the infusion fluid, because the addition of calcium gluconate will result in a deposit of calcium carbonate. If the calcium is given too quickly, bradycardia may result. When "normal" levels have been restored and feedings are being taken by mouth, further calcium may be administered for a few days by the oral route. Protracted hypocalcemia may be responsive to $1\alpha,25$-dihydroxyvitamin D.

SUMMARY

Hypocalcemia may be early or late in onset, the former being the result of transient hypoparathyroidism, the latter owing to phosphate retention. Clinical features are similar to those seen with hypoglycemia, ranging from jitteriness to lethargy. Diagnosis may be quicker by using the Q_oT_c interval on electrocardiography.

HYPERCALCEMIA

Idiopathic hypercalcemia has been described primarily in Britain. There are two types—mild and severe. The severe type can present in the neonatal period with intrauterine growth retardation, characteristic (elfin) facies, vomiting, and constipation. It has been associated with elevated plasma $1\alpha,25$-dihydroxyvitamin D levels. Cardiac murmurs may be associated with supravalvular aortic (and/or pulmonary) stenosis. Another form of hypercalcemia has been described in extremely low-birth-weight infants in association with low phosphate levels.

Treatment is primarily to eliminate vitamin D supplements and reduce calcium intake, but additional phosphate may be needed in extremely low-birth-weight infants. Steroid therapy to reduce calcium absorption or furosemide therapy to increase calcium excretion is rarely needed.

METABOLIC ACIDOSIS

INTRODUCTION

Any derangement in the delivery of oxygen to tissues for glucose metabolism is likely to result in the excessive production of lactic acid. This condition contributes to an increase in hydrogen ions, resulting in acidosis. In turn, metabolic acidosis may have far-reaching effects, most notably decreasing blood flow in the pulmonary vasculature as well as the skin, kidney, and gastrointestinal tract.

ETIOLOGY

A large number of disorders may produce metabolic acidosis as an end result, and one of the most important precipitating factors is cooling (see Chapter 5).

Knowledge of the more commonly associated disorders allows one to search for metabolic acidosis when such disorders occur or are suspected. These disorders include

1. Fetal distress and neonatal asphyxia
2. Hypovolemia and shock
3. Neonatal sepsis

4. Intracranial hemorrhage
5. Necrotizing enterocolitis
6. Renal abnormalities (tubular acidosis)
7. Various pulmonary disorders (e.g., respiratory distress syndrome) that result in low paO$_2$ (they may also depress the renal threshold for bicarbonate)
8. Inborn errors of metabolism (especially organic acid disorders)

There is also a form of metabolic acidosis that occurs late in premature infants and is related to protein intake.

DIAGNOSIS

The infant who requires prolonged resuscitation in the delivery room almost invariably has associated metabolic acidosis. The most striking feature seen throughout the neonatal period is pallor caused by intense vasoconstriction of the peripheral circulation. This tends to compound the problem of metabolic acidosis by delivering less oxygen to the tissues, creating a vicious cycle. A term newborn who has adequate pulmonary function can quickly compensate by blowing off carbon dioxide to bring the pH back toward normal. In so doing, tachypnea is usually observed.

Confirmation of metabolic acidosis is obtained by measuring blood gases and pH. The paO$_2$ is usually somewhat low, and the pCO$_2$ is either low-normal in uncompensated metabolic acidosis (with a low pH) or low in compensated metabolic acidosis (with pH in the normal range). With combined respiratory and metabolic acidosis (e.g., in respiratory distress syndrome), the pCO$_2$ may be elevated. Base deficit may be calculated from the Siggaard–Andersen nomogram when the values for pH and pCO$_2$ are known (see Appendix 4).

In a term infant who develops profound metabolic acidosis, especially in association with hypoglycemia and without predisposing illness, the diagnosis of an inborn error of metabolism should be considered.

MANAGEMENT

Any baby who has tachypnea and appears pale should be considered to have metabolic acidosis, if anemia has been excluded. Confirmation by determination of pH and pCO$_2$ may allow appropriate treatment to be given. Consideration should be given to the disorders listed as possible causal factors, and specific therapy should be administered when possible (e.g., blood or albumin for hypovolemia, antibiotics for sepsis). Increased oxygen concentration is frequently required to improve the paO$_2$ to a high-normal range.

In the extremely preterm infant, loss of bicarbonate in the urine commonly occurs. Testing of the urine for pH frequently reveals values of 7 to 8 and occasionally higher. Under these circumstances, addition of bicarbonate (or possibly acetate) to the infusion fluid is necessary.

Correction of a base deficit of less than 5 is usually not necessary. Base deficit can be corrected using 10% sodium bicarbonate based on the following formula:

$$\text{mEq sodium bicarbonate} = \text{wt (in kg)} \times \text{base deficit} \times 0.3$$

For instance, in a 2-kg infant with a base deficit of 10, the milliequivalents of bicarbonate would be $2 \times 10 \times 0.3 = 6$ mEq. If the pH is very low (below 7.20), half of the bicarbonate (3 mEq) may be given in a bolus by slow push (1 mEq/min—a clock or watch can be used) and the remainder in the fluid infusion over the next 1 or 2 hours. If the pH is not very low, the slower rate of infusion is probably preferable. Tris(hydroxymethyl)aminomethane (THAM) may also be used to correct acidosis, particularly if hypernatremia is present or imminent. It may produce respiratory arrest and hypoglycemia and is hyperosmolar. These disadvantages limit its use.

CAUTION: Remember that if the pH is low because of respiratory acidosis (high pCO_2), attention should be directed toward ventilation because the base deficit may be negligible. When pH is below 7.20 as a result of respiratory acidosis, it may limit pulmonary perfusion and produce metabolic acidosis. Under such circumstances, cautious administration of bicarbonate may be used while attention is paid to ventilation.

SUMMARY

Increased anaerobic metabolism produces metabolic acidosis in various clinical circumstances. The major signs in the baby are pallor and tachypnea. Blood pH and pCO_2 confirm the diagnosis. Correction of a base deficit (> 5) can be achieved with slow infusion of sodium bicarbonate. Attention should be paid to correction of underlying causes.

METABOLIC ALKALOSIS

Metabolic alkalosis is rarely encountered in the newborn period. It may be iatrogenic as a result of overadministration of base (usually sodium bicarbonate) or feeding of chloride-deficient formula; it may be the result of loss of hydrogen ion by vomiting (congenital hypertrophic pyloric stenosis); or it may be the result of depletion of total body potassium. If metabolic alkalosis is noted from pH and blood gas analysis, serum electrolyte levels should be evaluated.

DISORDERS OF MAGNESIUM METABOLISM

HYPERMAGNESEMIA

Prolonged use of magnesium sulfate when the mother is treated for toxemia of pregnancy or when it is used as a tocolytic may produce excessively high levels of magnesium (> 3 mg/dl) in the neonate. We have also encountered hypermagnesemia during total peripheral (intravenous) alimentation. Such levels may result in lethargy, intestinal (paralytic) ileus, meconium plug syndrome, and respiratory depression (occasionally requiring ventilator assistance).

HYPOMAGNESEMIA

A frequent accompaniment of hypocalcemia (with the clinical manifestations previously outlined), hypomagnesemia can occasionally be an isolated metabolic defect that produces jitteriness and convulsions.

OTHER ELECTROLYTE DISORDERS

HYPERNATREMIA

Overzealous use of sodium bicarbonate may result in hypernatremia. Severe diarrhea and nephrogenic diabetes insipidus may rarely be implicated, and dehydration in breast-fed infants has been associated. As at any age, hypernatremia may predispose to intracerebral bleeding. Convulsions may be the presenting feature. Serum sodium levels greater than 150 mEq/L are abnormal, and concentrations greater than 160 mEq/L are likely to have accompanying signs.

HYPONATREMIA

Hyponatremia may be the result of congestive failure, water intoxication (overload), inappropriate antidiuretic hormone secretion (secondary to asphyxia, meningitis, and so on), and salt-losing congenital adrenal hyperplasia (adrenogenital syndrome). Increased sodium loss in the urine may occur in premature infants with respiratory distress syndrome. Levels less than 130 mEq/L are seen frequently (without symptoms) in the neonatal period, usually because of failure to add electrolyte to the infusion fluid being given to premature infants. Levels below 120 mEq/L are likely to result in irritability and convulsions but may also produce lethargy or apnea.

HYPERKALEMIA

Relative hyperkalemia exists in almost all newborns in the first days of life, presumably as a result of breakdown of cells. After the first few days, such levels may be indicative of renal failure or salt-losing congenital adrenal hyperplasia.

The increased survival of extremely low-birth-weight infants (< 1000 g) has been accompanied by an increase in the number of babies who develop hyperkalemia. As more central samples are obtained, it is apparent that levels above 7 mEq/L may occur in the absence of oliguria and that cardiac arrhythmias may result. Higher levels reported some years ago to be normal in term babies were probably the result of hemolysis of the specimen.

HYPOKALEMIA

Hypokalemia is encountered infrequently but is usually the result of excessive loss via the kidney (with diuretic therapy) or intestines (diarrhea or ileostomy) or may be the result of failure to supplement intravenous fluids, particularly if excessive amounts of fluid have been given. It may also be seen with alkalemia (pH > 7.50).

INBORN ERRORS OF METABOLISM

An enormous number of genetically transmitted disorders exist that, by altering one small pathway of metabolism, may produce profound generalized effects. Most of these disorders are very rare and involve a deficiency of a single enzyme. The list of such disorders now numbers well over 1000. One or two of the more common inborn errors of metabolism may provide suitable examples (see also Screening Techniques section in Chapter 4).

PHENYLKETONURIA

Phenylketonuria is a disorder of amino acid metabolism, occurring with an incidence of approximately 1 in 10,000 children in the United States. Inheritance is autosomal-recessive, and the defect is a failure to convert phenylalanine to tyrosine. The accumulation of phenylalanine and other byproducts leads to mental retardation. Limitation of phenylalanine intake effectively prevents mental retardation in almost all cases. Damage to the fetus may occur if phenylalanine intake is not adequately controlled in a mother with phenylketonuria during pregnancy. Detection is possible by routine neonatal screening, using blood collected on filter paper after a day or two of milk-feeding. This screening is carried out using the Guthrie test, the principle of which is the enhancement of bacterial growth by elevated levels of phenylalanine.

GALACTOSEMIA

Galactosemia is another disorder that can be treated by dietary restriction. It is an inborn error of carbohydrate metabolism. The incidence is approximately 1 in 62,000. The main clinical features in the neonatal period are transient jaundice, digestive difficulties, hepatomegaly, and cataracts. The diagnosis may be suggested when urine is positive for reducing substances but is negative for glucose. A high percentage of cases of galactosemia present with *Escherichia coli* sepsis (see Chapter 15). The defect appears to be a deficiency of an enzyme that aids conversion of galactose-1-phosphate to glucose-1-phosphate. A screening test on small quantities of blood is now available. Treatment with limitation of lactose (and hence galactose) in the diet is usually successful if it is started before liver damage is advanced.

CRIGLER-NAJJAR SYNDROME

Crigler-Najjar syndrome is a rare disorder that is manifested by persistent unconjugated hyperbilirubinemia secondary to a deficiency of the enzyme glucuronyl transferase. In some cases, this deficiency is only partial and the enzyme can be stimulated by phenobarbital.

CYSTIC FIBROSIS (MUCOVISCIDOSIS)

Cystic fibrosis is another autosomal-recessive disorder; the incidence is approximately 1 in 1000 to 1 in 5000. The respiratory component rarely presents itself in the neonatal period. Meconium plug syndrome, meconium ileus, or meconium peritonitis may be the first clinical feature. Routine testing of meconium (to detect albumin) is of debatable value. Serum immunoreactive trypsin determination on dried blood spots has now proved to be a rather sensitive screening test. With discovery of the cystic fibrosis gene, prenatal and neonatal diagnosis can be more specific.

OTHER METABOLIC PROBLEMS

HYPOTHYROIDISM

Screening for congenital hypothyroidism is now available. Blood should preferably be sent for testing after the baby is 48 hours of age. Such testing is important, because the initial physical examination may be essentially normal (although large fontanels may be a clue). The most common symptoms during the first month of life are feeding difficulty, lethargy, umbilical hernia, thick tongue, constipation, and prolonged jaundice.

Abnormally low thyroxine values have been seen transiently in preterm, small-for-gestational age, and sick infants and may not be benign. In addition, hypothyroidism with associated goiter can be induced by excessive maternal ingestion of iodides (in cough medicines) or by cutaneous absorption of iodine. On the other hand, a baby may be protected from developing hypothyroidism for several months by breast-feeding.

HYPERTHYROIDISM

Hyperthyroidism is usually encountered in infants whose mothers have (or have had) thyrotoxicosis with exophthalmic goiter. The baby usually has some degree of exophthalmos, is restless, and has tachycardia. Hyperviscosity has also been associated (see Chapter 20). The disorder is self-limiting but may require drug therapy for 2 or 3 months. Propranolol has been advocated for this purpose.

HYPERAMMONEMIA

Although hyperammonemia has been recognized in association with congenital enzyme defects, it may also be a transient problem in preterm infants. It presents as an overwhelming illness, developing within the first 48 hours after birth. Mild respiratory distress progresses rapidly to deep coma, requiring assisted ventilation. Exchange transfusion, or peritoneal dialysis, or both seem to produce a good response if the diagnosis is made promptly.

VITAMIN DEFICIENCIES

In most term babies, vitamin deficiencies are very rarely encountered in the neonatal period. However, preterm infants are at greater risk.

Water-Soluble Vitamins

PYRIDOXINE DEFICIENCY (OR DEPENDENCY). Irritability and eventually convulsions may result from this disorder, which involves unusually high daily requirements of vitamin B_6. A diagnostic and therapeutic test is to give pyridoxine hydrochloride while performing electroencephalography: Abnormalities noted before pyridoxine injection disappear.

FOLATE AND VITAMIN B_{12}. A deficiency may occur when infants consume a small volume of formula.

VITAMIN C. Although vitamin C is present in adequate amounts in breast milk and most formulas, it is destroyed by heat. The preterm infant may have an increased requirement.

Fat-Soluble Vitamins

VITAMIN A. In at least one study, a relative deficiency of this vitamin was documented in preterm infants, with the suggestion that this deficiency may predispose to diseases involving the mucosal epithelium.

VITAMIN D. Because of decreased intake, rickets has been described in low-birth-weight infants taking formulas containing 400 IU of vitamin D per liter. A deficiency of vitamin D may also produce a tendency toward stress fractures of long bones and ribs.

VITAMIN E. More vitamin E is needed in formulas that are high in polyunsaturated fatty acids. Deficiency of vitamin E has been associated with hemolytic anemia in premature infants, and this condition may be accompanied by edema. This anemia may be exaggerated if iron is given before the deficiency is corrected. A deficiency of vitamin E has also been implicated in disorders in which oxygen toxicity has been involved (retinopathy of prematurity and bronchopulmonary dysplasia) because vitamin E acts as an antioxidant. There are conflicting results when vitamin E supplementation is given.

VITAMIN K. Deficiency of vitamin K produces hemorrhagic disease of the newborn (see Chapter 20).

The Committee on Nutrition of the American Academy of Pediatrics recommends "... that low-birth-weight infants receive an intramuscular injection of 1 to 2 mg of vitamin K at birth and a daily, oral multivitamin supplement providing the recommended daily allowance of vitamins for infants as established by the Food and Drug Administration" (Pediatrics 1977, 60:519).

BIBLIOGRAPHY

Hypoglycemia

Reid, M. McC., Reilly, B. J., Murdock, A. I., and Swyer, P. R.: Cardiomegaly in association with neonatal hypoglycemia. *Acta Paediatr.* 1971, 60:295.

Lilien, L. D., Pildes, R. S., Srinivasan, G., et al.: Treatment of neonatal hypoglycemia with minibolus and intravenous glucose infusion. *J. Pediatr.* 1980, 97:295–298.

Aynsley-Green, A., Polak, J. M., Bloom, S. R., et al.: Nesidioblastosis of the pancreas: Definition of the syndrome and the management of the severe neonatal hyperinsulinaemic hypoglycaemia. *Arch. Dis. Child.* 1981, 56:496–508.

Jaffe, R., Hashida, Y., and Yunis, E. J.: The endocrine pancreas of the neonate and infant. *Perspect. Pediatr. Pathol.* 1982, 7:137–165.

Editorial: Brain damage by neonatal hypoglycemia. *Lancet* 1989, i:882–883.

Collins, J. E., Leonard, J. V., Teale, D., et al.: Hyperinsulinemic hypoglycemia in small for dates babies. *Arch. Dis. Child.* 1990, 65:1118–1120.

Cornblath, M., Schwartz, R., Aynsley-Green, A., and Lloyd, J. K.: Hypoglycemia in infancy: The need for a rational definition. *Pediatrics* 1990, 85:834–837.

Hyperglycemia

Lilien, L. D., Rosenfield, R. L., Baccaro, M. M., and Pildes, R. S.: Hyperglycemia in stressed small premature neonates. *J. Pediatr.* 1979, 94:454–459.

Stonestreet, B. S., Rubin, L., Pollak, A., et al.: Renal functions of low birth weight infants with hyperglycemia and glucosuria produced by glucose infusions. *Pediatrics* 1980, 66:561–567.

Dellagrammaticas, H. D., and Papas, C. B.: Hyperglycemia and *Escherichia coli* sepsis in a preterm neonate (Letter). *Am. J. Dis. Child.* 1981, 135:186–187.

Coffey, J. D., Jr., and Killelae, D. E.: Transient neonatal diabetes mellitus in half sister. A sequel. *Am. J. Dis. Child.* 1982, 136:626–627.

Louik, C., Mitchell, A. A., Epstein, M. F., and Shapiro, S.: Risk factors for neonatal hyperglycemia associated with 10% dextrose infusion. *Am. J. Dis. Child.* 1985, 139:783–786.

Collins, J. W. Jr., Hoppe, M., Brown, K., et al.: A controlled trial of insulin infusion and parenteral nutrition in extremely low birth weight infants with glucose intolerance. *J. Pediatr.* 1991, 118:921–927.

Hypocalcemia

Tsang, R. C., Donovan, E. F., and Steichen, J. J.: Calcium physiology and pathology in the neonate. *Pediatr. Clin. North Am.* 1976, 23:611.

Giacoia, G. P., and Wagner, H. R.: Q_0T_c interval and blood calcium levels in newborn infants. *Pediatrics* 1978, 61:877.

Brown, D. R., and Salsburey, D. J.: Short-term biochemical effects of parenteral calcium treatment of early-onset neonatal hypocalcemia. *J. Pediatr.* 1982, 100:777–781.

Specker, B. L., Tsang, R. C., Ho, M. L., et al.: Low serum calcium and high parathyroid hormone levels in neonates fed "humanized" cow's milk–based formula. *Am. J. Dis. Child.* 1991, 145:941–945.

Hypercalcemia

Lyon, A. J., McIntosh, N., Wheeler, K., and Brooke, O. G.: Hypercalcaemia in extremely low birthweight infants. *Arch. Dis. Child.* 1984, 59:1141–1144.

Garabédian, M., Jacqz, E., Guillozo, H., et al.: Elevated plasma 1,25-dihydroxyvitamin D concentrations in infants with hypercalcemia and elfin facies. *N. Engl. J. Med.* 1985, 312:948–952.

Metabolic Acidosis

Svenningsen, N. W., and Lindquist, B.: Incidence of metabolic acidosis in term, preterm and small-for-gestational age infants in relation to dietary protein intake. *Acta Paediatr.* 1973, 62:1.

Rhodes, P. G., Hall, R. T., and Hellerstein, S.: Effects of single infusions of hypertonic sodium bicarbonate on body composition in neonates with acidosis. *J. Pediatr.* 1977, 90:789.

Schwartz, G. J., Haycock, G. B., Edelmann, C. M., and Spitzer, A.: Late metabolic acidosis—Reassessment of the definition. *J. Pediatr.* 1979, 95:102.

Winters, R. W.: Acid-base disorders. In *Principles of Pediatric Fluid Therapy*, 2nd ed. Little, Brown & Co., Boston, 1982, pp. 23–55.

Disorders of Magnesium Metabolism

Tsang, R. C., Strub, R., Brown, D. R., et al.: Hypomagnesemia in infants of diabetic mothers. Perinatal studies. *J. Pediatr.* 1976, 89:119.

Donovan, E. F., Tsang, R. C., Steichen, J. J., et al.: Neonatal hypermagnesemia—Effect on parathyroid hormone and calcium homeostasis. *J. Pediatr.* 1980, 96:305–310.

Green, K. W., Key, T. C., Coen, R., and Resnik, R.: The effects of maternally administered magnesium sulfate on the neonate. *Am. J. Obstet. Gynecol.* 1983, 146:29–33.

Giles, M. M., Laing, I. A., Elton, R. A., et al.: Magnesium metabolism in preterm infants: Effects of calcium, magnesium and phosphorus and of post-natal and gestational age. *J. Pediatr.* 1990, 117:147–154.

Other Electrolyte Disorders

Tarnow-Mordi, W. O., Shaw, J. C. L., Liu, D., et al.: Iatrogenic hyponatraemia of the newborn due to maternal fluid overload: A prospective study. *B.M.J.* 1981, 283:639–642.

Rowland, T. W., Zori, R. T., Lafleur, W. R., and Reiter, E. O.: Malnutrition and hypernatremic dehydration in breast-fed infants. *J.A.M.A.* 1982, 247:1016–1017.

Shaffer, S. G., Kilbride, H. W., Hayen, L. K., et al.: Hyperkalemia in very low birth weight infants. *J. Pediatr.* 1992, 121:275–279.

Shaffer, S. G., and Weismann D. N.: Fluid requirements in the preterm neonate. *Clin. Perinatol.* 1992, 19:233–250.

Wilkins, B. H.: Renal function in sick very low birthweight infants: 3. Sodium, potassium and water excretion. *Arch. Dis. Child.* 1992, 67:1154–1161.

Stefano, J. L., Norman, M. E., Morales, M. C., et al.: Decreased erythrocyte Na^+, K^+-ATPase activity associated with cellular potassium loss in extremely low birth weight infants with nonoliguric hyperkalemia. *J. Pediatr.* 1993, 122:276–284.

Inborn Errors of Metabolism

Symposium on Early Detection and Management of Inborn Errors. *Clin. Perinatol.* 1976, 3:1.

Aleck, K. A., and Shapiro, L. J.: Genetic-metabolic considerations in the sick neonate. *Pediatr. Clin. North Am.* 1978, 25:431.

Burton, B. K., and Nadler, H. L.: Clinical diagnosis of the inborn errors of metabolism in the neonatal period. *Pediatrics* 1978, 61:398.

Komrower, G. M.: Inborn errors of metabolism. *Pediatr. Rev.* 1980, 2:175–181.

Levy, H. L.: Phenylketonuria—1986. *Pediatr. Rev.* 1986, 7:269–275.

Bowling, F., Cleghorn, G., Chester, A., et al.: Neonatal screening for cystic fibrosis. *Arch. Dis. Child.* 1988, 63:196–198.

Editorial: Cystic fibrosis: Prospects for screening and therapy. *Lancet*, 1990, 335:79–80.

Ward, J. C.: Inborn errors of metabolism of acute onset in infancy. *Pediatr. Rev.* 1990, 11:205–216.

Schweitzer, S., Shin, Y., Jakobs, C., and Brodehl, J.: Long-term outcome in 134 patients with galactosemia. *Eur. J. Pediatr.* 1993, 152:36–43.

Other Metabolic Problems

Pearl, K. N., and Chambers, T. L.: Propranolol treatment of thyrotoxicosis in a premature infant. *B.M.J.* 1977, 2:738.

Ballard, R. A., Vinocur, B., Reynolds, J. W., et al.: Transient hyperammonemia of the preterm infant. *N. Engl. J. Med.* 1978, 299:920.

Bode, H. H., Vanjonack, W. J., and Crawford, J. D.: Mitigation of cretinism by breast-feeding. *Pediatrics* 1978, 62:13.

Chabrolle, J. P., and Rossier, A.: Goitre and hypothyroidism in the newborn after cutaneous absorption of iodine. *Arch. Dis. Child.* 1978, 53:495.

Editorial: Vitamin K and the newborn. *Lancet* 1978, i:755.

Heeley, A., Pugh, R. J. P., Clayton, B. E., et al.: Pyridoxal metabolism in vitamin B_6 responsive convulsions of early infancy. *Arch. Dis. Child.* 1978, 53:794.

Daneman, D., and Howard, N. J.: Neonatal thyrotoxicosis: Intellectual impairment and craniosynostosis in later years. *J. Pediatr.* 1980, 97:257–259.

O'Connor, M. K., Freyne, P. J., and Cullen, M. J.: Low-dose radioisotope scanning and quantitative analysis in the diagnosis of congenital hypothyroidism. *Arch. Dis. Child.* 1982, 57:490–494.

Tsang, R. C.: The quandary of vitamin D in the newborn infant. *Lancet* 1983, i:1370–1372.

Donn, S. M., and Banagale, R. C.: Neonatal hyperammonemia. *Pediatr. Rev.* 1984, 5:203–208.

Committee on Fetus and Newborn, American Academy of Pediatrics: Vitamin E and the prevention of retinopathy of prematurity. *Pediatrics* 1985, 76:315–316.

Pereira, G., and Zucker, A.: Nutritional deficiencies in the neonate. *Clin. Perinatol.* 1986, 13:175–189.

Sobel, E. H., and Saenger, P.: Hypothyroidism in the newborn. *Pediatr. Rev.* 1989, 11:15–20.

Glorieux, J., Dussault, J., and Van Vliet, G.: Intellectual development at age 12 years of children with congenital hypothyroidism diagnosed by neonatal screening. *J. Pediatr.* 1992, 121:581–584.

Meijer, W. J., Verloove-Vanhorick, S. P., Brand, R., and Van Den Brande, J. L.: Transient hypothyroxinaemia associated with developmental delay in very preterm infants. *Arch. Dis. Child.* 1992, 67:944–947.

18
NECROTIZING ENTEROCOLITIS

INTRODUCTION

The incidence of necrotizing enterocolitis (NEC) varies considerably, from fewer than 1% to 5% of neonatal intensive care unit admissions. In some nurseries, it seems to have become more common in the past 10 to 15 years. One postulate about the increased prevalence is that more babies who are predisposed to develop the disease who might otherwise have died are surviving.

ETIOLOGY AND PATHOPHYSIOLOGY

The idea that babies may be candidates for developing NEC has been proposed. Such babies are more likely to be premature and may have been subjected to some stress that results in ischemia of the bowel. The antecedent to ischemia is anything that produces significant acidosis (e.g., neonatal asphyxia, severe respiratory distress syndrome, sepsis), because the neonate responds to acidosis by diverting blood from skin, lungs, kidneys, and gastrointestinal tract to the vital organs (brain and heart). Other mechanisms contributing to decreased blood flow and oxygenation to the gut are

1. Persistent patent ductus arteriosus
2. Umbilical artery catheter obstructing blood flow to mesenteric arteries
3. Hypovolemia or anemia
4. Hyperviscosity (especially small for gestational age infants)
5. Shock (low blood pressure)
6. Pharmacologic doses of indomethacin (used to close patent ductus arteriosus)

It is possible that significant ischemia itself may result in infarction and subsequent necrosis of the bowel. Almost certainly, loss of the protective mucosal barrier occurs because of hypoxic injury. An intriguing recent finding is a decreased incidence of NEC in infants born to mothers who received glucocorticoid therapy, suggesting accelerated intestinal (as well as lung) maturity. At least three additional factors have been implicated.

INFECTION. A wide variety of organisms has been implicated, with enteric bacteria being the most common (particularly *Escherichia coli, Klebsiella,* and *Enterobacter cloacae*). Recent attention has been directed toward the role of endotoxin, enterotoxin, and anaerobic bacteria such as *Clostridium perfringens*. Several viruses have also been associated.

TYPE OF FEEDING. The integrity of the bowel wall (and resistance to infection) may be enhanced by macrophages in fresh breast milk. Hyperosmolar formula feedings have been incriminated as contributing to NEC. It seems most likely that feeding provides the metabolic substrate for bacteria to attack an already compromised intestinal tract. Proliferation of gas-forming organisms may produce pneumatosis intestinalis, with separation of the layers of intestine and either vascular compromise or perforation.

INFLAMMATION. Although ischemia is undoubtedly important, the idea that it may be a secondary rather than a primary contributing factor has recently gained support. Increasing evidence suggests that NEC should be considered a form of inflammatory bowel disease. Several inflammatory mediators, particularly platelet-activating factor, have been implicated in the pathogenesis of NEC.

DIAGNOSIS

Because of the poor results observed when the full syndrome has developed, every attempt should be made to make an early diagnosis. With an increased index of suspicion in high-risk groups (e.g., the asphyxiated premature infant), the initiation of treatment at the earliest indication may make definitive diagnosis impossible. The following features should suggest the diagnosis.

1. Birth weight of less than 1500 g
2. Previous hypoxia, acidosis, hypovolemia, and so on
3. Poor feeding
4. Apneic episodes
5. Abdominal distension (with radiographic confirmation of intestinal distension)
6. Prolonged gastric emptying (significant residual when baby is being gavage-fed)
7. Vomiting (may be bile stained)
8. Diarrheal stool, particularly if testing for reducing substance shows positive reaction of greater than 2 +

More dramatic, but late, features are

1. Increasing lethargy
2. Temperature instability
3. Pallor and shock
4. Blood-streaked or grossly bloody stool
5. Bleeding tendency
6. Signs of peritonitis
7. Radiographic features of
   a. Intramural gas (pneumatosis intestinalis, Figs. 18–1 and 18–2)
   b. Pneumoperitoneum (free air)
   c. Gas in the portal vein
   d. Persistent loop

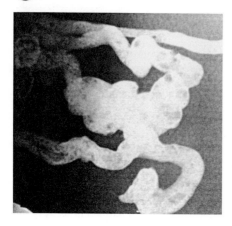

FIGURE 18–1. Radiograph of excised bowel in a baby with necrotizing enterocolitis, showing intramural air.

Recent evidence from large numbers of infants with NEC indicates that about 15% of subsequently documented cases do not display evidence of pneumatosis intestinalis. This makes the diagnosis even more difficult and suggests that adjunctive tests are needed to help differentiate equivocal cases from benign conditions. One possible approach, noted by the author and others, is the use of the acute-phase proteins C-reactive protein and α-acid glycoprotein (orosomu-

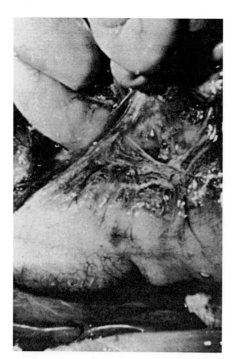

FIGURE 18–2. Operative photograph of the baby in Figure 18–1, showing bubbles of air on the surface of the bowel wall.

coid). Levels of these proteins increase with inflammation and necrosis, so that elevated levels (in the absence of documented sepsis) may indicate NEC.

MANAGEMENT

Cautious introduction of dilute enteral feedings may possibly prevent the development of NEC, and fresh breast milk has some theoretical advantages, but NEC has been seen in infants who have been fed only breast milk and in some who have not received any enteral feeding. Thus, all low-birth-weight infants (particularly those weighing < 1500 g) require careful observation for the features noted under Diagnosis.

An abdominal radiograph should be obtained whenever the possibility of NEC is raised. Because many features may also be seen with bacterial sepsis, a sepsis workup is usually performed at the same time. If any of the late features are noted, it is imperative that gastric feedings be discontinued, orogastric or nasogastric decompression be started, and (after cultures have been drawn) broad-spectrum antibiotics begun, with intravenous fluid therapy. The use of low-molecular-weight dextran has also been advocated.

In cases in which a bleeding tendency (evidence of disseminated intravascular coagulation), evidence of peritonitis, or radiographic evidence of pneumoperitoneum or portal vein gas is present, surgery is almost always necessary. Intestinal gangrene may possibly be diagnosed before surgery by use of paracentesis and lavage. Brown peritoneal fluid has been correlated with intestinal gangrene. When perforation has occurred, peritoneal drainage may be preferred in the very small, sick infant.

It was suggested in 1976 that NEC might be prevented in babies weighing less than 1500 g by giving an oral aminoglycoside (kanamycin) prophylactically. Subsequent studies have shown that although bowel flora may be altered, NEC is not prevented.

Antagonists to platelet-activating factor may be used in the future to prevent or lessen the severity of NEC.

SUMMARY

NEC seems to be a disorder of modern neonatal intensive care. It is linked primarily to ischemia of the bowel as a result of hypoxic stress in the low-birth-weight infant. However, term infants have also been affected. Bacterial infection, aided by milk-feeding, seems to compromise the bowel wall secondary to mucosal damage. The classic features are abdominal distension, bloody stools, and pneumatosis intestinalis (seen on radiography), but many other signs may allow early diagnosis. NEC is to be differentiated from bacterial sepsis. Treatment is primarily medical, with discontinuation of oral feeding, gastric decompression, intravenous fluid, and antibiotics. Surgical intervention may be necessary.

BIBLIOGRAPHY

Rowley, M. P., and Dahlenburg, G. W.: Gentamicin prophylaxis of neonatal necrotizing enterocolitis. *Lancet* 1978, ii:532.

Wexler, H. A.: Persistent loop sign in neonatal necrotizing enterocolitis: New indication for surgery. *Radiology* 1978, 126:201.

Brown, E. G, and Sweet, A. Y.: Neonatal necrotizing enterocolitis. *Pediatr. Clin. North Am.* 1982, 29:1149–1170.

Schwartz, M. Z., Hayden, C. K., Richardson, C. J., et al.: A prospective evaluation of intestinal stenosis following necrotizing enterocolitis. *J. Pediatr. Surg.* 1982, 17:764–770.

British Association for Perinatal Paediatrics and Public Health Laboratory Service Communicable Disease Surveillance Centre: Surveillance of necrotising enterocolitis, 1981–2. *B.M.J.* 1983, 287:824–826.

Cushing, A. H.: Necrotizing enterocolitis with *Escherichia coli* heat-labile enterotoxin. *Pediatrics* 1983, 71:626–630.

Kliegman, R. M., and Fanaroff, A. A.: Necrotising enterocolitis. *N. Eng. J. Med.* 1984, 310:1093–1103.

Bauer, C. R., Morrison, J. C., Poole, W. K., et al.: A decreased incidence of necrotizing enterocolitis after prenatal glucocorticoid therapy. *Pediatrics* 1984, 73:682–688.

Kuhl, G., Wille, L., Bokenius, M., and Seyberth, H. W.: Intestinal perforation associated with indomethacin treatment in premature infants. *Eur. J. Pediatr.* 1985, 143:213–216.

Philip, A. G. S., Sann, L., and Bienvenu, F.: Acute phase proteins in neonatal necrotizing enterocolitis. *Acta Paediatr. Scand.* 1986, 75:1032–1033.

Isaacs, D., North, J., Lindsell, D., and Wilkinson, A. R.: Serum acute phase reactants in necrotizing enterocolitis. *Acta Paediatr. Scand.* 1987, 76:923–927.

Stoll, B. J., and Kliegman, R. M. (eds): Necrotizing Enterocolitis. *Clin. Perinatol.* 1994, 21:205–462.

19

INTRACRANIAL HEMORRHAGE

INTRODUCTION

Starting in the 1970s, our ability to detect neonatal intracranial hemorrhage improved remarkably, initially using computed tomographic scans and subsequently using cephalic ultrasonography. Further advances in our understanding have come from positron-emission tomography scans and magnetic resonance imaging and spectroscopy.

There are several different types of intracranial hemorrhage, which may be broadly classified as (1) subarachnoid, (2) subdural, (3) intraventricular or periventricular, (4) intracerebral, (5) intracerebellar, and (6) brainstem.

Currently, periventricular hemorrhage (PVH) is the most important form of intracranial hemorrhage to consider. In the early 1980s, it was seen in approximately 40% of very-low-birth-weight infants, but figures closer to 25% or less have been seen more recently. As other causes of neonatal mortality decrease in frequency, severe PVH assumes increasing importance.

ETIOLOGY

The primary causes are birth trauma (e.g., breech delivery or difficult forceps delivery) and hypoxic insult. Subarachnoid and subdural hemorrhage are more likely to be seen in term infants, whereas PVH is most likely to be seen in very preterm infants. Trauma is likely to produce subdural and intracerebellar hemorrhage, whereas hypoxia is associated more often with other forms of intracranial hemorrhage. The various causes have been summarized in Table 19–1. Intraventricular or periventricular hemorrhage (IVH/PVH) was originally considered to be a problem of venous hypertension, but later investigations suggested that rupture of capillaries (or the precursors of capillaries) may occur on the arterial rather than the venous side. Hypoxia, or events leading to hypoxia, may result in elevations or surges of arterial blood pressure. The capillaries (or immature vessels) situated in the region of the germinal matrix seem to be particularly susceptible to hypoxia and hypertension, with abolition of contractility (loss of autoregulation) allowing pressure to be transmitted directly, causing rupture of vessels. In addition to early gestation, babies who are also small for gestational age seem to be predisposed to develop IVH. The risk of hemorrhage in tiny babies seems to be decreased by cesarean section

TABLE 19–1. TYPES AND CAUSES OF INTRACRANIAL HEMORRHAGES

Type of Hemorrhage	Causes
Subarachnoid	
Generalized	Asphyxia; hemostatic failure
Convexity	Hemostatic failure–consumptive coagulopathy; increased venous pressure
Subdural	Asphyxia; hemostatic failure (e.g., hemophilia); forceps delivery (underlying fracture)
Intra(peri)ventricular	Asphyxia—loss of autoregulation; increased venous pressure: increases (surges) of arterial pressure; poorly supported blood vessels
Intracerebral	
Localized	Asphyxia (associated with periventricular hemorrhage)
Diffuse	Electrolyte disturbance (hypernatremia)
Intracerebellar	Asphyxia; face masks—cranial compression, increased venous pressure; complicated delivery—occipital osteodiastasis

delivery. In the era before modern neonatal intensive care, the incidence of intraventricular hemorrhage was estimated at approximately 1 in 1000 live births. Evidence from a number of centers indicates that the greater the degree of prematurity, the higher the frequency of PVH. In the early 1980s, the incidence in babies at 33 to 34 weeks' gestation was roughly 5% and increased to about 25% at 29 to 32 weeks' gestation, 50% at 27 to 28 weeks' gestation, and 75% at 26 weeks' or less gestation. In the early 1990s, these figures were considerably lower.

Other factors that may contribute to intracranial hemorrhage are thrombocytopenia, a generalized hypocoagulable state, tight nuchal cord, distortion of the cranial vault, hypernatremia, and vasodilator substances (prostaglandins and increased $paCO_2$).

DIAGNOSIS

The advent of computed tomographic scans and the subsequent widespread application of cephalic ultrasonography have dramatically altered our ability to diagnose intracranial hemorrhage in the neonate (see pp. 371 to 373). Before the introduction of these techniques, the primary method of detecting intracranial hemorrhage was to use clinical signs, such as rapid deterioration, persistent metabolic acidosis, poor peripheral perfusion (shock), a falling hematocrit value, temperature instability (fever has been noted in some cases of IVH), and convulsions (seizures), which are an ominous sign and which may present as decerebrate posturing.

Despite increasing inspired oxygen concentration, it may be difficult to maintain an adequate arterial oxygen tension. Fullness and tenseness of the anterior fontanel may be prominent, but not in all cases. Apnea is a common, but nonspecific, feature in babies not receiving assisted ventilation. Despite such classic features, there is a depressingly poor correlation with evidence of hemorrhage by computed tomographic scan (Lazzara and colleagues, 1980). However, abnormal eye signs and seizures were not seen in the absence of hemorrhage. More recently, PVH (documented by ultrasound) was associated with roving eye movements and a tight popliteal angle (Dubowitz and colleagues, 1981).

Although subarachnoid and subdural hemorrhages have traditionally been considered to occur shortly after delivery, PVH was considered most likely to occur on the second and third days. Ultrasonographic studies now indicate that 50% of PVH occur in the first 24 hours and 85% or more occur by the end of the third day.

An important point to remember is that hemorrhage may not cause injury by itself. It is more likely that hemorrhage serves as a marker for ischemic damage. This has been demonstrated by use of positron-emission tomographic scans. Cephalic ultrasonography performed prior to discharge may also reveal cystic changes consistent with periventricular leukomalacia.

MANAGEMENT

Prevention is undoubtedly the key to management. Prevention of preterm birth, together with elimination of obstetric trauma and intrauterine or extrauterine hypoxia, would effectively resolve the problem of intracranial hemorrhage. There has been controversy about the role of correction of coagulation defects, either by administering plasma factors or by using exchange transfusion. The routine prophylactic use of either of these measures in low-birth-weight babies cannot be recommended, but in the presence of an obvious bleeding tendency (e.g., oozing from heel-stick puncture sites), correction by the most effective and available method is desirable. There is conflicting evidence about the role of sodium bicarbonate in IVH, and it is unlikely to be associated when given carefully and slowly. Avoidance of elevated pCO_2 values and possibly hyperventilating infants of very low birth weight may decrease cerebral vasodilation.

Pharmacologic agents have also been used to prevent PVH, either prenatally or postnatally (e.g., phenobarbital, vitamin K, ethamsylate, indomethacin). The most convincing evidence of an effect with a drug administered prenatally to prevent PVH concerns the use of phenobarbital, although postnatally administered phenobarbital does not seem to be effective (despite some initially encouraging results). There is also evidence of a beneficial effect after prenatal corticosteroid therapy to stimulate lung maturity. For instance, in a recent multicenter study, early IVH/PVH (at 6 hours) occurred in 9% of extremely low-birthweight infants when the mother had received steroids, but in 17% of those whose mothers had not received steroids.

Postnatally, ethamsylate and, more recently, indomethacin have been shown to decrease the incidence of PVH. In 209 babies with birth weights of 600 to 1250 g who did not have PVH at 5 to 11 hours after birth, all hemorrhages, particularly severe hemorrhages, were significantly reduced by low-dose indomethacin (0.1 mg/kg/dose) given on each of the first 3 days, compared with 222 placebo controls. There is conflicting evidence concerning vitamin E.

When PVH is documented using ultrasonography in the first week after birth, it can be followed with weekly scans to detect posthemorrhagic hydrocephalus. If no ventricular dilation occurs in the first month, it is unlikely to occur later. Some infants have ventricular dilation that does not progress and requires no treatment. This has been termed ventriculomegaly. Other infants have progressive dilation with either evidence of increased intracranial pressure or a rapidly increasing head circumference (true hydrocephalus). Initially, this condition may be treated with some form of ventricular drainage, either sequential lumbar punctures (successful in some cases), or ventriculostomy drainage. Dark brown ventricular fluid becomes increasingly less brown. In some cases, the ventricles remain decompressed, but in others, they begin to dilate again, which is usually an indication that a ventriculoperitoneal shunt is required. The cerebrospinal fluid glucose values frequently remain low for some time after hemorrhage has occurred.

In the case of subdural hemorrhage, repeated subdural taps may be necessary. In severe forms, manifested by coma and brainstem dysfunction, neurosurgical operative intervention is required. This is also true for some cases of intracerebellar hemorrhage that present in the same way.

OUTLOOK

The follow-up of infants with germinal matrix hemorrhage or mild IVH is usually very good. More extensive IVH/PVH is more likely to have associated ischemic injury, with periventricular leukomalacia, or to result in posthemorrhagic hydrocephalus. Most infants who require intervention have some neurologic deficit. Intraparenchymal hemorrhage in the white matter close to the ventricular wall is likely to produce spastic diplegia (involving the lower extremities). More extensive lesions may involve all four extremities, but small porencephalic cysts are sometimes quite benign.

SUMMARY

There are several forms of intracranial hemorrhage, but all are primarily the result of either obstetric trauma or intrauterine or extrauterine hypoxia. The most important form is PVH, which occurs in a high percentage of very-low-birth-weight infants; the incidence of PVH increases with decreasing gestational age. Diagnosis has been greatly enhanced by the use of cephalic ultrasonography, which can be performed at the bedside. Prevention remains the best approach to treatment. The major complication of PVH is posthemorrhagic hydrocephalus, which may respond to sequential lumbar punctures or ventriculostomy. Survivors are likely to have a normal neurologic outcome, except for those with large intraparenchymal hemorrhages or posthemorrhagic hydrocephalus requiring intervention.

BIBLIOGRAPHY

Pomerance, J. J., and Richardson, C. J.: Hyperpyrexia as a sign of intraventricular hemorrhage in the neonate. *Am. J. Dis. Child.* 1973, 126:854.

Hambleton, G., and Wigglesworth, J. S.: Origin of intraventricular hemorrhage in the preterm infant. *Arch. Dis. Child.* 1976, 51:651.

Finberg, L.: The relationship of intravenous infusions and intracranial hemorrhage: A commentary. *J. Pediatr.* 1977, 91:777.

Lazzara, A., Ahmann, P., Dykes, F., et al.: Clinical predictability of intraventricular hemorrhage in preterm infants. *Pediatrics* 1980, 65:30.

Alvarez-Garijo, J. A.: Subdural hematomas in neonates. Surgical treatment. *Childs Nerv. Syst.* 1981, 8:31–38.

Dubowitz, L. M. S., Levene, M. I., Morante, A., et al.: Neurologic signs in neonatal intraventricular hemorrhage: A correlation with real-time ultrasound. *J. Pediatr.* 1981, 99:127–133.

Volpe, J. J.: Anterior fontanel: Window to the neonatal brain (Editorial). *J. Pediatr.* 1982, 100:395–398.

Editorial: Ischaemia and haemorrhage in the premature brain. *Lancet* 1984, ii:847–848.

Allan, W. C., and Philip, A. G. S.: Neonatal cerebral pathology diagnosed by ultrasound. *Clin. Perinatol.* 1985, 12:195–218.

Ment, L. R.: Prevention of neonatal intraventricular hemorrhage (Editorial). *N. Engl. J. Med.* 1985, 312:1385–1387.

Philip, A. G. S., Allan, W. C., Tito, A. M., and Wheeler, L. R.: Intraventricular hemorrhage in preterm infants: Declining incidence in the 1980s. *Pediatrics* 1989, 84:797–801.

Bada, H. S., Korones, S. B., Perry, E. H., et al.: Mean arterial blood pressure changes in premature infants and those at risk for intraventricular hemorrhage. *J. Pediatr.* 1990, 117:607–614.

Kaempf, J. W., Porreco, R., Molina, R., et al.: Antenatal phenobarbital for the prevention of periventricular and intraventricular hemorrhage: A double-blind randomized, placebo-controlled, multihospital trial. *J. Pediatr.* 1990, 117:933–938.

Krishnamoorthy, K. S., Kuban, K. C. K., Leviton, A., et al.: Periventricular-intraventricular hemorrhage: Sonographic localization, phenobarbital and motor abnormalities in low birth weight infants. *Pediatrics* 1990, 85:1027–1033.

Marro, P. J., Dransfield, D. A., Mott, S. H., and Allan, W. C.: Post-hemorrhagic hydrocephalus: Use of an intravenous-type catheter for cerebro-spinal fluid drainage. *Am. J. Dis. Child.* 1991, 145:1141–1146.

Philip, A. G. S., and Allan, W. C.: Does cesarean section protect against intraventricular hemorrhage in preterm infants? *J. Perinatol.* 1991, 11:3–9.

Van de Bor, M., Den Ouden, L., and Guit, G. L.: Value of cranial ultrasound and magnetic resonance imaging in predicting neurodevelopmental outcome in preterm infants. *Pediatrics* 1992, 90:196–199.

Leviton, A., Kuban, K. C., Pagano, M., et al.: Antenatal corticosteroids appear to reduce the risk of postnatal germinal matrix hemorrhage in intubated low birth weight newborns. *Pediatrics* 1993, 91:1083–1088.

Ment, L. R., Oh, W., Ehrenkranz, R. A., et al.: Low-dose indomethacin and prevention of intraventricular hemorrhage: A multicenter randomized trial. *Pediatrics* 1994, 93:543–550.

Ment, L. R., Oh, W., Ehrenkranz, R. A., et al.: Antenatal steroids, delivery-mode and intraventricular hemorrhage in preterm infants. *Am. J. Obstet. Gynecol.* 1995, 172:795–800.

See also Chapter 8.

20
BLOOD DISORDERS

Hemolytic disease of the newborn is discussed in Chapter 10, bleeding (hemorrhage) is discussed under Neonatal Emergencies in Chapter 24, and thrombocytopenia is discussed under Petechiae and Purpura in Chapter 32.

Three other problems require special attention because of their frequency or potential frequency. These are (1) anemia of prematurity, (2) hemorrhagic disease of the newborn, and (3) hyperviscosity (high-hematocrit) syndrome.

ANEMIA OF PREMATURITY

INTRODUCTION

Most premature infants develop some degree of anemia in the first weeks of life because the usual stimulus of erythropoietin seems to be lacking in this period. The usual form of anemia in the premature infant is a normocytic normochromic anemia, but occasionally, a hemolytic anemia develops in association with edema.

ETIOLOGY

During the first 6 to 8 weeks of life, the premature neonate's bone marrow seems to be lying dormant, apparently because of ineffective erythropoietin production. Blood volume during this time increases in proportion to the weight in an attempt to maintain a level of approximately 80 ml/kg. On the basis of hemodilution alone (excluding red cell breakdown), one can quickly understand how anemia develops.

In the 1-kg infant with a hematocrit value of 50% (hemoglobin, approximately 16 g/dl) and a blood volume of 80 ml/kg, there are 40 ml of red cells. By the time the infant weighs 2 kg, the same 40 ml of red cells will be in approximately 160 ml of blood, giving a hematocrit value of 25% (unless blood has been transfused). Less commonly, a hemolytic anemia of prematurity is produced by a lack of vitamin E in the diet of the premature infant.

DIAGNOSIS

This problem should be anticipated in all premature infants, and, in addition to clinical manifestations (pallor, tachypnea, and poor weight gain), the hemoglobin and/or hematocrit value should be checked weekly. The blood smear and reticulocyte count are additional investigations to confirm the diagnosis.

With anemia induced by vitamin E deficiency, associated edema may be present. Haptoglobin levels are not helpful for confirming hemolysis during the neonatal period, because these levels are normally very low.

MANAGEMENT

The administration of iron alone to the premature infant in the first weeks of life does not prevent anemia of prematurity and, in the absence of an adequate vitamin E intake, may accentuate the tendency to hemolysis. It is therefore important to introduce an adequate intake of vitamin E before the administration of iron. There appears to be no good reason to give oral iron supplements to premature infants in the first 4 to 6 weeks of life, except when erythropoietin is used (see later). It is probably unnecessary to give such supplements until reticulocytosis begins. The breakdown of red cells releases iron for storage that can be incorporated into reticulocytes. Ingested iron seems to be ineffectively utilized in the first weeks of life but should be introduced before 2 months of age in a dosage of 2 to 4 mg/kg/day of elemental iron.

If anemia is severe (hemoglobin < 7 g/dl), particularly in the presence of clinical manifestations other than pallor, it may be necessary to give the baby a blood transfusion. Evidence suggests that transfusion may improve weight gain in infants with severe anemia but seems to provide no clinical advantage in infants with mild anemia (hemoglobin < 10 g/dl). With chronic lung disease, it seems wise to maintain the hematocrit value above about 35%.

Two strategies may help minimize the need for blood transfusion. The first has always been available, to allow the preterm infant to benefit from placental transfusion, which increases the blood volume, particularly the volume of red blood cells. Placental transfusion is accomplished by delaying umbilical cord clamping, with the baby below the level of the placenta. However, the transfer of blood may depend on the initiation of respiration, which may make delayed cord clamping impractical unless special arrangements are made.

The second strategy is the use of recombinant human erythropoietin and has only recently become available. Although this therapy is undoubtedly beneficial in decreasing the need for late transfusions, it is not helpful in the first few days of life, when transfusions are required to replace blood removed for laboratory tests during acute illness. The ideal dose is still being evaluated, but several injections are needed several times a week for several weeks. Neutropenia may develop but may not be related to therapy. Even though the drug is expensive, it is less expensive in preterm neonates than in older people because the dose used is small. The use of recombinant human erythropoietin, which is not a blood product, to avoid transfusions is particularly appreciated by

Jehovah's Witness families. When this material is used, iron supplementation is necessary.

SUMMARY

Anemia of prematurity is most frequently secondary to ineffective hematopoiesis after delivery, which results in anemia by hemodilution as the baby's blood volume increases. Vitamin E deficiency may produce a hemolytic anemia, and this vitamin should be given in the early weeks of life before iron supplementation is started. Occasionally, blood transfusion is required, but the need may be decreased by the use of recombinant human erythropoietin.

HEMORRHAGIC DISEASE OF THE NEWBORN

INTRODUCTION AND INCIDENCE

Hemorrhagic disease of the newborn is a disorder of coagulation caused by a deficiency of vitamin K. Today in most nurseries, vitamin K is given routinely to all newborn infants, although some nurseries administer it only rarely. Approximately 1 in 200 babies who do not receive this supplement develop a bleeding disorder. Obviously this problem can (and should) be prevented. Recent evidence, from both Great Britain and the United States, indicates that this problem continues to rear its ugly head, despite the ease with which it can be prevented. The reluctance to administer vitamin K was reinforced by a claim that intramuscular vitamin K was associated with childhood cancer; this claim was subsequently refuted.

ETIOLOGY

Vitamin K is necessary for synthesis of prothrombin and other coagulation factors in the liver. The fetus obtains this vitamin from the maternal circulation, but the newborn infant has to await appropriate bacterial colonization of the intestine before vitamin K is synthesized. Mothers who have received phenytoin have infants who are particularly prone to this disorder. Infants who are breast-fed without receiving vitamin K at birth may be more likely to develop hemorrhagic disease after 5 to 6 weeks because of lower levels of vitamin K in human milk than in commercial infant formula.

DIAGNOSIS

The most frequent clinical manifestation is bleeding from the gut, but there may be a generalized bleeding tendency that is most likely to occur on the second or third day of life. Late-onset disease may present with intracranial bleeding. In cases of early-onset gastrointestinal bleeding, it may be necessary

TABLE 20–1. COMPARISON OF HEMORRHAGIC DISEASE OF THE NEWBORN AND DISSEMINATED INTRAVASCULAR COAGULATION

	Coagulation Times				Factors and Fragments					
	Bleeding	Clotting	Prothrombin	Partial Thromboplastin	Thrombin	Fibrin Split Products	Factor V	Fibrinogen	Platelets	RBC Fragments
Hemorrhagic disease	N	↑	↑↑↑	↑	N	–	N	N	N	–
DIC	?↑	±	±↑	↑	↑	+	↓	?↓	?↓	?+

DIC = disseminated intravascular coagulation. N = normal; RBC = red blood cell.
? = often; ± = variable; ↑ = increased; ↓ = decreased; + = present.

to rule out the possibility of swallowed maternal blood. The prothrombin time is greatly prolonged, but the platelet count is normal (in contrast to disseminated intravascular coagulation). See Table 20–1 for comparison of hemorrhagic disease and disseminated intravascular coagulation.

MANAGEMENT

Prevention by routine administration of 0.5 to 1.0 mg of vitamin K (usually vitamin K_1) is desirable. Large doses of water-soluble vitamin K analogues were associated in the past with hyperbilirubinemia secondary to hemolysis of red cells. Active bleeding may be treated with 1 to 2 mg of vitamin K given intravenously. If bleeding is severe, transfusion with fresh whole blood (or fresh-frozen plasma with packed cells) may be necessary to restore blood volume and provide clotting factors.

SUMMARY

Hemorrhagic disease of the newborn is easily prevented. Vitamin K should be given routinely to all infants. The most common feature is bleeding on the second or third day of life, usually from the gut.

HYPERVISCOSITY SYNDROME

INTRODUCTION AND INCIDENCE

Hyperviscosity in the newborn infant is almost always associated with a high venous hematocrit value. Undoubtedly, considerable variation exists, but the incidence may be as high as 5% of all term infants (in Denver, which is 1 mile above sea level). In certain subpopulations (e.g., infants who are small for gestational age), the incidence is even higher. Alternative terms that have been used are plethora, polycythemia, and erythrocythemia.

ETIOLOGY

Many factors affect viscosity in the adult, but in the neonate, hematocrit value is the single most important factor, although temperature may also play a role. There is a linear increase in viscosity with increasing hematocrit value up to about 65% (venous), but a sharp increase occurs after this value.

Elevated hematocrit levels (and hence hyperviscosity) are seen with conditions predisposing to chronic hypoxia, which may also result in intrauterine growth retardation. In addition, an excessive transfer of blood from the placenta to the baby (placental transfusion) or between twins (twin-twin transfusion or parabiotic syndrome) may produce high hematocrit values. Infants with Down's syndrome and those of diabetic mothers may also be predisposed to high hematocrit and/or viscosity levels. Hyperviscosity has also been described with neonatal thyrotoxicosis.

DIAGNOSIS

In addition to a plethoric appearance, five groups of associated clinical features exist.

CYANOSIS. It may be severe enough to cause difficulty in distinguishing it from cyanotic congenital heart disease. Acrocyanosis (peripheral cyanosis) may also occur after 4 hours of age, despite adequate warming.

RESPIRATORY SIGNS. Both tachypnea and dyspnea have been reported, presumably because of decreased pulmonary perfusion. Chest x-ray study may show findings similar to those of retained lung fluid syndrome.

CENTRAL NERVOUS SYSTEM SIGNS. These are primarily jitteriness or lethargy (possibly with truncal hypotonia), but seizures and apneic spells may occur.

JAUNDICE. Because of the increased number of red blood cells, proportionally more red cell destruction and release of bilirubin may occur. This situation is particularly likely to cause problems if the baby is born prematurely (preterm).

NECROTIZING ENTEROCOLITIS. Infants who are small for gestational age and have associated hyperviscosity have been noted to develop necrotizing enterocolitis more frequently (see also Chapter 18).

The diagnosis can be confirmed by doing a microhematocrit determination on a warm heel-stick sample (cold heel samples can give erroneously high values). If the peripheral hematocrit value is higher than 70%, a venous sample should be obtained, and if the value is higher than 65%, the baby may be classified as having the high-hematocrit syndrome. For accurate characterization of this phenomenon as hyperviscosity syndrome, a viscosity study is necessary. Rapid changes occur in the first several hours after birth, and the hematocrit value may be considerably higher at 4 to 6 hours than at 24 hours after birth.

MANAGEMENT

After the diagnosis is established, a decision has to be made about treatment. If the baby is asymptomatic (a high hematocrit value detected on routine evaluation), active intervention may not be necessary. If the baby is symptomatic, it is usually considered wise to perform either phlebotomy with colloid (albumin) infusion or a partial exchange transfusion with plasma. Despite numerous recent investigations, it is still not clear if active intervention is needed in all cases. Some follow-up studies suggest that neurologic abnormalities are more common among nonexchanged asymptomatic infants, but others question whether differences exist even in symptomatic infants. Recent evidence supports the idea that decreased cerebral blood flow is secondary to increased arterial oxygen content rather than hyperviscosity.

If the decision is made to perform phlebotomy or partial exchange, one usually plans to decrease the hematocrit 10 to 15% (4 to 5 g/dl of hemoglobin). For a partial exchange transfusion with plasma, one may use the following formula to approximate the volume to be exchanged:

$$\text{Exchange volume (ml)} = \frac{\text{wt (kg)} \times 80 \times \text{desired fall in hematocrit}}{\text{hematocrit m}}$$

where 80 is the approximate blood volume in milliliters per kilogram and hematocrit m is the mean of initial and desired hematocrit.

SUMMARY

Hyperviscosity is associated with a high hematocrit level and is most commonly seen after chronic intrauterine hypoxia or excessive transfer of blood from the placenta. Clinical presentations may include cyanosis, respiratory difficulty, jitteriness, lethargy, jaundice, and abdominal distension. A venous hematocrit level of greater than 65% is diagnostic and can be treated with a partial exchange transfusion using plasma.

Two other problems that occur in the early neonatal period also deserve mention.

FETOMATERNAL HEMORRHAGE

Although the fetal and maternal circulations are considered to be separate in the placenta, a few fetal cells usually pass into the maternal circulation. If large numbers of fetal cells cross over to the maternal circulation, a profound anemia with resultant shock may occur in the neonate (see Chapter 24, under Neonatal Emergencies). If large numbers of cells pass chronically, the anemia may produce heart failure and result in hydrops fetalis. When a baby is born with anemia or hydrops, the possibility of fetomaternal hemorrhage should be considered. Before delivery, one may suspect fetomaternal hemorrhage in the presence of third trimester bleeding, decreased fetal movement, or when the uterus and its contents have been subjected to trauma. Diagnosis is by evaluation of maternal blood, looking for fetal cells (the Kleihauer-Betke technique). An estimate of the amount of blood lost by the fetus is derived by multiplying the percentage of fetal cells in maternal blood by 50 ml. Alpha-fetoprotein levels may also be valuable in detecting fetomaternal hemorrhage.

DISORDERED COAGULATION

Several circumstances suggest abnormal coagulation. Disseminated intravascular coagulation may produce a picture of bleeding and is described in Chapter 24 (Neonatal Emergencies section). Most neonates have a hypercoagulable state, but this may be very pronounced and may lead to thrombotic episodes in the presence of a severe deficiency of protein C. When thrombosis occurs, venous hematocrit level might be elevated, but a protein C level should be determined.

For further discussion of hemorrhage in the newborn with the physiology of normal hemostasis, see Pramanik, 1992.

BIBLIOGRAPHY

Anemia of Prematurity

Stockman, J. A. III, and Oski, F. A.: RBC values in low-birth-weight infants during the first seven weeks of life. *Am. J. Dis. Child.* 1980, 134:945–946.

Blank, J. P., Sheagren, T. G., Vajaria, J., et al.: The role of RBC transfusion in the premature infant. *Am. J. Dis. Child.* 1984, 138:831–833.

Dickerman, J. D.: Anemia in the newborn infant. *Pediatr. Rev.* 1984, 6:131–138.

Stockman, J. A. III, and Clark, D. A.: Weight gain: A response to transfusion in selected preterm infants. *Am. J. Dis. Child.* 1984, 138:828–830.

Dallman, P. R.: Anemia of prematurity: The prospects for avoiding blood transfusions by treatment with recombinant human erythropoietin. *Adv. Pediatr.* 1993, 40:385–403.

Shannon, K.: Recombinant erythropoietin in anemia of prematurity: Five years later. *Pediatrics* 1993, 92:614–617.

Hemorrhagic Disease of the Newborn

Lane, P. A., Hathaway, W. E., Githens, J. H., et al.: Fatal intracranial hemorrhage in a normal infant secondary to vitamin K deficiency. *Pediatrics* 1983, 72:562–564.

O'Connor, M. E., Livingstone, D. S., Hannah, J., and Wilkins, D.: Vitamin K deficiency and breast feeding. *Am. J. Dis. Child.* 1983, 137:601–602.

Verity, C. M., Carswell, F., and Scott, G. L.: Vitamin K deficiency causing infantile intracranial haemorrhage after the neonatal period. *Lancet* 1983, 1:1439–1440.

McNinch, A. W., and Tripp, J. H.: Haemorrhagic disease of the newborn in the British Isles: Two year prospective study. *B.M.J.* 1991, 303:1105–1109.

Ekelund, H., Finnstrom, O., Gunnarskog, J., et al.: Administration of vitamin K to newborn infants and childhood cancer. *B.M.J.* 1993, 307:89–91.

Klebanoff, M. A., Reed, J. S., Mitts, J. L. and Shiona, P. H.: The risk of childhood cancer after neonatal exposure to vitamin K. *N. Engl. J. Med.* 1993, 329:905–908.

Hyperviscosity Syndrome

Bussman, Y. L., Tillman, M. L., and Pagliara, A. S.: Neonatal thyrotoxicosis associated with hyperviscosity syndrome. *J. Pediatr.* 1977, 90:266.

Shohat, M., Merlob, P., and Reisner, S. H.: Neonatal polycythemia: I. Early diagnosis and incidence relating to time of sampling. *Pediatrics* 1984, 73:7–10.

Oh, W.: Neonatal polycythemia and hyperviscosity. *Pediatr. Clin. North Am.* 1986, 33:523–532.

Black, V. D.: Neonatal hyperviscosity syndromes. *Curr. Probl. Pediatr.* 1987, 17:73–130.

Norman, M., Fagrell, B., and Herin, P.: Skin microcirculation in neonatal polycythaemia and effects of hemodilution: Interaction between haematocrit, vasomotor activity and perfusion. *Acta Paediatr. Int. J. Paediatr.* 1993, 82:672–677.

Fetomaternal Hemorrhage

Lachman, E., Hingley, S. M., Bates, G., et al.: Detection and measurement of fetomaternal haemorrhage: serum alpha-fetoprotein and the Kleihauer technique. *B.M.J.* 1977, 1:1372.

Fay, R. A.: Feto-maternal haemorrhage as a cause of fetal morbidity and mortality. *Br. J. Obstet. Gynaecol.* 1983, 90:443–446.

Elliott, J. P.: Massive fetomaternal hemorrhage treated by intravascular transfusion. *Obstet. Gynecol.* 1991, 78:520–523.

Marions, L., and Thomassen, P.: Six cases of massive feto-maternal bleeding causing intrauterine fetal death. *Acta Obstet. Gynecol. Scand.* 1991, 70:85–88.

Disordered Coagulation

Manco-Johnson, M. J., Abshire, T. C., Jacobson, J. L., and Marler, R. A.: Severe neonatal protein C deficiency: Prevalence and thrombotic risk. *J. Pediatr.* 1991, 119:793–798.

Pramanik, A. K.: Bleeding disorders in neonates. *Pediatr. Rev.* 1992, 13:163–173.

21
DRUGS AND THE FETUS AND NEONATE

EFFECTS OF TRANSPLACENTAL PASSAGE

Before considering specific aspects of the effects of drugs on the fetus, one should take a moment to consider the factors that affect placental transfer of a drug. These are as follows:

1. Lipid solubility and degree of ionization
2. Protein binding
3. Molecular weight
4. Placental blood flow
5. Placental maturation
6. Placental metabolism of drugs

It is quite apparent from considering the variety of factors that affect placental transfer that this is not a simple process. Because of this, some of the information on pharmacokinetics of a given drug is noticeably deficient. An attempt will be made to summarize the effects on the fetus.

TERATOGENIC EFFECTS

Although it had long been realized that drugs given to the mother might produce abnormalities of the fetus as a result of alterations in embryogenesis, it was not until the so-called thalidomide disaster in the very early 1960s that attention was focused on this problem (Taussig, 1962). Thalidomide had been considered a very safe sedative or hypnotic, but the appearance of a constellation of defects, with limb-reduction deformities (phocomelia) most prominent, resulted in a sweeping reappraisal of all drugs used in pregnancy. It became apparent that certain animal studies alone were not enough to determine the toxicity (or potential toxicity) of a given drug. On the other hand, certain drugs, when given to animal models, produce deformity with considerable ease. Because of this effect, each drug must be carefully evaluated individually. In recent years, the new subspecialty of dysmorphology has been emerging. Radiation and other environmental factors (e.g., methyl mercury and polychlorinated biphenyls in fish) need to be considered, as well as drugs.

Many patterns of malformation emerged as distinct entities. One of the first of these was a pattern of malformation observed in offspring of chronic *alcoholic* mothers. The major features associated with the fetal alcohol syndrome are shown in Table 21–1. Recently, it has been suggested that *toluene* may produce an embryopathy that is very similar to that produced by alcohol. *Warfarin* sodium (Coumadin) has also been implicated in the syndrome of chondrodysplasia punctata. This syndrome has external features of flattening of the nose, hypertelorism, and frontal bossing and radiologically shows stippling in cartilaginous areas of the skeleton, especially the epiphyses. Another syndrome has been associated with *hydantoin*, with craniofacial anomalies, nail and digital hypoplasia, prenatal onset of growth deficiency, and mental deficiency as external features. *Trimethadione* has been associated with V-shaped eyebrows, epicanthus, low-set ears, palatal anomaly, irregular teeth, speech difficulty, and developmental delay. The frequency of problems (87% in one review) suggests that trimethadione and related drugs should be avoided during pregnancy. Yet another antiepileptic drug, namely *valproic acid*, has been implicated in the production of birth defects. An increased incidence of several malformations, including spina bifida, tracheomalacia, genital anomalies, and congenital heart defects, has been observed. Teratogenesis is also seen with the use of *retinoic acid* preparations used to treat acne. Such examples indicate that there may be critical time periods during which a drug may produce striking anomalies, whereas at other times, minimal or no effect is observed. Unfortunately, embryogenesis, and consequently teratogenesis, occurs at a time when many

TABLE 21-1. PRINCIPAL FEATURES OF THE FETAL ALCOHOL SYNDROME*

Feature	Very Common†	Common‡
CNS Dysfunction		
Intellectual	Mild to moderate mental retardation	
Neurologic	Microcephaly	Poor coordination, hypotonia
Behavioral	Irritability in infancy	Hyperactivity in childhood
Growth Deficiency		
Prenatal	<2 SD for length and weight	
Postnatal	<2 SD for length and weight	Disproportionate decrease in adipose tissue
Facial Characteristics		
Eyes	Short palpebral fissures	
Nose	Hypoplastic philtrum	Short, upturned
Maxilla		Hypoplastic
Mouth	Thinned upper vermilion, retrognathia in infancy	Micrognathia or relative prognathia (in adolescence)

*Adapted from: Clarren, S. K., and Smith, D. W.: The fetal alcohol syndrome. *N. Engl. J. Med.* 1978, 298:1063.
†> 80% of patients.
‡> 50% of patients.
CNS = central nervous system; SD = standard deviation.

women are unaware of their pregnancy and therefore are unable to take steps to discontinue or avoid specific drugs. Antiemetics are probably the most widely used drugs in pregnancy and were investigated carefully in recent years. Bendectin (doxylamine-pyridoxine combination), in particular, seemed to be exonerated, but despite this, it was removed from the market by the manufacturer because of legal claims to the contrary. Although it is unlikely that antiemetics cause congenital abnormalities in most pregnancies, it is possible that in some cases, there is a genetic predisposition that causes teratogenesis. Considerable concern was generated by the association of congenital malformations of babies born to fathers exposed to a defoliant named Agent Orange, used in the Vietnam war. The association is now considered somewhat tenuous.

OTHER HARMFUL EFFECTS

Some of the antimicrobial agents have produced classic problems in the fetus and newborn. Long-acting *sulfonamide* drugs, for example, compete for albumin-binding sites and may consequently displace bilirubin from those binding sites, producing bilirubin toxicity (kernicterus) at lower levels of bilirubin than are normally considered toxic. *Tetracyclines* may interfere with growth or may result in staining of the teeth. *Smoking*, probably as a result of the release of carbon monoxide, results in some degree of fetal growth retardation, which seems to be more severe in those who are heavy smokers. *Phenytoin* can possibly result in a hemorrhagic tendency in the newborn, perhaps as a result of its effect on folic acid metabolism. This problem seems to be treatable with vitamin K. *Aspirin* taken within 2 weeks of delivery may affect coagulation. The hypoglycemic agent *chlorpropamide* has been associated with hypoglycemia in the neonate. *Antithyroid drugs*, including radioactive iodine, may ablate the fetal (and hence neonatal) thyroid. *Reserpine* given to the mother may result in neonatal nasal stuffiness. Perhaps more alarming than all of these (in which the effect of a drug during the pregnancy is observed in the neonatal period) is the association of vaginal cancer in adolescent girls whose mothers had received *diethylstilbestrol* in early pregnancy. Those drugs that may still be used in mothers that have effects on the fetus and neonate are listed in Table 21–2. Drugs of addiction form a special category and are considered later in this chapter under Problems of the Neonate (see p. 252).

NONPROVEN ASSOCIATION

Although it is obvious that each drug has to be considered carefully, it is nevertheless tempting to associate abnormalities with drugs that may have been ingested during the pregnancy. If the drug is one commonly ingested, then an abnormality is more likely to be linked with it. On this basis, it was felt several years ago that *antihistamine drugs* were very likely teratogens. Unfortunately, because of the problem of vomiting in early pregnancy, a great many antihistamines are used to prevent vomiting, and the association with any given anomaly is not clear at this time. Similarly, in an era when diuretics of the *thiazide group*

TABLE 21-2. COMMON DRUGS (AVAILABLE TO BE GIVEN TO THE MOTHER DURING PREGNANCY) THAT MAY HAVE DELETERIOUS EFFECTS ON THE FETUS AND NEWBORN

Pharmacologic Agent	Effect on Fetus or Neonate
Alcohol	Fetal alcohol syndrome (see Table 21-1)
Aspirin	Bleeding (impaired platelet function)
Barbiturates	Withdrawal effects (activates liver enzymes)
Chloramphenicol	Circulatory collapse
Chloroquine	Hemolysis (susceptible individuals)
Diazepam (Valium)	Respiratory depression; withdrawal effects
General anesthetics	Respiratory depression
Iodides (cough medicines)	Goiter
Magnesium sulfate	Respiratory or neuromotor depression
Narcotics	Respiratory depression; withdrawal effects
Oral contraceptives	Limb defects
Phenytoin (Dilantin)	Cleft palate; bleeding ($\downarrow$ vitamin K)
Progestins (Provera)	Heart and genital defects; VATER association
Quinine	Thrombocytopenia
Reserpine	Stuffy nose
Smoking (? nicotine)	Decreased growth; premature delivery (caused by antepartum hemorrhage)
Sulfonamides (long-acting)	Displacement of bilirubin from albumin
Tetracyclines	Decreased growth; staining of teeth
Thiocarbamides (Thiouracil)	Goiter; thyroid suppression
Trimethadione	Embryopathy (see text)
Warfarin (Coumadin)	Embryopathy (see text); bleeding

VATER = vertebral defects, imperforate anus, tracheoesophageal fistula, and radial and renal dysplasia.

were being liberally used, an association with thrombocytopenia in the newborn was made. Subsequently, this was shown to be an unlikely association. More recently, *amphetamines* have been linked with cardiovascular malformations, but this, too, has been strongly disputed. It may be necessary to have a genetic disposition to react to a certain drug. There was recent concern that *caffeine* might be teratogenic, and *diazepam* (Valium) was linked to the production of cleft lip. Further evaluation of these agents shows that it is extremely unlikely that either one of them is implicated in the production of abnormalities.

DRUGS IN LABOR

It is apparent that several drugs given in labor may produce problems of similar if not greater magnitude than those produced by drugs given during pregnancy. When *analgesia* is given at the wrong time with respect to time of delivery, neonatal respiratory depression may result. Similar effects may be observed with *general anesthesia*. Certain agents used for *regional anesthesia*, in particular the amide group of anesthetics, such as lidocaine, mepivacaine, and prilocaine, may result in maternal hypotension and consequent reduction in uteroplacental blood flow. In addition, epidural or paracervical block anesthesia may result in profound neonatal depression. Another agent that may result in neonatal respiratory depression is *diazepam* (Valium). Yet another agent associated with this problem is *magnesium sulfate* given to the mother in preeclamptic toxemia (see Hypermagnesemia section in Chapter 17). *Agents used to induce labor* (oxytocin and prostaglandins) have been associated with hyperbilirubinemia. Whether or not this is a direct effect is debatable because one report showed a difference between the use of oxytocin to augment labor and oxytocin to induce labor. More recent evidence disputes the association.

POTENTIAL BENEFITS

Although it is obvious that the emphasis so far has been on the deleterious effects that drugs may have on the fetus and neonate, there may be some potential benefits from their use. One example is the use of *vitamin K* when given to the mother, which may prevent hemorrhagic disease of the newborn. Although this was an effective means of eliminating the problem, excessive dosages became popular and resulted in more harm than good. Many infants traded their hemorrhagic disease of the newborn for hyperbilirubinemia. Because of this, it is now unusual for vitamin K to be administered to mothers before delivery. Another agent found to be valuable in the neonatal period has been used with effect when given to the mother before delivery. *Phenobarbital* has been used to prevent hyperbilirubinemia in situations in which this problem was anticipated (see also Chapter 10). The mechanism of action is probably complicated but includes enzyme induction in the liver. Barbiturates may also exert a protective effect for the brain when given *before* asphyxia (i.e., given to the mother). There are at least two other groups of drugs that may profoundly influence the outcome of pregnancy.

INHIBITORS OF UTERINE ACTIVITY. Suppression of labor with terbutaline, magnesium sulfate, or other tocolytic agents may prevent premature delivery (see Chapter 1) and the problem of prematurity (see Chapter 12).

SURFACTANT INDUCERS. In 1972, Liggins and Howie first described the use of *betamethasone,* administered more than 24 hours before delivery, in reducing the frequency or severity of respiratory distress syndrome. Evidence has continued to accumulate supporting the benefits of this mode of therapy (or of *dexamethasone*) while finding few contraindications. Another agent shown to have a similar effect in the experimental animal (and more recently in humans) is *aminophylline* (or theophylline). *Heroin* may have a similar effect (see Chapter 9 for references).

PROBLEMS OF THE NEONATE

Before some of the specific problems encountered by the neonate are considered it should be emphasized that the pharmacokinetics of a given drug depend on four major factors: (1) absorption, (2) distribution, (3) metabolism, and (4) excretion.

The factors governing absorption are not dissimilar to those affecting placental transfer and include molecular size, blood flow, and the properties of membranes across which the drug must pass. Other limiting factors for the newborn infant are an immature liver, which may take time to "turn on" specific enzyme systems; a limited number of binding sites on albumin, which may mean competition with bilirubin; and a decreased glomerular filtration rate. There is a gradual increase in glomerular filtration rate during the first days of life. During that time, drugs that are excreted via the kidney need not be given as frequently as in the older infant and child. Another problem encountered by the neonate (which differs from those encountered by the fetus) is drugs excreted in breast milk. Although, for the most part, drugs are excreted in small quantities and consequently do not have an adverse effect on the infant, some agents may be potentially harmful. In addition to antithyroid drugs mentioned under the section on Breast-Feeding, other agents that may be harmful are narcotics and analgesics, some oral contraceptives, certain anticoagulants, hypnotics, and tranquilizers (Table 21–3). Other drugs of abuse should also be avoided (e.g., cocaine, amphetamine), and antineoplastic agents (particularly doxorubicin) are also contraindicated. Attention has also been focused on environmental contaminants, e.g., strontium 90, dichlorodiphenyltrichloroethane (DDT), and mercury.

The number of drugs that need to be used in the neonatal period is quite

TABLE 21–3. DRUGS FOUND IN BREAST MILK*

Drugs to Be Avoided
Some anticoagulants (e.g., phenindione, ethyl biscoumacetate)
Antimetabolites
Some cathartics (e.g., phenolphthalein)
Chloramphenicol
Chlorpromazine (and other phenothiazine drugs)
Diazepam
Dihydrotachysterol
Ergot alkaloids
Iodides
Lithium carbonate
Metronidazole
Radioactive drugs (therapeutic use)
Tetracycline
Thiouracil (questionable)

Drugs That Are Usually Safe
Antibiotics (most, not chloramphenicol or tetracycline)
Antidiarrheals
Antihistamines
Aspirin (occasional)
Epinephrine
Heparin
Insulin
Propranolol
Warfarin

Adapted from: Giacoia, G. P., and Catz, C. S.: Drugs and pollutants in breast milk. *Clin. Perinatol.* 1979, 6:181.

small, and the major drugs used are listed in the Minipharmacopeia in Chapter 37. The harmful effects of drugs administered to the mother may obviously be duplicated in the neonate when such effects are observed soon after administration. (For example, sulfonamides and tetracyclines are carefully avoided in the neonatal period.) In addition, it should be emphasized that chloramphenicol has potential toxicity related to its dosage, primarily because chloramphenicol must be metabolized in the body before elimination. Because different infants have different rates of metabolism, it is advisable to know what level of chloramphenicol is circulating in the serum at a given time to avoid the gray baby syndrome (Weiss, 1960). The excretion of theophylline and caffeine (methylxanthines) is markedly different in the neonate, with great variability among babies. Accurate determinations of circulating levels may be needed to avoid toxicity.

Another potential source of problems for the neonate may be the environment. For example, apparently innocuous materials, such as umbilical catheters and containers of blood products, may release plasticizer that can be deposited in neonatal tissues. Cleaning agents (phenolic detergents) have been incriminated in a higher frequency of hyperbilirubinemia. Benzyl alcohol was used as a preservative in a number of preparations administered to neonates and was implicated in deaths from gasping syndrome in very-low-birth-weight infants (Brown et al., 1982, and Gershanik et al., 1982). Inhalant epinephrine, packaged in a way similar to vitamin E, has produced a picture resembling neonatal sepsis, and a new intravenous preparation of vitamin E produced an unusual symptom complex, with several deaths. Constant vigilance is required to prevent the introduction of potentially toxic products into the neonate's world, which is already fraught with danger.

DRUG WITHDRAWAL

In some communities, the drugs of addiction are in widespread use, and it is consequently important to remember the possibility of withdrawal effects on the neonate in the first days of life. Although methadone was introduced to replace heroin in the early 1970s, drug withdrawal in the neonate was not avoided. The effects on the neonate are quite similar with these two agents. The most striking features are a coarse, flapping tremor and irritability, which may be accompanied by muscular rigidity. In addition, vomiting, diarrhea, a high-pitched cry, sneezing, and yawning are often present, and excessive sweating may also be seen. Despite a tendency to increased sucking, these babies may be inefficient feeders. Convulsions are occasionally seen and may be more common with methadone. One interesting observation that resulted from careful study of these babies was that infants born to heroin-addicted mothers rarely developed respiratory distress syndrome, whereas the same cannot be said for those born to methadone-addicted mothers. A similar but less pronounced picture may be observed in withdrawal from chronic barbiturate use. It has been suggested that the onset of such withdrawal is later than that with the narcotic agents. Withdrawal has also been reported with alcohol, diazepam, and possibly amphetamine. The percentage of babies showing withdrawal symptoms seems to vary from one hospital to another but probably represents about 30% of babies born to addicted mothers. Several agents have been used to treat signs of narcotic withdrawal, including phenobarbital, chlorpromazine, paregoric, and diazepam, with paregoric apparently the most effective in narcotic withdrawal. Many of these babies are born small for gestational age, but whether this is caused by poor nutrition or a more direct effect is unclear. The long-term outlook for such infants may depend more on management of the parents than that of the children. In recent years, the possibility of exposure to multiple drugs seems to be increasing in some communities. Such polydrug exposure may lead to difficulties in diagnosis and may interfere with later parent-infant interaction, resulting in a continuum of impairment.

During the past decade, the most widely used drug of abuse (apart from alcohol and tobacco) seems to have been cocaine. Its impact on perinatal health has crossed both socioeconomic and racial lines and has increased enormously the hospital costs for exposed neonates.

It appears safe to conclude that placental dysfunction due to cocaine's vasoconstrictive activity increases risk for intra-uterine growth retardation and prematurity; fetal disruption due to acute cocaine-induced vascular compromise places the fetus at risk for structural anomalies; and neurotoxicity due to cocaine's action at the post synaptic junction places the infant at risk for neurobehavioral abnormalities. (Chasnoff, 1991)

Some of these babies do not display overt signs of withdrawal, and without routine surveillance, their exposure may not be detected in the nursery. Cocaine depresses interactive behavior in babies and limits their ability to organize responses to stimuli. When substance abuse is suspected, urine is frequently sent for toxicology evaluation, but the results may be negative if the substance is not used within 3 days of delivery. Studies using meconium or hair samples have provided positive evidence of abuse when the results of urine testing have been negative.

BIBLIOGRAPHY

Teratogenic Effects

Taussig, H. B.: A study of the German outbreak of phocomelia. The thalidomide syndrome. *J.A.M.A.* 1962, 180:1106.
Apt, L., and Gaffney, W. L.: Ocular teratogens: A commentary. *J. Pediatr.* 1975, 87:844.
Warkany, J.: A warfarin embryopathy? (Commentary) *Am. J. Dis. Child.* 1975, 129:287.
Feldman, G. L., Weaver, D. D., and Lovrien, E. W.: Fetal trimethadione syndrome: Report of an additional family and further delineation of this syndrome. *Am. J. Dis. Child.* 1977, 131:1389.
Committee on Radiology, American Academy of Pediatrics: Radiation of pregnant women. *Pediatrics* 1978, 61:117.
Doering, P. L., and Stewart, R. B.: The extent and character of drug consumption during pregnancy. *J.A.M.A.* 1978, 239:843.
Rothman, K. J., and Louik, C.: Oral contraceptives and birth defects. *N. Engl. J. Med.* 1978, 299:522.
Smithells, R. W.: Drugs, infections, and congenital abnormalities. *Arch. Dis. Child.* 1978, 53:93.

Aarskog, D.: Maternal progestins as a possible cause of hypospadias. *N. Engl. J. Med.* 1979, 300:75.

Spielberg, S. P.: Pharmacogenetics and the fetus (Editorial). *N. Engl. J. Med.* 1982, 307:115–116.

Leeder, J. S., Spielberg, S. P., and MacLeod, S. M.: Bendectin: The wrong way to regulate drug availability *Can. Med. Assoc. J.* 1983, 129:1085–1087.

Lipson, A.: Agent Orange and birth defects. *N. Engl. J. Med.* 1983, 309:491–502.

Erickson, J. D., Mulinare, J., McLain, P. W., et al.: Vietnam veterans' risk for fathering babies with birth defects. *J.A.M.A.* 1984, 252:903–912.

Fein, G. G., Jacobson, J. L., Jacobson, S. W., et al.: Prenatal exposure to polychlorinated biphenyls: Effects on birth size and gestational age. *J. Pediatr.* 1984, 105:315–320.

Jones, K. L.: Fetal alcohol syndrome. *Pediatr. Rev.* 1986, 8:122–126.

Hoyme, H. E.: Teratogenically induced fetal anomalies. *Clin. Perinatol.* 1990, 17:547–567.

D'Souza, S. W., Robertson, I. G., Donnai, D., and Mawer, G.: Fetal phenytoin exposure, hypoplastic nails and jitteriness. *Arch. Dis. Child.* 1991, 66:320–324.

Autti-Ramo, I., Gaily, E., and Granstrom, M.-L.: Dysmorphic features in offspring of alcoholic mothers. *Arch. Dis. Child.* 1992, 67:712–716.

Pearson, M. A., Hoyme, H. E., Seaver, L. H., and Rimsza, M. E.: Toluene embryopathy: Delineation of the phenotype and comparison with fetal alcohol syndrome. *Pediatrics* 1994, 93:211–215.

Other Harmful Effects

Herbst, A. L., Scully, R. E., Robboy, S. J., and Welch, W. R.: Complications of prenatal therapy with diethylstilbestrol. *Pediatrics* 1978, 62(Suppl):1151.

Committee on Drugs, American Academy of Pediatrics: Anticonvulsants and pregnancy. *Pediatrics* 1979, 63:331.

Stuart, M. J., Gross, S. J., Elrad, H., and Graeber, J. E.: Effects of acetylsalicylic-acid ingestion on maternal and neonatal hemostasis. *N. Engl. J. Med.* 1982, 307:909–912.

Neiburg, P., Marks, J. S., McLaren, N. M., and Remington, P. L.: Fetal tobacco syndrome. *J.A.M.A.* 1985, 253:2998–2999.

Berlin, C. M. Jr.: Effects of drugs on the fetus. *Pediatr. Rev.* 1991, 12:282–287.

Donnenfeld, A. E., Pulkkinen, A., Palomaki, G. E., et al.: Simultaneous fetal and maternal cotinine levels in pregnant women smokers. *Am. J. Obstet. Gynecol.* 1993, 168:781–782.

Nonproven Association

Merenstein, G. B., O'Loughlin, E. P., and Plunkett, D. C.: Effects of maternal thiazides on platelet counts of newborn infants. *J. Pediatr.* 1970, 76:766.

Briggs, G. G., Samson, J. H., and Crawford, D. J.: Lack of abnormalities in a newborn exposed to amphetamine during gestation. *Am. J. Dis. Child.* 1975, 129:249.

Linn, S., Solomon, S. C., Monson, R. R., et al.: No association between coffee consumption and adverse outcomes of pregnancy. *N. Engl. J. Med.* 1982, 306:141–154.

Kurppa, K., Holmberg, P. C., Kuosma, E., and Saxen, L.: Coffee consumption during pregnancy and selected congenital malformations: A nationwide case-control study. *Am. J. Public Health* 1983, 73:1397–1399.

Rosenberg, L., Mitchell, A. A., Parsells, J. L., et al.: Lack of relation of oral clefts to diazepam use during pregnancy. *N. Engl. J. Med.* 1983, 309:1282–1285.

Drugs in Labor

Morishima, H. O., Heymann, M. A., Rudolph, A. M., and Barrett, C. T.: Toxicity of lidocaine in the fetal and newborn infant lamb and its relationship to asphyxia. *Am. J. Obstet. Gynecol.* 1972, 112:72.

Yeh, S. Y., Paul, R. H., Cordero, L., and Hon, E. H.: A study of diazepam during labor. *Obstet. Gynecol.* 1974, 43:363.

Committee on Drugs, American Academy of Pediatrics: Effect of medication during labor and delivery on infant outcome. *Pediatrics* 1978, 62:403.

Johnson, J. D., Aldrich, M., Angelus, P., et al.: Oxytocin and neonatal hyperbilirubinemia: Studies of bilirubin production. *Am. J. Dis. Child.* 1984, 138:1047–1050.

Potential Benefits

Trolls, D.: Decrease of total serum-bilirubin concentration in newborn infants after pheno-barbitone treatment. *Lancet* 1968, ii:705.

Brann, A. W., and Montalvo, J. M.: Barbiturates and asphyxia. *Pediatr. Clin. North Am.* 1970, 17:851–863.

Liggins, G. C., and Howie, R. N.: A controlled trial of antepartum glucocorticoid treatment for prevention of the respiratory distress syndrome in premature infants. *Pediatrics* 1972, 50:515.

Leonardi, M. R., and Hankins, G. D. V.: What's new in tocolytics. *Clin. Perinatol.* 1992, 19:367–384.

Problems of the Neonate

Weiss, C. F., Glazko, A. J., and Weston, J. K.: Chloramphenicol in the newborn infant: A physiologic explanation of its toxicity when given in excessive doses. *N. Engl. J. Med.* 1960, 262:787.

Hillman, L. S., Goodwin, S. L., and Sherman, W. R.: Identification and measurement of plasticizer in neonatal tissues after umbilical catheters and blood products. *N. Engl. J. Med.* 1975, 292:381.

Aranda, J. V., and Turmen, T.: Methylxanthines in apnea of prematurity. *Clin. Perinatol.* 1979, 6:87.

Committees on Fetus and Newborn and on Drugs, American Academy of Pediatrics: Benzyl alcohol: Toxic agent in neonatal units. *Pediatrics* 1983, 72:356–358.

Ernst, J. A., Williams, J. M., Glick, M. R., and Lemons, J. A.: Osmolality of substances used in the intensive care nursery. *Pediatrics* 1983, 72:347–352.

Solomon, S. L., Wallace, E. M., Ford-Jones, E. L., et al.: Medication errors with inhalant epinephrine mimicking an epidemic of neonatal sepsis. *N. Engl. J. Med.* 1984, 310: 166–170.

Lorch, V., Murphy, M. D., Hoersten, L. R., et al.: Unusual syndrome among premature infants: Association with a new intravenous vitamin E product. *Pediatrics* 1985, 75: 598–602.

Committee on Drugs, American Academy of Pediatrics: The transfer of drugs and other chemicals into human milk. *Pediatrics*, 1994, 93:137–150.

Drug Withdrawal

Pierog, S., Chandavasu, O., and Wexler, I.: Withdrawal symptoms in infants with fetal alcohol syndrome. *J. Pediatr.* 1977, 90:630.

Rementeria, J. L., and Bhatt, K.: Withdrawal symptoms in neonates from intrauterine exposure to diazepam. *J. Pediatr.* 1977, 90:123.

Eriksson, M., Larsson, G., Windbladh, B., and Zetterstrom, R.: The influence of amphetamine addiction on pregnancy and the newborn infant. *Acta Paediatr.* 1978, 67:95.

Brown, W. J., Buist, N. R. M., Gipson, H. T., et al.: Fatal benzyl alcohol poisoning in a neonatal intensive care unit (Letter). *Lancet* 1982, 1:1250.

Gershanik, J., Boecler, B., Ensley, H., et al.: The gasping syndrome and benzyl alcohol poisoning. *N. Engl. J. Med.* 1982, 307:1384–1388.

Sweet, A. Y.: Narcotic withdrawal syndrome in the newborn. *Pediatr. Rev.* 1982, 3:285–291.

Committee on Drugs, American Academy of Pediatrics: Neonatal drug withdrawal. *Pediatrics* 1983, 72:895–902.

Chasnoff, I. J.: Cocaine and pregnancy: Clinical and methodologic issues. *Clin. Perinatol.* 1991, 18:113–123.

Doberczak, T. M., Kandall, S. R., and Wilets, I.: Neonatal opiate abstinence syndrome in term and preterm infants. *J. Pediatr.* 1991, 118:933–937.

McCalla, S., Minkoff, H. L., Feldman, J., et al.: The biologic and social consequences of perinatal cocaine use in an inner-city population: Results of an anonymous cross-sectional study. *Am. J. Obstet. Gynecol.* 1991, 164:625–630.

Phibbs, C. S., Bateman, D. A., and Schwartz, R. M.: The neonatal costs of maternal cocaine use. *J.A.M.A.* 1991, 266:1521–1526.

Chasnoff, I. J., Griffith, D. R., Freier, C., and Murray, J.: Cocaine/polydrug use in pregnancy: Two year follow-up. *Pediatrics* 1992, 89:284–289.

Ostrea, E. M., Jr., Romero, A., and Yeed, H.: Adaptation of the meconium drug test for mass screening. *J. Pediatr.* 1993, 122:152–154.

Vega, W. A., Kolody, B., Hwang, J., and Noble, A.: Prevalence and magnitude of perinatal substance exposures in California. *N. Engl. J. Med.* 1993, 329:850–854.

22

NEONATAL AND PERINATAL MORTALITY

DEFINITIONS

The following definitions are based on the recommendations for terminology of a World Health Organization Working Party (1975). Births and perinatal deaths to be included in statistics should only include those fetuses and infants who are delivered weighing 500 g or more. Those weighing less than 500 g are considered to be abortuses, although recently many babies less than this weight have survived. In the absence of a measured birth weight, a body length of 25 cm is considered to be equivalent to 500 g. When neither weight nor length is available, a gestational age of 22 weeks is considered to be equivalent to 500 g.

LIFE AT BIRTH: Life is considered to be present at birth when the infant breathes or shows any other evidence of life, such as beating of the heart, pulsation of the umbilical cord, or definite movement of the voluntary muscles.

STILLBIRTH: The process of birth when no evidence of life exists at or after birth.

EARLY NEONATAL DEATH: Death of a liveborn infant during the first 7 completed days of life.

LATE NEONATAL DEATH: Death of a liveborn infant after 7 but before 28 completed days of life.

MORTALITY RATES: Stillbirth (or fetal death) rate is defined as the number of stillborn infants/1000 total births (stillborn plus live births). *Early neonatal mortality rate* is defined as the number of early neonatal deaths/1000 live births. *Perinatal mortality rate* is defined as the number of stillborn infants and early neonatal deaths/1000 total births (stillbirths plus live births). It has been suggested that for international comparison, a *standard* rate should be applied, which calls for inclusion of infants weighing 1000 g and over. If birth weight is not known, a body length (crown to heel) of 35 cm or a gestational age of 28 completed weeks should be taken as equivalent to 1000-g birth weight. It is hoped that by use of this standard rate, a truer degree of comparability will be obtained.

INFANT MORTALITY RATE: This is defined as the number of deaths during the first year per 1000 live births. This figure may be divided into neonatal deaths and postneonatal deaths. At present, it may be important to look at infant deaths rather than to concentrate on neonatal deaths because many very-low-birth-weight infants (and some term infants) may be kept alive for longer than 28 days but may die before discharge from the nursery. A more realistic approach may be to think of survival rather than mortality. For further details, see Appendix 9.

RELATION TO LOW-BIRTH-WEIGHT RATE

Low birth weight is defined as less than 2500 g and includes weights over 500 g. Although not always a true reflection of prematurity or immaturity, the low-birth-weight rate inevitably is reflected in the perinatal mortality. Experience throughout the world indicates that higher neonatal mortality is associated with increased numbers of low-birth-weight infants, whether or not such low-birth-weight babies are born appropriate or small for gestational age. It therefore becomes apparent that any measure that contributes to a decrease in the low-birth-weight rate will result in an overall decrease in the neonatal and perinatal mortality. As an example, in Sweden and Japan, two countries with extremely low neonatal and perinatal mortality rates, the low-birth-weight rates were 4.1 and 5.3, respectively, in the early 1970s, at a time when the rates in the United States were approximately 7 for all races and 13 in the black population. These rates have not changed substantially in the United States during the past two decades.

FACTORS INFLUENCING PERINATAL MORTALITY

A great many factors influence the outcome of any given pregnancy. It is not possible to cover all aspects adequately in a discussion of this kind. Nevertheless, it seems appropriate to mention some of the more important variables.

PREVIOUS OBSTETRIC LOSS. Whenever a previous pregnancy has resulted in either spontaneous abortion, stillbirth, or early neonatal death, the chances of one of these events happening in a subsequent pregnancy are greatly increased.

SOCIOECONOMIC FACTORS. This is not a clearly defined association, but one that is undoubtedly present. The low socioeconomic groups demonstrate higher neonatal and perinatal mortality rates.

NUTRITIONAL INFLUENCE. This factor has only recently received the attention it deserves and is most likely intimately involved with the socioeconomic category. Prepregnancy nutrition as well as nutrition during pregnancy seems to affect the outcome.

MATERNAL AGE. Both teenage pregnancy and pregnancy in women later in the childbearing period are associated with increased perinatal mortality.

UNMARRIED STATE. The preceding three factors appear to be implicated in the known association of high rates of low-birth-weight infants with the unmarried state. Certain nonspecific stress factors may also play a role.

LIBERAL ABORTION LAWS. By reducing the number of unwanted and high-risk pregnancies (in some of the categories already stated), some countries have noted improvement in neonatal and perinatal mortality, although other factors may have been working concomitantly.

MATERNAL MEDICAL PROBLEMS. Disorders such as diabetes mellitus, cardiovascular disease, chronic pulmonary disease, and renal disease, are all associated with a greater risk to the pregnancy.

OBSTETRIC PROBLEMS. Both stillbirths and neonatal deaths are affected by such disorders as toxemia, postterm delivery, placenta previa, abruptio placentae, and prolapsed cord.

MULTIPLE PREGNANCY. The incidence of premature delivery and hence low-birth-weight babies is increased with multiple pregnancy, and there is therefore the inevitable rise in perinatal mortality.

SPECIFIC EFFECTS ON THE FETUS. Traumatic delivery is likely to result in asphyxia, infection may result in premature (preterm) delivery in an infant with a compromised defense mechanism, and congenital malformations may precipitate early delivery or be incompatible with survival.

CAUSES OF NEONATAL DEATH

Currently, a limited number of problems commonly account for neonatal death. Extreme prematurity (immaturity) usually implies a neonate weighing less than 750 g and/or less than 26 weeks' gestation and is associated with a high mortality risk, although survival has increased considerably in recent years. The respiratory distress syndrome (hyaline membrane disease) accounted for a further sizable proportion of deaths of somewhat larger and more mature babies, who nevertheless are usually less than 32 weeks' gestation, but with the availability of exogenous surfactant, deaths from respiratory distress syndrome are uncommon. Intraventricular hemorrhage accounts for a large number of deaths in this category, although this number has been decreasing as we learn about ways to prevent it. Neonatal infection continues to play a significant role in neonatal deaths and may be due to pneumonia, sepsis, meningitis, or viral syndromes. Approximately 20 to 30% of neonatal deaths are accounted for by congenital malformations that are incompatible with life, and this percentage may be increasing as other causes decrease. Asphyxia continues to be implicated in a number of intrapartum or early neonatal deaths.

FACTORS CONTRIBUTING TO THE DECLINE IN PERINATAL MORTALITY

As stated earlier, anything that contributes to a lowering of the low-birth-weight rate is likely to have a similar effect on perinatal mortality. The following factors contribute to such a decline.

REGIONALIZATION. Particularly when infants are transported to a center in utero, the chances that the infant will receive appropriate specialized care are improved.

FETAL MONITORING. In many centers, the use of electronic fetal heart rate monitoring, in association with fetal scalp blood sampling, has had a demonstrable impact on neonatal and perinatal deaths, particularly in circumstances that might formerly have resulted in intrapartum deaths. Although fetal monitoring is clearly valuable in high-risk pregnancies, there is still debate about the cost-benefit ratio in low-risk pregnancies.

EARLY DELIVERY WITH PREMATURE (PROLONGED) RUPTURE OF MEMBRANES. Because of the known increase in infection rates after prolonged rupture of the membranes beyond 24 hours (and certainly after 36 hours), there has been increasing emphasis in recent years on delivery of babies under such circumstances, particularly from 34 weeks' gestation onward. This trend has probably diminished the number of neonatal infections, with a subsequent reduction in neonatal mortality, although some centers prefer expectant management.

DECLINE IN BREECH DELIVERY. Although considerable controversy remains about the best method for delivering a baby who is in the breech presentation, many obstetricians have been persuaded that breech delivery is more likely to be traumatic, particularly in the primigravida or if the baby is of low birth weight. Both preterm and primigravid breech presentations are frequently delivered by cesarean section today, but by careful selection, vaginal delivery may frequently carry no higher risk (see Chapter 1).

PREVENTION AND TREATMENT OF THE RESPIRATORY DISTRESS SYNDROME. The use of prenatal corticosteroids to enhance the production and utilization of surfactant, in conjunction with the measures currently available in most neonatal intensive care units (continuous positive airway pressure, assisted ventilation, and exogenous surfactant), has resulted in a declining mortality associated with this problem. Respiratory distress syndrome was once the leading cause of death in newborn infants, but it is now becoming just one of a number of diverse problems causing death (see Chapter 9).

PREVENTION OF MECONIUM ASPIRATION SYNDROME. The aggressive approach to the baby born through meconium-stained amniotic fluid and the prevention of postterm delivery have undoubtedly resulted in a decline in the number of deaths from meconium aspiration syndrome in some areas (see Chapter 9). However, not all aspiration can be prevented.

PREVENTION OF ERYTHROBLASTOSIS FETALIS. One of the most remarkable changes in the past 20 years is the dramatic decline in the number of babies dying as the result of rhesus incompatibility. This is now an extremely rare cause of perinatal mortality (see Chapter 10).

SUPPRESSION OF PREMATURE LABOR. Although it is not always possible (or advisable) to suppress labor in the absence of ruptured membranes, β-sympathomimetic drugs and other tocolytic agents have undoubtedly contributed to prolongation of pregnancy in many instances. More recent studies have helped to define the groups of women who may respond to such tocolysis (see also Chapter 1).

MANAGEMENT OF PERSISTENT PULMONARY HYPERTENSION. During the late 1980s and early 1990s, many larger infants (> 2 kg) with severe persistent pulmonary hypertension (see Chapter 9) were treated with extracorporeal membrane oxygenation. Undoubtedly, many babies survived because of treatment with extracorporeal membrane oxygenation, although it is possible that some would have survived without it. At present, additional strategies are the use of exogenous surfactant and high-frequency ventilation, and nitric oxide therapy is rapidly emerging as an alternative therapy.

FUTURE IMPROVEMENT

Although progress in obstetrics and pediatrics continues, several areas continue to deserve attention. If these important aspects are dealt with, it seems likely that perinatal mortality could be reduced to a so-called irreducible minimum.

FAMILY PLANNING

It was mentioned earlier that teenage pregnancies result in both a higher low-birth-weight rate and a higher perinatal mortality. It seems eminently reasonable that if, in fact, pregnancies could be deferred until the mother were in her 20s, a considerable reduction in both of these rates could be achieved. Because of social and ideologic considerations, this phenomenon already seems to have taken place to a considerable extent in China. Although the information is hard to verify outside the major cities, it appears that teenage pregnancy is almost unheard of, and that the low-birth-weight rate and perinatal mortality are also now extremely low in that country. This is also true of Japan.

ENCOURAGING BETTER NUTRITION

Better nutrition has already been mentioned as an important factor in neonatal and perinatal mortality. For instance, in Guatemala, when diets were supplemented with two different forms of caloric supplementation, the birth weights of the offspring increased. There is a distinct impression that differences in birth weight between different ethnic groups may be much smaller than currently stated. The primary differential may reside in the adequacy of the diet provided to the pregnant mother. The marked differences in infant mortality between the designations "white" and "nonwhite" in the United States are almost certainly the result of socioeconomic factors, with nutrition playing a very important part.

ENCOURAGING FETAL GROWTH

The problem of low birth weight occurs not only in the premature infant (preterm) but also in the infant who has intrauterine growth retardation. Another term for this is fetal malnutrition, or the placental insufficiency syndrome (see pp. 208 to 212). When intrauterine growth retardation has been identified, it would seem more logical to improve the intrauterine environment (if possible) rather than deciding that delivery to an extrauterine existence was preferable. To improve the supply of substrate for growth, infusions of glucose and lipid have been given to mothers, with positive effects on fetal growth. Another technique reported to have had some success is intermittent abdominal decompression. This technique appears to improve the perfusion of the uterus during such decompressions. The use of agents that would selectively improve uterine blood flow is another promising approach.

DISCOURAGING SMOKING

As noted earlier (p. 248), smoking increases the low-birth-weight rate, probably by causing more intrauterine growth retardation. It may also be implicated in a higher frequency of pregnancy complications. This seems to be particularly true of teenage pregnancies. After birth, children of smokers are more prone to respiratory illness in the first year, presumably as a result of passive smoking. For all these reasons, smoking is to be discouraged in the pregnant woman.

PREVENTING PREMATURITY

Several different approaches show some promise. In particular, the work of Papiernick in France suggests that better understanding of uterine contractions may allow mothers to modify their lifestyle so as to avoid contractions (see Cole, 1985). Social conditions will need to change in several ways in the United States if advances are to be made (e.g., longer work leave, provision of home help).

The multiplicity of factors contributing to fetal and neonatal mortality makes this subject one that is difficult to summarize. Perhaps the best closing message is the hope, "Every baby a wanted baby, and every baby a healthy baby."

BIBLIOGRAPHY

Alberman, E.: Prospects for better perinatal health. *Lancet* 1980, i:189.
Bauman, K. E., and Anderson, A. E.: Legal abortions and trends in fetal and infant mortality rates in the United States. *Am. J. Obstet. Gynecol.* 1980, 136:194–202.
Garn, S. M., Johnston, M., Ridella, S. A., and Petzold, A. S.: Effect of maternal cigarette smoking on Apgar scores. *Am. J. Dis. Child.* 1981, 135:503–506.
Philip, A. G. S., Little, G. A., Polivy, D. R., and Lucey, J. F.: Neonatal mortality risk for the eighties: The importance of birth weight/gestational age groups. *Pediatrics* 1981, 68:122–130.
Kitchen, W. H., Yu, V. Y. H., Lissenden, J. V., and Bajuk, B.: Collaborative study of very-low-birthweight infants: Techniques of perinatal care and mortality. *Lancet* 1982, i:1454–1455.

Koops, B. L., Morgan, L. J., and Battaglia, F. C.: Neonatal mortality risk in relation to birth weight and gestational age: Update. *J. Pediatr.* 1982, 101:969–977.

Paneth, N., Kiely, J. L., Wallenstein, S., et al.: Newborn intensive care and neonatal mortality in low-birth-weight infants: A population study. *N. Engl. J. Med.* 1982, 307:149–155.

Wallace, H. M., Goldstein, H., and Ericson, A.: Comparison of infant mortality in the United States and Sweden. *Clin. Pediatr.* 1982, 21:156–162.

Williams, R. L., and Chen, P. M.: Identifying the sources of the recent decline in perinatal mortality rates in California. *N. Engl. J. Med.* 1982, 306:207–214.

David, R. J., and Siegel, E.: Decline in neonatal mortality, 1968 to 1977: Better babies or better care? *Pediatrics* 1983, 71:531–540.

Editorial: Inquiries into perinatal and later childhood deaths. *Lancet* 1983, ii:83–84.

Naeye, R. L.: The investigation of perinatal deaths (Editorial). *N. Engl. J. Med.* 1983, 309:611–612.

Prentice, A. M., Watkinson, M., Whitehead, R. G., et al.: Prenatal dietary supplementation of African women and birth-weight. *Lancet* 1983, i:489–491.

Zuckerman, B., Alpert, J. J., Dooling, E., et al.: Neonatal outcome: Is adolescent pregnancy a risk factor? *Pediatrics* 1983, 71:489–493.

Olshan, A. F., Shy, K. K., Luthy, D. A., et al.: Cesarean birth and neonatal mortality in very low birth weight infants. *Obstet. Gynecol.* 1984, 64:267–270.

Cole, C. H.: Prevention of prematurity: Can we do it in America? *Pediatrics* 1985, 76:310–312.

McCormick, M. C.: The contribution of low birth weight to infant mortality and childhood morbidity. *N. Engl. J. Med.* 1985, 312:82–90.

Leon, D. A., Vagero, D., and Otterblad-Olausson, P.: Social class differences in infant mortality in Sweden: Comparison with England and Wales. *B.M.J.* 1992, 305:687–691.

Paz, J. E., Otano, L., Gadow, E. C., and Castilla, E. E.: Previous miscarriage and stillbirth as risk factors for other unfavorable outcomes in the next pregnancy. *Br. J. Obstet. Gynecol.* 1992, 90:808–812.

Phelan, J. P. (ed.): Prevention of Prematurity. *Clin. Perinatol.* 1992, 18:275–487.

Hack, M., and Fanaroff, A.: Outcomes of extremely immature infants—A perinatal dilemma. *N. Engl. J. Med.* 1993, 329:1649–1650.

Wegman, M. E.: Annual summary of vital statistics—1993. *Pediatrics* 1994, 94:792–803 (see also similar summaries published annually).

Philip, A. G. S.: Neonatal mortality: Is further improvement possible? *J. Pediatr.* 1995, 126:427–433.

23
MILESTONES IN NEONATOLOGY

Care of the neonate is constantly being modified, and one occasionally has to be reminded that what we frequently take for granted was not long ago "hot news." The events listed below are intended as a review of some of the more important news items during this time. Because "there is nothing new" in medicine, the dates given below are not necessarily the earliest that a given procedure, technique, or approach was used.

1958

1. Phototherapy reported from England.[1]
2. Second report on careful evaluation of the newborn in the delivery room and a scoring system.[2]
3. Improved survival of premature newborn infants by increasing environmental temperature.[3]
4. Pulsed echo ultrasonographic diagnosis introduced into obstetrics.[4]

1959

1. Reports on infants of diabetic mothers from Scotland and the United States.[5, 6]
2. Cytogenetics starts with first association of chromosomal abnormality with clinical disorder.[7]
3. Surfactant deficiency reported in association with respiratory distress syndrome (hyaline membrane disease).[8]

1960

1. The term *neonatology* is coined.[9]
2. Report of new autosomal trisomy syndrome.[10]
3. Chloramphenicol toxicity (gray baby syndrome) related to dosage.[11]
4. Chronic pulmonary syndrome reported in small premature infants with distinctive x-ray study changes.[12]

1961

1. Attention drawn to fetal malnutrition (intrauterine growth retardation).[13]
2. Relationship of thalidomide to congenital defects recognized.[14]

1962

1. Early diagnosis and treatment of congenital dislocation of the hip joint in the newborn emphasized.[15, 16]

1963

1. Decreased mortality in respiratory distress syndrome with early administration of intravenous glucose and sodium bicarbonate.[17]
2. Intrauterine transfusion of the fetus in hemolytic disease described in New Zealand.[18]
3. Early feeding begun in premature infants.[19, 20]

1964

1. Description of symptomatic neonatal hypoglycemia.[21]
2. Attention drawn to necrotizing enterocolitis in premature infants.[22]

1965

1. Pulmonary hypoperfusion described as basis for pathophysiology of respiratory distress syndrome.[23]
2. Reports of successful use of assisted ventilation to treat respiratory disorders in newborn infants.[24, 25]
3. Suprapubic bladder aspiration described in neonates.[26]
4. Expanded congenital rubella syndrome described.[27]

1966

1. Use of Rh immune globulin (anti-D) to prevent Rh incompatibility.[28, 29]
2. Concept of transitional care nursery described.[30]
3. Prediction of continued development in neonatal intensive care and transfer to regional centers.[31]

1967

1. Birth weight–gestational age classification described.[32]
2. Chronic lung disease following respirator therapy described in United States and England.[33, 34]
3. Use of immunoglobulin M (IgM) to detect chronic intrauterine infection described.[35]
4. Dangers of hyperosmolar solutions producing central nervous system damage cited.[36]

1968

1. Phototherapy used to prevent hyperbilirubinemia of prematurity in United States.[37]
2. Neurologic assessment of gestational age by workers in Paris appears in English.[38]
3. First report of anomalies in infants born to alcoholic mothers in France (reported in French).[39]

1969

1. Continuous positive airway pressure introduced as treatment for respiratory distress syndrome (published in 1971).[40]
2. Microtechniques for blood gases become more generally available.[41]
3. Relevance of early extrauterine nutrition to subsequent brain development in the human newborn stressed.[42, 43]

1970

1. Recognition of electrical hazards in neonatal care.[44]
2. Importance of parent-infant interaction stressed.[45, 46]
3. Use of phenobarbital to reduce hyperbilirubinemia in neonate.[47]
4. Scoring system for gestational age assessment described.[48]
5. Technique for nasojejunal feeding described.[49]

1971

1. Echocardiography introduced for noninvasive assessment of cardiac disease.[50]
2. Description of clinical use of lecithin-to-sphingomyelin ratio on amniotic fluid in predicting respiratory distress syndrome.[51]
3. Hexachlorophene associated with neuropathologic lesions in newborn experimental animals.[52]

4. High-caloric peripheral intravenous alimentation described in premature infants.[53]

5. Causal relationship between elevated p_aO_2 and retrolental fibroplasia emphasized by American Academy of Pediatrics.[54]

1972

1. Use of prenatal corticosteroids (betamethasone) to prevent respiratory distress syndrome described (New Zealand).[55]

2. α-Fetoprotein in amniotic fluid used to predict neural tube defects (Scotland).[56]

3. Transcutaneous measurement of blood pO_2 developed in West Germany.[57]

4. Hexachlorophene use restricted by Food and Drug Administration.[58]

5. Foam stability test (shake test) for rapid assessment of risk of respiratory distress syndrome.[59]

6. Continuous negative chest wall pressure described for respiratory distress syndrome, using negative pressure respirator.[60]

1973

1. Nasal device (prongs) for delivering continuous positive airway pressure described.[61]

2. Device for delivering continuous negative external pressure within an incubator described.[62]

3. Group B streptococci established as new challenge in neonatal infections.[63]

4. Brazelton evaluation of newborn adaptive behavior and responsiveness published.[64]

5. Xanthines introduced for the treatment of apnea.[65]

6. Independent recognition of fetal alcohol syndrome in United States.[66]

1974

1. Aggressive approach to suctioning meconium from airway to prevent meconium aspiration syndrome described.[67, 68]

2. Rediscovery of association between vitamin E deficiency and retrolental fibroplasia.[69]

3. Mass screening program for neonatal hypothyroidism begun in Quebec, Canada.[70]

1975

1. Transillumination of the chest to detect pneumothorax and pneumomediastinum.[71]

2. Computed tomography used to detect neonatal intracranial lesions (e.g., hydrocephalus).[72]

3. First examination by subboard of Neonatal-Perinatal Medicine of the American Board of Pediatrics.

4. Tolazoline used to successfully treat persistent fetal circulation—first report,[73] but may have been successful earlier.[74]

5. Prostaglandin E used to maintain patency of ductus arteriosus in cases of cyanotic congenital heart disease.[75]

1976

1. Transcutaneous supplementation of fatty acids with sunflower seed oil.[76]

2. First report of infantile botulism syndrome.[77]

3. Pharmacologic closure of the ductus arteriosus in preterm infant by prostaglandin inhibition described.[78, 79]

1977

1. Association of *Chlamydia trachomatis* with distinctive pneumonia syndrome in young infants.[80]

2. Report of high incidence of unsuspected intracranial hemorrhage in very-low-birth-weight infants detected by computed tomographic scan.[81]

3. Demonstration of shunting through the ductus arteriosus using "double-site" transcutaneous pO_2 monitoring in Japan (first reported in Japanese).[82]

4. Noninvasive intracranial pressure monitoring using a fiberoptic device reported to be potentially valuable in many clinical situations.[83]

5. Report of miniaturized electrode to measure transcutaneous pCO_2.[84]

1978

1. Treatment of posthemorrhagic hydrocephalus by serial lumbar punctures in a series of infants.[85]

2. Fetoscopy used to detect neural tube defects and to obtain pure fetal blood.[86, 87]

3. Description of transient hyperammonemia of prematurity producing coma and responding to treatment.[88]

1979

1. First reports of ultrasound to detect cerebral hemorrhage (and other brain damage) at the bedside.[89]

2. Syndrome of chronic lung disease in prematurity reported to be associated with cytomegalovirus infection.[90]

1980

1. Use of artificial surfactant reported from Japan, with dramatic improvement in babies with respiratory distress syndrome.[91]
2. Transcutaneous bilirubinometry reported from Japan.[92]

1981

1. Granulocyte transfusion to treat neonatal sepsis reported from Italy.[93]
2. Increased levels of maternal hemoglobin A_{1c} associated with congenital malformations in diabetic pregnancies.[94]
3. Prevention (decrease) of intraventricular hemorrhage in preterm infants using pharmacologic agents described in the United States and the United Kingdom.[95, 96]
4. Attention drawn to the need for careful evaluation of regional neonatal intensive care.[97]
5. High-frequency ventilation reported to be beneficial in human newborn infants.[98]

1982

1. Association of benzyl alcohol (used as a preservative) with a gasping syndrome in very-low-birth-weight infants. Widely separated centers suggest that this may be lethal.[99, 100]
2. Attention called to our poor understanding of bilirubin toxicity despite many years of "knowledge."[101]
3. Nuclear magnetic resonance imaging and phosphorus spectroscopy introduced to neonatology.[102, 103]
4. Resurgence of interest in chorionic villus biopsy to make early prenatal diagnosis[104, 105] (probably began in late 1960s and mid 1970s).
5. First report of high survival rate after treatment with extracorporeal membrane oxygenation in a series of moribund infants.[106]

1983

1. Positron-emission tomography demonstrates that small periventricular hemorrhages in very-low-birth-weight infants may be associated with extensive ischemic cerebral injury.[107]
2. Report of the use of human surfactant obtained from amniotic fluid in the treatment of respiratory distress syndrome.[108]
3. Publication of a joint manual by the American College of Obstetricians and Gynecologists and American Academy of Pediatrics (first meeting, November 1978; work on manual started, 1980).[109]
4. "Baby Doe" regulations (dealing with treatment of handicapped infants)

promulgated by federal government; ruled invalid on procedural grounds; revised.[110]

5. Report of physiologic repair of hypoplastic left heart syndrome. Preliminary work as early as 1979; first report with normal 6-month follow-up.[111]

1984

1. Reappraisal of the etiology of retrolental fibroplasia.[112]

2. New intravenous vitamin E preparation associated with neonatal deaths (hepatic, renal, and hematopoietic toxicity).[113]

3. Acceptance of high degree of protection against hepatitis B by combining immune globulin and vaccine.[114]

4. Association of intrauterine infection with human parvovirus B19 and hydrops fetalis.[115]

1985

1. First documentation in the newborn of transfusion-related acquired immunodeficiency syndrome (AIDS) due to infection with human T-cell lymphotropic virus type III, now called human immunodeficiency virus.[116]

2. Report of noninvasive method for measuring neonatal cerebral oxygenation at the bedside using near infrared light; dubbed the NIROS-scope.[117]

3. Documentation of bright light in the neonate's environment contributing to retinopathy of prematurity.[118]

4. Report of cocaine use in pregnancy and its neurobehavioral effects on infants.[119]

1986

1. Series of intravascular fetal blood transfusions reported from United Kingdom and United States.[120, 121]

2. Pulse oximetry gains increasing acceptance in neonatal intensive care.[122]

3. Minimal enteral feeding (hypocaloric feeding) reported to improve later tolerance of feeds in small babies.[123, 124]

1987

1. Application of the polymerase chain reaction (described in 1985) to prenatal diagnosis.[125, 126]

2. Attention drawn to the neonate's ability to perceive pain.[127]

1988

1. Report of metalloporphyrins to treat neonatal jaundice published.[128]
2. Human Genome Project initiated.[129, 130]
3. Preliminary report published of improved outcome with cryotherapy for severe retinopathy of prematurity.[131]
4. Trials of recombinant human erythropoietin initiated for the treatment of anemia of prematurity.[132]

1989

1. Second randomized trial of extracorporeal membrane oxygenation versus conventional therapy reported, showing better outcome of the former in severe persistent pulmonary hypertension.[133]
2. Organization of large-scale multicenter trials of exogenous surfactants (Exosurf and Survanta) begun.[134, 135]
3. Isolation of the cystic fibrosis gene reported.[136]
4. Description of the use of liquid ventilation with perfluorocarbons in preterm infants.[137]

1990

1. Report of tight prepregnancy control decreasing the incidence of congenital malformations in infants of diabetic mothers.[138] (May have been documented as early as 1983.)
2. Successful in utero repair of congenital diaphragmatic hernia in the fetus reported.[139]
3. Food and Drug Administration approves use of Exosurf.

1991

1. Food and Drug Administration approves use of Survanta.
2. Reduction of neural tube defects using folic acid supplementation reported from large multicenter study.[140]

1992

1. Reports from two centers of the successful treatment of severe persistent pulmonary hypertension of the newborn by use of inhaled nitric oxide.[141, 142]
2. Report of the effects of famine affecting the third generation, with decreased birth weights in offspring of mothers exposed in utero.[143]
3. Description of association between feeding breast milk to preterm infants and higher intelligence quotient at 7½ to 8 years.[144]

1993

1. New serotype of group B streptococcus (type V) reported to be responsible for neonatal sepsis.[145]

2. Publication of "Towards Improving the Outcome of Pregnancy: The Nineties and Beyond," which was sponsored by the March of Dimes but had input from multiple organizations concerned with perinatal health.[146]

3. Description of methods to measure severity of illness or neonatal mortality risk with acronyms CRIB (clinical risk index for babies) and SNAP (score for neonatal acute physiology).[147, 148]

1994

1. Use of antenatal corticosteroids to reduce morbidity and mortality from respiratory distress syndrome, intraventricular hemorrhage, and other complications of prematurity strongly endorsed by the National Institutes of Health consensus development conference on "Effect of Corticosteroids for Fetal Maturation on Perinatal Outcomes."[149]

2. A 1993 judgment that emergency treatment had to be provided on request for an anencephalic infant upheld by the United States Court of Appeals.[150]

REFERENCES

1. Cremer, R. J., Perryman, P. W., and Richards, D. H.: Influence of light on the hyperbilirubinemia of infants. *Lancet* 1958, i:1094.
2. Apgar, V., Holaday, D. A., James, L. S., et al.: Evaluation of the newborn infant—Second report. *J.A.M.A.* 1958, 168:1985.
3. Silverman, W. A., Fertig, J. W., and Berger, A. P.: The influence of the thermal environment upon the survival of newly born premature infants. *Pediatrics* 1958, 22:876.
4. Donald, I., MacVicar, J., and Brown, T. G.: Investigation of abdominal masses by pulsed ultrasound. *Lancet* 1958, i:1188.
5. Farquhar, J. W.: The child of the diabetic woman. *Arch. Dis. Child.* 1959, 34:76.
6. Gellis, S. S., and Hsia, D. Y. Y.: The infant of the diabetic mother. *Am. J. Dis. Child.* 1959, 97:1.
7. Jacobs, P. A., Baikie, A. G., Brown, W. M. C., and Strong, J. A.: The somatic chromosomes in mongolism. *Lancet* 1959, i:710.
8. Avery, M. E., and Mead, J.: Surface properties in relation to atelectasis and hyaline membrane disease. *Am. J. Dis. Child.* 1959, 97:517.
9. Shaffer, A. J.: *Diseases of the Newborn*, 1st ed. W. B. Saunders, Philadelphia, 1960.
10. Patau, K., Smith, D. W., Therman, E., et al.: Multiple congenital anomaly caused by an extra chromosome. *Lancet* 1960, i:790.
11. Weiss, C. F., Glazko, A. J., and Weston, J. K.: Chloramphenicol in the newborn infant: A physiologic explanation of its toxicity when given in excessive doses. *N. Engl. J. Med.* 1960, 262:787.
12. Wilson, M. J., and Mikity, V. G.: A new form of respiratory disease in premature infants. *Am. J. Dis. Child.* 1960, 99:489.
13. Warkany, J., Monroe, B. B., and Sutherland, B. S.: Intrauterine growth retardation. *Am. J. Dis. Child.* 1961, 102:249.

14. Taussig, H. B.: A study of the German outbreak of phocomelia. The thalidomide syndrome. *J.A.M.A.* 1962, 180:1106.
15. von Rosen, S.: Diagnosis and treatment of congenital dislocation of the hip joint in the newborn. *J. Bone Joint Surg.* 1962, 44B:284.
16. Barlow, T. G.: Early diagnosis and treatment of congenital dislocation of the hip. *J. Bone Joint Surg.* 1962, 44B:292.
17. Usher, R.: Reduction of mortality from respiratory distress syndrome of prematurity with early administration of intravenous glucose and sodium bicarbonate. *Pediatrics* 1963, 32:966.
18. Liley, A. W.: Intrauterine transfusion of foetus in haemolytic disease. *B.M.J.* 1963, 2:1107.
19. Haworth, J. C., and Ford, J. D.: The effect of early and late feeding and glucagon upon blood sugar and serum bilirubin levels of premature babies. *Arch. Dis. Child.* 1963, 38:328.
20. Smallpiece, V., and Davies, P. A.: Immediate feeding of premature infants with undiluted breast milk. *Lancet* 1964, ii:1349.
21. Cornblath, M., Wybregt, S. H., Baens, G. S., and Klein, R. I.: Studies of carbohydrate metabolism in the newborn infant: VIII. Symptomatic neonatal hypoglycemia. *Pediatrics* 1964, 33:388.
22. Berdon, W. E., Grossman, H., Baker, D. H., et al.: Necrotizing enterocolitis in the premature infant. *Radiology* 1964, 83:879.
23. Chu, J., Clements, J. A., Cotten, E., et al.: The pulmonary hypoperfusion syndrome. *Pediatrics* 1965, 35:733.
24. Stahlman, M. T., Young, W. C., Gray, J., and Shepard, F. M.: The management of respiratory failure in the idiopathic respiratory distress syndrome of prematurity. *Ann. N.Y. Acad. Sci.* 1965, 121:930.
25. Thomas, D. V., Fletcher, G., Sunshine, P., et al.: Prolonged respirator use in pulmonary insufficiency of the newborn. *J.A.M.A.* 1965, 193:183.
26. Nelson, J. D., and Peters, P. C.: Suprapubic aspiration of urine in premature and term infants. *Pediatrics* 1965, 36:132.
27. Rausen, A. R., London, R. D., Mizrahi, A., and Cooper, L. Z.: Generalized bone changes and thrombocytopenic purpura in association with intrauterine rubella. *Pediatrics* 1965, 36:264.
28. Clarke, C. A., Donohoe, W. T. A., McConnell, R. B., et al.: Prevention of Rh-haemolytic disease: Results of the clinical trial. A combined study of centers in England and Baltimore. *B.M.J.* 1966, 2:907.
29. Freda, V. J., Gorman, J. G., and Pollack, W.: Suppression of the primary Rh immune response with passive Rh IgG immunoglobulin. *N. Engl. J. Med.* 1967, 277:1022.
30. Desmond, M. M., Rudolph, A. J., and Phitaksphraiwan, P.: The transitional care nursery. *Pediatr. Clin. North Am.* 1966, 13:651.
31. Segal, S.: Neonatal intensive care: A prediction of continuing development. *Pediatr. Clin. North Am.* 1966, 13:1149. Transfer of a premature or other high-risk newborn infant to a referral hospital. *Pediatr. Clin. North Am.* 1966, 13:1195.
32. Battaglia, F. C., and Lubchenco, L. O.: A practical classification of newborn infants by weight and gestational age. *J. Pediatr.* 1967, 71:159.
33. Northway, W. H., Jr., Rosan, R. C., and Porter, D. Y.: Pulmonary disease following respiratory therapy of hyaline membrane disease: Bronchopulmonary dysplasia. *N. Engl. J. Med.* 1967, 276:357.
34. Hawker, J. M., Reynolds, E. O. R., and Taghizadeh, A.: Pulmonary surface tension and pathological changes in infants dying after respirator treatment for severe hyaline membrane disease. *Lancet* 1967, ii:75.
35. Alford, C. A., Shaefer, J., Blankenship, W. J., et al.: A correlative immunologic, microbiologic and clinical approach to the diagnosis of acute and chronic infections in newborn infants. *N. Engl. J. Med.* 1967, 277:437.
36. Finberg, L.: Dangers to infants caused by changes in osmolar concentrations. *Pediatrics* 1967, 40:1030.
37. Lucey, J. F., Ferreiro, M., and Hewitt, J. R.: Prevention of hyperbilirubinemia of prematurity by phototherapy. *Pediatrics* 1968, 41:1047.

38. Amiel-Tison, C.: Neurological evaluation of the maturity of newborn infants. *Arch. Dis. Child.* 1968, 43:89.
39. Lemoine, P., Harousseau, H., Borteyru, J. P., et al.: Les enfants de parents alcoöliques: anomalies observées. *Quest. Med.* 1968, 25:476.
40. Gregory, G. A., Kitterman, J. A., Phibbs, R. H., et al.: Treatment of idiopathic respiratory distress syndrome with continuous positive airway pressure. *N. Engl. J. Med.* 1971, 284:1333.
41. Committee on Fetus and Newborn, American Academy of Pediatrics: History of oxygen therapy and retrolental fibroplasia. James, L. S., and Lanman, J. T. (eds.), *Pediatrics* 1976, 57(Suppl):624.
42. Winick, M., and Rosso, R.: The effect of severe early malnutrition on cellular growth of human brain. *Pediatr. Res.* 1969, 3:181.
43. Dobbing, J.: Undernutrition and the developing brain: The relevance of animal models to the human problem. *Am. J. Dis. Child.* 1970, 120:411.
44. Chernick, V., and Raber, M.: Electrical hazards in the newborn nursery. *J. Pediatr.* 1970, 77:143.
45. Barnett, E. R., Leiderman, P. H., Grobstein, R., and Klaus, M.: Neonatal separation: The maternal side of interactional deprivation. *Pediatrics* 1970, 45:197.
46. Klaus, M., and Kennel, J.: Mothers separated from their newborn infants. *Pediatr. Clin. North Am.* 1970, 17:1015.
47. Stern, L., Khanna, N. N., Levy, G., and Yaffe, S. J.: Effect of phenobarbital on hyperbilirubinemia and glucuronide formation in newborns. *Am. J. Dis. Child.* 1970, 120:26.
48. Dubowitz, L. M. S., Dubowitz, V., and Goldberg, C.: Clinical assessment of gestational age in the newborn infant. *J. Pediatr.* 1970, 77:1.
49. Rhea, J. W., and Kilby, J. O.: A nasojejunal tube for infant feeding. *Pediatrics* 1970, 46:36.
50. Winsberg, F.: Echocardiography of the fetal and newborn heart. *Invest. Radiol.* 1972, 7:152.
51. Gluck, L., Kulovich, M. V., Borer, R. C., et al.: Diagnosis of the respiratory distress syndrome by amniocentesis. *Am. J. Obstet. Gynecol.* 1971, 109:440.
52. Gaines, T. B., and Kimbrough, R. D.: The oral and dermal toxicity of hexachlorophene in rats. *Toxicol. Appl. Pharmacol.* 1971, 19:375.
53. Benda, G. I., and Babson, S. G.: Peripheral intravenous alimentation of the small premature infant. *J. Pediatr.* 1971, 79:494.
54. Committee on Fetus and Newborn, American Academy of Pediatrics: *Standards and Recommendations for Hospital Care of Newborn Infants,* 5th ed. American Academy of Pediatrics, Evanston, 1971.
55. Liggins, G. C., and Howie, R. N.: A controlled trial of antepartum glucorticoid treatment for prevention of the respiratory distress syndrome in premature infants. *Pediatrics* 1972, 50:515.
56. Brock, D. J. H., and Sutcliffe, R. G.: Alpha-fetoprotein in antenatal diagnosis of anencephaly and spina bifida. *Lancet* 1972, ii:197.
57. Huch, R., Huch, A., and Lubbers, D. W.: Transcutaneous measurements of blood pO_2 (tcPO_2): Method and applications in perinatal medicine. *J. Med. Perinatol.* 1973, 1:183.
58. Lockhart, J. D., and Simmons, H. E.: Hexachlorophene decisions at the FDA. *Pediatrics* 1973, 51:430.
59. Clements, J. A., Platzker, A. C., Tierney, D. F., et al.: Assessment of the risk of the respiratory distress syndrome by a rapid new test for surfactant in amniotic fluid. *N. Engl. J. Med.* 1972, 268:1077.
60. Chernick, V., and Vidyasagar, D.: Continuous negative chest wall pressure in hyaline membrane disease: One year experience. *Pediatrics* 1972, 49:753.
61. Kattwinkel, J., Fleming, D., Cha, C. C., et al.: A device for administration of continuous positive airway pressure by the nasal route. *Pediatrics* 1973, 52:131.
62. Bancalari, E., Gerhardt, T., and Monkus, E.: Simple device for producing continuous negative pressure in infants with IRDS. *Pediatrics* 1973, 52:167.
63. McCracken, G. H., Jr.: Group B streptococci: The new challenge in neonatal infections. *J. Pediatr.* 1973, 82:703.

64. Brazelton, T. B.: Neonatal Behavioral Assessment Scale. *Clin. Dev. Med.* No. 50. SIMP, J. B. Lippincott, Philadelphia, 1973.
65. Kuzemko, J. A., and Paala, J.: Apneic attacks in the newborn treated with aminophylline. *Arch. Dis. Child.* 1973, 48:404.
66. Jones, K. L., Smith, D. W., Ulleland, C. N., et al.: Pattern of malformations in offspring of chronic alcoholic mothers. *Lancet* 1973, i:1267.
67. Gregory, G. A., Gooding, C. A., Phibbs, R. H., and Tooley, W. H.: Meconium aspiration in infants: Prospective study. *J. Pediatr.* 1974, 85:848.
68. Ting, P., and Brady, J. P.: Tracheal suctioning in meconium aspiration. *Am. J. Obstet. Gynecol.* 1975, 122:767.
69. Johnson, L., Schaffer, D., and Boggs, T. R.: The premature infant, vitamin E deficiency and retrolental fibroplasia. *Am. J. Clin. Nutr.* 1974, 27:1158. (See also Owens and Owens, *Am. J. Ophthalmol.* 1949, 32:1.)
70. Dussault, J. H., Coulombe, P., Laberge, C., et al.: Preliminary report on a mass screening program for neonatal hypothyroidism. *J. Pediatr.* 1975, 86:670.
71. Kuhns, L. R., Bednarek, F. J., Wyman, M. L., et al.: Diagnosis of pneumothorax or pneumomediastinum in the neonate by transillumination. *Pediatrics* 1975, 56:355.
72. Houser, O. W., Smith, J. B., Gomez, M. R., and Baker, H. L.: Evaluation of intracranial disorders in children by computerized transaxial tomography: A preliminary report. *Neurology* 1975, 25:607.
73. Koronees, S. B., and Eyal, F. B.: Successful treatment of "persistent fetal circulation" with tolazoline. *Pediatr. Res.* 1975, 9:367.
74. Goetzman, B. W., Sunshine, P., Johnson, J. D., et al.: Neonatal hypoxia and pulmonary vasospasm. Response to tolazoline. *J. Pediatr.* 1976, 89:617.
75. Elliot, R. B., Starling, M. B., and Neutze, J. M.: Medical manipulation of the ductus arteriosus. *Lancet* 1975, i:140.
76. Freidman, Z., Shochat, S. J., Maisels, M. J., et al.: Correction of essential fatty acid deficiency in newborn infants by cutaneous application of sunflower seed oil. *Pediatrics* 1976, 58:650.
77. Pickett, J., Berg, B., Chaplin, E., and Brunstetter-Shafer, M.: Syndrome of botulism in infancy: Clinical and electrophysiological study. *N. Engl. J. Med.* 1976, 295:770.
78. Friedman, W. F., Hirschklau, M. J., Printz, M. P., et al.: Pharmacologic closure of patent ductus arteriosus in the premature infant. *N. Engl. J. Med.* 1976, 295:526.
79. Heymann, M. A., Rudolph, A. M., and Silverman, N. H.: Closure of the ductus arteriosus by prostaglandin inhibition. *N. Engl. J. Med.* 1976, 295:530.
80. Beem, M. D., and Saxon, E. M.: Respiratory tract colonization and distinctive pneumonia syndrome in infants infected with *Chlamydia trachomatis. N. Engl. J. Med.* 1977, 296:306.
81. Papile, L. A., Burstein, J., Burstein, R., and Koffler, H.: Incidence and evolution of sub-ependymal and intraventricular hemorrhage: A study of infants with birthweights less than 1500 grams. *J. Pediatr.* 1978, 92:529.
82. Yamanouchi, I., and Igarashi, I.: Ductal shunt in premature infants observed by tcPO$_2$ measurements. In *Transcutaneous Blood Gas Monitoring, Birth Defects.* Original Article Series, Vol. 15(4), AR Liss, New York, 1979.
83. Vidyasagar, D., and Raju, T. N. K.: A simple non-invasive technique of measuring intracranial pressure in the newborn. *Pediatrics* 1977, 59(Suppl):957.
84. Huch, A., Huch, R., Seiler, D., et al.: Transcutaneous pCO$_2$ measurement with a miniaturized electrode. *Lancet* 1977, i:982.
85. Papile, L. A., Koffler, H., Burstein, R., and Kopps, B.: Non-surgical treatment of acquired hydrocephalus: Evaluation of serial lumbar puncture (Abstract). *Pediatr. Res.* 1978, 12:554.
86. Rodeck, C. H., and Campbell, S.: Early prenatal diagnosis of neural tube defects by ultra-sound guided fetoscopy. *Lancet* 1978, i:1128.
87. Rodeck, C. H., and Campbell, S.: Sampling pure fetal blood by fetoscopy in second trimester of pregnancy. *B.M.J.* 1978, 2:728.
88. Ballard, R. A., Vinocur, B., Reynolds, J. W., et al.: Transient hyperammonemia of the preterm infant. *N. Engl. J. Med.* 1978, 299:920.

89. Pape, K., Blackwell, R. J., Cusick, G., et al.: Ultrasound detection of brain damage in preterm infants. *Lancet* 1979, i:1261.
90. Ballard, R. A., Drew, W. L., Hufnagle, K. G., and Riedel, P. A.: Acquired cytomegalovirus infection in preterm infants. *Am. J. Dis. Child.* 1979, 133:482.
91. Fujiwara, T., Maeta, H., Chida, S., et al.: Artificial surfactant therapy in hyaline membrane disease. *Lancet* 1980, i:55.
92. Yamanouchi, I., Yamauchi, Y., and Igarashi, I.: Transcutaneous bilirubinometry: Preliminary studies of non-invasive transcutaneous bilirubin meter in the Okayama National Hospital. *Pediatrics* 1980, 65:195.
93. Laurenti, F., Ferro, R., Isacchi, G., et al.: Polymorphonuclear leukocyte transfusion for the treatment of sepsis in the newborn infant. *J. Pediatr.* 1981, 98:118–123.
94. Miller, E., Hare, J. W., Cloherty, P. J., et al.: Elevated maternal hemoglobin A_{1c} in early pregnancy and major congenital anomalies in infants of diabetic mothers. *N. Engl. J. Med.* 1981, 304:1331–1334.
95. Donn, S. M., Roloff, D. W., and Goldstein, G. W.: Prevention of intraventricular hemorrhage in preterm infants by phenobarbitone. *Lancet* 1981, ii:215–217.
96. Morgan, M. E. I., Benson, J. W. T., and Cooke, R. W. I.: Ethamsylate reduces the incidence of periventricular hemorrhage in very low-birth-weight babies. *Lancet* 1981, ii:830–831.
97. Sinclair, J. C., Torrance, G. W., Boyle, M. H., et al.: Evaluation of neonatal intensive-care programs. *N. Engl. J. Med.* 1981, 305:489–494.
98. Marchak, B. E., Thompson, W. K., Duffty, P., et al.: Treatment of RDS by high-frequency oscillatory ventilations: A preliminary report. *J. Pediatr.* 1981, 99:287–292.
99. Gershanik, J., Boechler, B., Ensley, H., et al.: The gasping syndrome and benzyl alcohol poisoning. *N. Engl. J. Med.* 1982, 307:1384–1388.
100. Brown, W. J., Buist, N. R. M., Gipson, H. T., et al.: Fetal benzyl alcohol poisoning in a neonatal intensive care unit (Letter). *Lancet* 1982, i:1250.
101. Lucey, J. F.: Bilirubin and brain damage—A real mess. *Pediatrics* 1982, 69:381–382.
102. Levene, M. I., Whitelaw, A., Dubowitz, V., et al.: Nuclear magnetic resonance imaging of the brain in children. *B.M.J.* 1982, 285:774–776.
103. Cady, E. B., Costello, A. M. deL., Davidson, M. J., et al.: Non-invasive investigation of cerebral metabolism in newborn infants by phosphorus nuclear magnetic resonance spectroscopy. *Lancet* 1983, i:1059–1062.
104. Old, J. M., Ward, R. H. T., Petrou, M., et al.: First-trimester fetal diagnosis for haemoglobinopathies: Three cases. *Lancet* 1982, ii:1413–1416.
105. Gosden, J. R., Mitchell, A. R., Gosden, C. M., et al.: Direct vision chorion biopsy and chromosome-specific DNA probes for determination of fetal sex in first-trimester prenatal diagnosis. *Lancet* 1982, ii:1416–1419.
106. Barlett, R. H., Andrews, A. F., Toomasian, J. M., et al.: Extracorporeal membrane oxygenation for newborn respiratory failure: Forty-five cases. *Surgery* 1982, 92:425–433.
107. Volpe, J. J., Herscovitch, P., Perlman, J. M., and Raichie, M. E.: Positron emission tomography in the newborn: Extensive impairment of regional cerebral blood flow with intraventricular hemorrhage and hemorrhagic intracerebral involvement. *Pediatrics* 1983, 72:589–601.
108. Hallman, M., Merritt, T. A., Schneider, H., et al.: Isolation of human surfactant from amniotic fluid and a pilot study of its efficacy in respiratory distress syndrome. *Pediatrics* 1983, 71:473–482.
109. American Academy of Pediatrics/American College of Obstetricians and Gynecologists: *Guidelines for Perinatal Care.* American Academy of Pediatrics, Elk Grove Village, IL, 1983.
110. *Federal Register,* January 12th, 1984, 49:1622–1654.
111. Norwood, W. I., Lang, P., and Hansen, D. D.: Physiologic repair of aortic atresia—hypoplastic left heart syndrome. *N. Engl. J. Med.* 1983, 308:23–26.
112. Lucey, J. F., and Dangman, B.: A reexamination of the role of oxygen in retrolental fibroplasia. *Pediatrics* 1984, 73:82–96.
113. Phelps, D. L.: E-Ferol: What happened and what now? *Pediatrics* 1984, 74:1114–1116.

114. Immunization Practices Advisory Committee: Post-exposure prophylaxis of hepatitis B. *MMWR Morbid. Mortal. Weekly Rep.* 1984, 33:285–290.
115. Brown, T., Anand, A., and Ritchie, L. D.: Intrauterine parvovirus infection associated with hydrops fetalis. *Lancet* 1984, ii:1033.
116. Wykoff, R. F., Pearl, E. R., and Saulsbury, F. T.: Immunologic dysfunction in infants infected through transfusion with HTLV-III. *N. Engl. J. Med.* 1985, 132:294–296.
117. Brazy, J. E., Lewis, D. V., Mitnick, M. H., and Jöbsis, F. F.: Non-invasive monitoring of cerebral oxygenation in preterm infants: Preliminary observations. *Pediatrics* 1985, 75:217–225.
118. Glass, P., Avery, G. B., Subramanian, K. N. S., et al.: Effect of bright light in the hospital nursery on the incidence of retinopathy of prematurity. *N. Engl. J. Med.* 1985, 313:401–404.
119. Chasnoff, I. J., Burns, W. J., Schnoll, S. H., et al.: Cocaine use in pregnancy. *N. Engl. J. Med.* 1985, 313:666–669.
120. Berkowitz, R. L., Chitkara, U., Goldberg, J. D., et al.: Intravascular transfusion in utero: The percutaneous approach. *Am. J. Obstet. Gynecol.* 1986, 154:622–623.
121. Nicolaides, K. H., Soothill, P. W., Rodeck, C. H., et al.: Rh disease: Intravascular fetal blood transfusion by cordocentesis. *Fetal Diagn. Ther.* 1986, I:185–192.
122. Jennis, M. S., and Peabody, J. L.: Pulse oximetry: An alternative method for the assessment of oxygenation in newborn infants. *Pediatrics* 1987, 79:524–528.
123. Lucas, A., Bloom, R., and Aynsley-Green, A.: Gut hormones and minimal enteral feeding. *Acta Paediatr.* 1986, 75:719–721.
124. Dunn, L., Hulman, S., Weiner, J., and Kliegman, R.: Beneficial effects of early hypocaloric enteral feeding on neonatal gastro-intestinal function: Preliminary report of a randomized trial. *J. Pediatr.* 1988, 112:622–629.
125. Orkin, S. H.: Genetic diagnosis by DNA analysis: Progress through amplification. *N. Engl. J. Med.* 1987, 317:1023–1025.
126. Eisenstein, B. I.: The polymerase chain reaction: A new method of using molecular genetics for medical diagnosis. *N. Engl. J. Med.* 1990, 322:178–183.
127. Anand, K. J. S., and Hickey, P.R.: Pain and its effects in the human neonate and fetus. *N. Engl. J. Med.* 1987, 317:1321–1329.
128. Kappas, A., Drummond, G. S., Manola, T., et al.: Sn-Protoporphyrin use in the management of hyperbilirubinemia in term newborns with direct Coombs-positive ABO incompatibility. *Pediatrics* 1988, 81:485–497.
129. Editorial: Mapping the human genome. *Lancet* 1987, i:1121–1222.
130. Watson, J. D.: The Human Genome Project: Past, present and future. *Science* 1990, 248:44–51.
131. Cryotherapy for Retinopathy of Prematurity Co-operative Group: Multicenter trial of cryotherapy for retinopathy of prematurity: Preliminary results. *Pediatrics* 1988, 81:697–706.
132. Stockman, J. A. III.: Erythropoietin: Off again, on again. *J. Pediatr.* 1988, 112:906–908.
133. O'Rourke, P. P., Crone, R. K., Vacanti, J. P., et al.: Extracorporeal membrane oxygenation and conventional medical therapy in neonates with persistent pulmonary hypertension of the newborn: A prospective randomized study. *Pediatrics* 1989, 84:957–963.
134. Mercier, C. E., and Soll, R. F.: Clinical trials of natural surfactant extract in respiratory distress syndrome. *Clin. Perinatol.* 1993, 20:711–735.
135. Corbet, A.: Clinical trials of synthetic surfactant in the respiratory distress syndrome of premature infants. *Clin. Perinatol.* 1993, 20:737–760.
136. Rommens, J. M., Riordan, J. R., Kerem, B-S., et al.: Identification of the cystic fibrosis gene: I. Chromosome walking and jumping; II. Cloning and characterization of complementary DNA; III. Genetic analysis. *Science* 1989, 245:1059–1080.
137. Greenspan, J. S., Wolfson, M. R., Rubenstein, S. D., and Shaffer, T. H.: Liquid ventilation of human preterm neonates. *J. Pediatr.* 1990, 117:106–111 (and *Lancet*, November 4, 1989).
138. Steel, J. M., Johnstone, F. D., Hepburn, D. A., and Smith, A. F.: Can prepregnancy care of diabetic women reduce the risk of abnormal babies? *B.M.J.* 1990, 301:1070–1074.
139. Harrison, M. R., Adzick, N. S., Longaker, M. T., et al.: Successful repair in utero of a

fetal diaphragmatic hernia after removal of herniated viscera from the left thorax. *N. Engl. J. Med.* 1990, 322:1582–1584.

140. Wald, N.: For the Medical Research Council Vitamin Study Research Group: Prevention of neural tube defects: Results of the Medical Research Council Vitamin Study. *Lancet* 1991, 338:131–137.
141. Roberts, J. D., Polaner, D. M., Lang, P., and Zapol, W. M.: Inhaled nitric oxide in persistent pulmonary hypertension of the newborn. *Lancet* 1992, 340:818–819.
142. Kinsella, J. P., Neish, S. R., Shaffer, E., and Abman, S. H.: Low dose inhalational nitric oxide therapy in persistent pulmonary hypertension of the newborn. *Lancet* 1992, 340:819–820.
143. Lumey, L. H.: Decreased birthweights in infants after maternal in utero exposure to the Dutch famine of 1944–1945. *Paediatr. Perinat. Epidemiol.* 1992, 6:240–253.
144. Lucas, A., Morley, R., Cole, T. J., et al.: Breast milk and subsequent intelligence quotient in children born preterm. *Lancet* 1992, 339:261–264.
145. Rench, M. A., and Baker, C. J.: Neonatal sepsis caused by a new group B streptococcal serotype. *J. Pediatr.* 1993, 122:638–640.
146. Little, G. A., and Merenstein, G. B.: Toward improving the outcomes of pregnancy, 1993: Perinatal regionalization revisited. *Pediatrics,* 1993, 92:611–612.
147. The International Neonatal Network: The CRIB (clinical risk index for babies) score: A tool for assessing initial neonatal risk and comparing performance of neonatal intensive care units. *Lancet* 1993, 342:193–198.
148. Richardson, D. K., Gray, J. E., McCormick, M. C., et al.: Score for neonatal acute physiology: A physiologic severity index for neonatal intensive care. *Pediatrics* 1993, 91:617–623.
149. McCarthy, M.: U.S. recommendations for antenatal corticosteroids. *Lancet* 1994, 343:726.
150. Annas, G. J.: Asking the courts to set the standard of emergency care—The case of Baby K. *N. Engl. J. Med.* 1994, 330:1542–1545.

Clinical Presentations and Their Assessment

In the following discussions, it is assumed that careful clinical evaluation precedes any other investigation. In many cases, it will be necessary to refer to other sections of the book. Where a specific diagnosis is involved, the references will usually be found in the other sections.

24

NEONATAL EMERGENCIES

There are many situations in which it is important to recognize the problem and act promptly. The following clinical presentations require a specific course of action, which should be accomplished without delay. Less urgent problems are discussed in subsequent chapters. (The contents of this chapter should be carefully reviewed by anyone who is likely to encounter these problems.)

BIRTH ASPHYXIA
(see also Chapter 2)

Birth asphyxia may be defined as the failure of a newborn infant to establish adequate respiration after birth, with associated biochemical disturbance (profound metabolic or mixed acidemia, hypoxemia, and hypercarbia). This emergency can be lessened by anticipation of the need for resuscitation. Evidence of placenta previa, abruptio placentae, prolapsed cord, and major abnormalities of fetal heart rate monitoring (particularly with decreased fetal scalp pH) should alert the perinatal staff to the need for active intervention. In the absence of spontaneous respiration, it is important to immediately visualize the vocal cords using a laryngoscope. If the view is obscured by fluid, it should be suctioned, either with a DeLee trap or wall suction. A suitably sized endotracheal tube should be inserted (2.5 to 3.5 mm) to a depth that allows breath sounds to be heard on both sides of the chest (approximately 1 cm beyond the vocal cords). After bag-to-tube ventilation restores a normal color, the baby should be checked for about 10 seconds approximately every 1 to 2 minutes to see if there is any spontaneous respiratory activity. If there is no spontaneous breathing effort within 30 minutes of active resuscitation, the baby will almost certainly either die or have profound neurologic damage. Thus, further resuscitation is inappropriate under such circumstances, even though it is very difficult to stop if the baby is pink.

In the presence of heavily meconium-stained amniotic fluid, it is important not to stimulate the baby but to suck out any material in the trachea under direct laryngoscopic visualization before attempting to ventilate the lungs. The same procedure should be followed when blood is present.

When narcotic administration can be documented as the cause of depressed respiration, naloxone (Narcan) should be given in a dose of 0.1 mg/kg.

Failure of gasping to proceed to regular respiration may indicate complete nasal obstruction, which is most likely due to choanal atresia. The nasal obstruc-

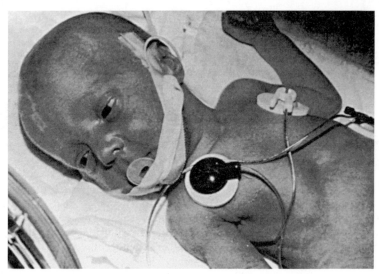

FIGURE 24–1. Emergency treatment of congenital choanal atresia with an oral airway.

tion can be bypassed by use of an oral airway or an orotracheal tube (Figs. 24–1 and 24–2). Another problem that may present as airway obstruction is retrognathia. In this condition, the mandible is underdeveloped; the posterior displacement of the tongue (glossoptosis) can be corrected by positioning and gravity, in most cases by placing the baby on the abdomen. Pulling forward on the mandible or inserting an oral airway may be necessary.

True asphyxia usually results in multiple organ involvement. In addition to effects on the brain (and possible seizure activity), the kidney is frequently

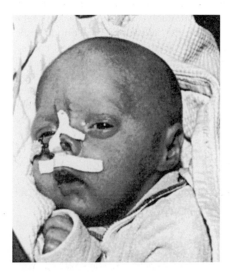

FIGURE 24–2. Nasal tubes in place after surgical correction of congenital choanal atresia.

affected, with marked decrease in urine output and increased serum creatinine levels. Cardiac contractility may be compromised, there may be pulmonary vasoconstriction (producing persistent pulmonary hypertension), and the gut may also be dysfunctional.

Although not widely used, serum hypoxanthine concentrations have been shown to reflect the degree of asphyxia.

SUDDEN DETERIORATION ("CRASH" OR "CRUMP")

Many babies (both premature and full term) initially appear quite well but later demonstrate rather rapid deterioration of their condition. It is perhaps easiest to consider the problem under two headings:

BABY ON ASSISTED VENTILATION. The major considerations are:

1. Faulty ventilation: caused by blockage of an endotracheal tube, a displaced tube, disconnected ventilator, and other mechanical problems
2. Pneumothorax: detect by transillumination or x-ray study
3. Intracranial hemorrhage: detect by full fontanel, falling hematocrit value metabolic acidosis, and so on or by ultrasonography (if available)
4. Sepsis or meningitis

BABY BREATHING SPONTANEOUSLY. The major considerations are:

1. Overwhelming infection: bacterial or viral
2. Massive hemorrhage: such as subcapsular hematoma of liver
3. Congenital heart disease: precipitated by closure of ductus arteriosus
4. Necrotizing enterocolitis
5. Metabolic problem: such as hyperammonemia, organic acidemia
6. Perforated viscus (e.g. gastric perforation, which may also occur on assisted ventilation)

Physical examination, complete blood count, blood gases and pH, x-ray study (or transillumination) of chest and abdomen, and electrocardiography usually indicate the need (and direction) for further investigation and treatment.

SHOCK

Shock is characterized by extreme pallor and poor perfusion (with slow capillary refill) and is usually the result of hypovolemia (decreased blood volume). When it is noticed in the delivery room, it is most frequently the result of significant third-trimester bleeding, with bleeding from the fetal side of the placenta. Hypovolemia is now considered to occur frequently with third-trimester bleeding. It may also be the result of bleeding of the fetus into the mother via the placenta (fetomaternal hemorrhage). This may also occur more commonly than was considered previously and can be documented by use of the Kleihauer technique. A third problem presenting in the delivery room (or operating room) is blood loss resulting from cutting of the placenta (either accidentally or intentionally) at cesarean section.

Shock occurring later in the neonatal period may be the result of sepsis, hemorrhage (discussed later in this chapter), necrotizing enterocolitis, or dehydration (resulting from vomiting and diarrhea).

The treatment of shock is directed at replacing blood volume. In almost all cases, the best replacement fluid is whole blood. However, whole blood may not be immediately available, and it may be necessary to use any kind of fluid, preferably colloid (albumin), to improve perfusion. In some cases, it may be more convenient to use fresh-frozen plasma, with or without added packed red blood cells. In an extreme emergency, unmatched blood (usually type O Rh-negative) should be given because the risk of administering such blood is minor when faced with imminent death. Dehydration should be treated with electrolyte solutions. Hypotension may also require treatment with pressor agents (e.g., dopamine).

OTHER CAUSES OF EXTREME PALLOR

In addition to hypovolemia and other causes of shock (as just noted), one should also remember the following:

SEVERE METABOLIC ACIDOSIS. This may be confirmed by determining pH and pCO_2. If the base deficit is large, sodium bicarbonate may be given. An emergency dose is 2 mEq/kg, but further calculation may be required (see Chapter 17).

SEVERE ANEMIA. This is most likely to occur in hemolytic disease of the newborn, usually Rh incompatibility. Some of these babies are hypervolemic but not all. Red blood cells may be urgently needed to provide oxygen-carrying capacity. Severe anemia may also be a manifestation of congenital leukemia, but it is usually accompanied by subcutaneous nodules, thrombocytopenia, and petechiae or purpura. Emergency treatment usually is not required.

CARDIAC DYSFUNCTION. Any disorder that decreases cardiac output is likely to result in pallor because peripheral perfusion is decreased. When palpating peripheral pulses is difficult, in the absence of other apparent reasons for shock, one should consider the possibility of hypoplastic left heart syndrome. This and other cardiac dysfunctions may be detected with echocardiography. Pressor agents may be needed.

NEONATAL COLD INJURY (EXTREME HYPOTHERMIA). Although this problem is rarely seen in the United States, it is not uncommon in Great Britain and has even been seen in subtropical climates. Physicians should be aware of its existence. The baby is usually seen because of lethargy and poor feeding. The face, feet, and hands are quite pink (even red) in contrast to the marked pallor of the trunk. The body is obviously cold, and core temperature does not register on the usual thermometer. A low-reading thermometer is required, and the baby should be placed in an incubator with the temperature just above that of the baby. An intravenous infusion of glucose is started, and the incubator temperature is usually raised slowly (approximately 0.5 to 1°C/hr) until a normal body temperature has been achieved, although recent reports indicate that rapid rewarming may decrease mortality. Thrombocytopenia and pulmonary hemorrhage are potential complications.

EXTREME CYANOSIS

The baby who has persistent deep cyanosis after birth despite resuscitation or who develops rapidly worsening cyanosis in the neonatal period requires careful evaluation and appropriate management. Four major groups of disorders are to be considered. These are

1. *Cyanotic congenital heart disease* (pp. 96 to 100)
2. *An acute pulmonary problem:* most frequently tension pneumothorax (pp. 119 to 121) or diaphragmatic hernia (pp. 91 to 93)
3. *Persistent pulmonary hypertension:* often called persistent fetal (or transitional) circulation (pp. 122 to 124)
4. *Hyperviscosity* (or high hematocrit) syndrome (pp. 242 to 243)

A chest radiograph is extremely valuable in helping to distinguish between pulmonary disorders. Pneumothorax can often be detected with thoracic transillumination, and this procedure should be performed first, together with a hematocrit determination on venous blood. If these results are normal, a hyperoxia test may be performed (see p. 376), but if the pO_2 remains low, it may be impossible to distinguish between heart disease and persistent pulmonary hypertension. Electrocardiography should be performed, and a pediatric cardiologist, who frequently performs echocardiography first but may move directly to cardiac catheterization, should be consulted immediately. If pulmonary hypertension is diagnosed by exclusion, it may be possible to see marked improvement with assisted ventilation, particularly if respiratory alkalosis can be achieved, but other therapy (e.g., pressors, tolazoline, magnesium sulfate) may be required.

These manipulations should be carried out only in an intensive care nursery. In particular, tolazoline can result in generalized vasodilation, with hypotension requiring dopamine therapy (may be started first). If these measures fail, high-frequency ventilation, extracorporeal membrane oxygenation, or nitric oxide therapy may be needed later.

CARDIOPULMONARY ARREST

Strictly speaking, the term cardiopulmonary arrest means that there is absence of both cardiac action and spontaneous breathing movements. In practice in the newborn infant, a heart rate of less than 50 to 60 beats/min, in association with ineffective respiratory activity, is an indication to perform cardiopulmonary resuscitation. If two people are available, one may perform external cardiac massage while the other attends to endotracheal intubation and bag-to-tube ventilation. However, it is difficult to intubate during cardiac massage, and it may be necessary to discontinue it briefly. If only one person is available, a few beats of external cardiac massage should be given before moving directly to intubation. After taping the tube in place, it is difficult (but not impossible) to do one-handed cardiac massage while attempting to bag ventilate with the other.

Two-handed cardiac massage is performed by using one hand under the back as a firm support and pressing over the lower sternum with two fingers of the other hand. Alternatively, the thumbs may be placed one on top of the other over the lower third of the sternum while wrapping the fingers around the trunk and exerting a squeezing action. The sternum should be depressed approximately 2 cm with each compression. If the baby is attached to a heart rate monitor (with an oscilloscope), the effectiveness of cardiac massage can be visualized. The one-handed technique is similar to the alternative two-handed technique, with one thumb over the sternum and the fingers wrapped around the chest. Compression should be 100 to 120 beats/min and, when combined with respirations of 40 to 60/min, give a ratio of 3:1 to 2:1 if attempts to synchronize resuscitation efforts are made.

When ventilation has been established, it may be necessary to supplement cardiopulmonary efforts with pharmacologic agents, such as sodium bicarbonate.

DYSRHYTHMIA (ARRHYTHMIA)

Some irregularities of heart rate do not require emergency treatment, but others do. Particularly when the heart rate is rapid, it is important to obtain an electrocardiograph to evaluate the type of dysrhythmia. Sinus arrhythmia (variation with respiration) is commonly observed in neonates, but when the heart rate is above 200 beats/min, one must suspect supraventricular tachycardia. Normal P waves are not detectable on the electrocardiograph. Frequently, atrial tachycardia is paroxysmal, but there is the danger of precipitating cardiac failure if it persists for several hours. It is worth using a maneuver based on the diving reflex, in which ice cold water was originally used but has been modified to instead use ice cubes. One ice cube is placed in contact with the nose, and another is gently rubbed back and forth across the upper lip. Even if this maneuver is successful (but certainly if it is not), it may be necessary to use digoxin or propranolol to maintain (or obtain) a normal sinus rhythm. In recent years, rapid resolution of supraventricular tachycardia is usual with administration of adenosine by rapid bolus injection intravenously (initial dose, 0.05 mg/kg). Because this drug has a very short half-life, maintenance medication is usually required. Direct-current cardioversion is needed on rare occasion (2 to 10 Wsec/kg).

If the atrial rate is above 300 beats/min, atrial flutter is usually the reason, and a characteristic saw-toothed appearance is seen on the electrocardiograph. This condition is rare in the newborn infant, but it may be treated with digoxin, quinidine, or cardioversion.

Another uncommon dysrhythmia is congenital complete heart block producing marked bradycardia (see also p. 305). This condition is generally asymptomatic, but when it is associated with findings suggesting syncope, an emergency pacemaker may be needed.

Ventricular arrhythmia may also occur and is frequently associated with major disease but usually resolves spontaneously.

BLEEDING (HEMORRHAGE)

The type of bleeding that is usually classified as an emergency is generalized, but certain kinds of localized bleeding may also cause consternation and require prompt management.

GENERALIZED BLEEDING (DIFFUSE AND OOZING FROM PUNCTURE WOUNDS)

Generalized bleeding may be the result of hereditary or acquired coagulopathies. If the baby appears well, bleeding is most likely to be the result of a hereditary coagulation defect (clotting factor deficiency), hemorrhagic disease of the newborn (vitamin K deficiency), or immune-mediated thrombocytopenia. If the baby appears sick, bleeding is most likely the result of disseminated intravascular coagulation, which may be triggered by various events, including sepsis, hypoxia, and tissue factors released into the circulation (e.g., with necrotizing enterocolitis, dead twin fetus). Disseminated intravascular coagulation is best treated by supportive care (to restore blood pressure) and attention to underlying disorders. Heparin does not seem to be beneficial.

Comparatively few laboratory investigations usually differentiate these conditions. These are (1) hemoglobin or hematocrit determination, (2) peripheral blood smear, (3) platelet count, (4) prothrombin time, (5) partial thromboplastin time, and (6) fibrinogen (and maybe fibrin split products) determination. Whether or not vitamin K has been given earlier, it seems wise to administer another 1 mg intravenously. Except when one suspects that platelet antibodies may be present, the basis for therapy is 10 ml/kg of platelet concentrate because this also supplies a minimal hemostatic level of all coagulation factors. However, a more readily available alternative would be a similar volume of fresh-frozen plasma or fresh whole blood. If the platelet count is greater than 30,000/mm^3, it is not necessary to treat thrombocytopenia. The risk of intracranial hemorrhage is apparently increased below this level. In the presence of isoimmune thrombocytopenia, maternal platelets should be transfused (if available and if the platelet count is below 30,000/mm^3 at birth). Approximately two units of washed maternal platelets should be used (in < 40 ml). If mother's blood is not available, random platelets are used. If the platelet count is below 20,000/mm^3 6 or 8 hours later, an exchange transfusion to remove antibody is necessary. Platelets from random donors can be used as well, knowing that survival is short but that antibody may be mopped up; steroids may also be considered, and intravenous immunoglobulin is another alternative (1 g/kg for 3 days).

LOCALIZED BLEEDING

1. Bleeding from the gastrointestinal tract may be caused by swallowed maternal blood, or it may be fetal in origin. The Apt test can be used to differentiate bright red blood that is vomited or passed rectally, (see p. 380). If blood is fetal, it may be caused by vitamin K deficiency, a gastric (stress) ulcer, or a hereditary coagulation defect. Management depends on the baby's condition—watchful waiting may be indicated, or the measures for generalized bleeding may be initiated.

2. Bleeding from a circumcision (or a large hematoma) in a well infant usually indicates a hereditary clotting defect.

3. Bleeding from the umbilical cord usually indicates ineffective clamping or ligation (especially after catheter insertion).

4. Bleeding into and around the umbilical cord seems to be particularly common with hereditary factor XIII deficiency (as well as factor VIII).

5. Bleeding into the brain is most likely in the very premature infant (intraventricular hemorrhage, see pp. 233 to 236) and is the result of hypoxia and immature cerebral blood vessels.

6. Bleeding into the liver is usually the result of trauma at delivery, with subcapsular hematoma formation, which may produce blueness of the abdominal wall. Blood transfusion is urgently required.

ACUTE ABDOMINAL DISTENSION
(see also p. 312)

Three major reasons for rapidly developing abdominal distension exist: (1) bacterial sepsis, (2) necrotizing enterocolitis, and (3) intestinal obstruction (principally volvulus).

With sepsis producing ileus there may be other clinical manifestations, such as apnea, lethargy, and temperature instability (see Chapter 15). Valuable information can be obtained from a white blood cell count and differential, erythrocyte sedimentation rate (mini-ESR), and C-reactive protein. Blood, urine, and cerebrospinal fluid cultures should precede broad-spectrum antibiotic therapy.

With necrotizing enterocolitis, there may be associated loose stools with or without blood (see Chapter 18), and an abdominal radiograph is suggestive (thickened bowel wall or dilated loops) or diagnostic (intramural air). Treatment is to stop feedings by mouth and give antibiotics directed at gram-negative organisms.

In cases of intestinal obstruction, the abdominal radiograph is very valuable. If the obstruction seems to be complete, the possibility of volvulus is high, and early surgical exploration is required if necrosis of the bowel is to be prevented.

Other reasons for acute abdominal distension are a perforated viscus and, especially if the baby is on a respirator, pneumoperitoneum (without perforation). Free air in the abdomen can be detected by either transillumination or x-ray study. Ileus may also be caused by hypermagnesemia.

ASCITES PRODUCING RESPIRATORY EMBARRASSMENT

With massive ascites, movement of the diaphragm may be compromised. If this action produces respiratory difficulty, fluid should be removed by needle aspiration (paracentesis abdominis).

BLUENESS OF THE ABDOMINAL WALL

In certain cases of abdominal distension, there is also a bluish discoloration of the abdominal wall. This usually indicates a surgical problem with hemorrhage into the abdominal cavity, but it may also be the result of obstruction of the inferior vena cava. Perhaps the most likely diagnoses are spontaneous rupture of a viscus (e.g., stomach), subcapsular hemorrhage of the liver, and perforation secondary to necrotizing enterocolitis.

BILE-STAINED VOMITUS
(see also pp. 309 to 310)

Vomitus that contains bile indicates intestinal obstruction beyond the level of the ampulla of Vater. When associated with abdominal distension, it suggests a relatively low obstruction (lower ileum and colon). Bile-stained vomitus is almost invariably associated with conditions requiring surgery, and the baby should be evaluated by a pediatric surgeon.

FREQUENT OR CONTINUOUS CONVULSIONS
(see also pp. 319 to 320)

Whenever convulsive activity is difficult to control, the most likely reasons are hypoxic (or ischemic) encephalopathy, intracranial hemorrhage, and either congenital abnormality or infection of the central nervous system. Metabolic causes (e.g., hypocalcemia and hypoglycemia) usually respond quickly to specific therapy directed at the metabolic problem, except for hyperglycinemia.

When convulsions are frequent or continuous, there is the danger of producing a vicious cycle, with the increased intracranial pressure decreasing the cerebral blood flow and producing further ischemic damage and brain swelling. Seizures in infants of low birth weight carry a particularly grim prognosis (90% mortality in one series).

Phenobarbital is usually the first drug of choice, and 20 mg/kg intravenously is the usual dosage needed to achieve therapeutic levels. This may be given in two divided doses several hours to as little as 30 minutes apart (depending on continued seizure activity) or as a single dose if assisted ventilation is being used. Even 30 mg/kg as a single dose may not depress respiration. Phenytoin (Dilantin) is an alternative (or additive) drug, in a similar dosage.

Although diazepam (Valium) may cause respiratory arrest and can displace bilirubin from albumin, it may be useful (given intravenously in a dosage of 0.3 to 0.5 mg/kg) to bring seizures under control acutely, especially if the baby is already on assisted ventilation. Paraldehyde may also be necessary in difficult cases in a dosage of 0.3 ml/kg given rectally (this is made up to a total volume approximately 10 times the amount of paraldehyde, i.e., about 10 ml in a 3-kg infant). When brain swelling is present (or anticipated), it may be useful to use mannitol or glycerol immediately and dexamethasone to maintain the effect. However, there is little documented evidence of the effectiveness of these agents. With assisted ventilation, it may be valuable to hyperventilate the baby, and fluids should be somewhat restricted.

If delivery was difficult in a term baby, without evidence of hypoxia, subdural hematoma may produce convulsions. Subdural taps may be both diagnostic and therapeutic. When it is available, computed tomographic scan (or ultrasonography) may provide a noninvasive diagnosis of intracranial hemorrhage, including subdural hemorrhage (see p. 371).

SWELLING OF THE SCROTUM

Scrotal swelling that transilluminates easily is almost invariably caused by a hydrocele. However, when scrotal swelling fails to transilluminate, it may be caused by an inguinal hernia or torsion of the spermatic cord (testicular torsion). If a hernia cannot be reduced, it may be difficult to differentiate between these two conditions. Both require immediate surgical intervention. Testicular torsion occurs more frequently than is generally recognized and may be bilateral. In the neonate, it is usually asymptomatic apart from the swelling, which is the result of marked induration and massive enlargement of the scrotal contents. Occasionally, a dimple is seen in the scrotum, and there may be an ecchymotic patch overlying the twisted structures.

CONGENITAL ABNORMALITIES REQUIRING EMERGENCY MANAGEMENT

Most congenital abnormalities do not require immediate attention, but several abnormalities need a specific course of action.

1. *Airway obstruction,* caused by conditions such as choanal atresia and retrognathia (see earlier this chapter), should be relieved using either an oral airway or an endotracheal tube.

2. *Esophageal atresia,* with or without tracheoesophageal fistula (p. 89), gives rise to excessive amounts of mucus. No attempt to feed the baby orally should be made. X-ray studies can be carried out using air, rather than dye, as contrast.

3. *Diaphragmatic hernia,* as mentioned earlier, may produce progressive cyanosis. When chest x-ray study shows this disorder, an orogastric tube should be passed to decompress the stomach and prevent further passage of air into the

intestines. If the baby is to be transported to a center, an endotracheal tube should be inserted, in case assisted ventilation is required (see also pp. 91 to 92).

4. *Gastroschisis or ruptured omphalocele,* in which intestines are exposed on the surface of the skin, should be covered with warm saline soaks, paying particular attention to trying to prevent kinking of the bowel (to minimize vascular compromise). If a special skinlike polymer membrane is available, it can be used to cover an omphalocele, which might rupture without such protection. An intravenous infusion should be started because there is a large surface from which fluid (and protein) may be lost. Careful attention should be given to thermoregulation (see also pp. 44 to 48).

5. *Membrane-covered neural tube defects* should have a sterile dressing placed over them to prevent trauma, which might result in breakdown of the membrane.

6. *Ectopia vesicae (exstrophy of the bladder)* appears as if a specific form of emergency treatment should be carried out, but it is generally not amenable to early repair.

7. *Ambiguous genitalia* are most frequently caused by congenital adrenal hyperplasia (discussed on pp. 348 to 350).

BIBLIOGRAPHY

Birth Asphyxia

Hey, E.: Resuscitation at birth. *Br. J. Anaesth.* 1977, 49:25.
Pietz, J., Guttenberg, N., and Gluck, L.: Hypoxanthine: A marker for asphyxia. *Obstet. Gynecol.* 1988, 72:762–766.
Van Bel, F., and Walther, F. J.: Myocardial dysfunction and cerebral blood flow velocity following birth asphyxia. *Acta Paediatr.* 1990, 79:756–762.
Berseth, C. L., and McCoy, H. H.: Birth asphyxia alters neonatal intestinal motility in term neonates. *Pediatrics* 1992, 90:669–673.

Sudden Deterioration

Ballard, R. A., Vinocur, B., Reynolds, J. W., et al.: Transient hyperammonemia of the preterm infant. *N. Engl. J. Med.* 1978, 299:920.
French, C. E., and Waldstein, G.: Subcapsular hemorrhage of the liver in the newborn. *Pediatrics* 1982, 69:204–208.
Tan, C. E. L., Kiely, E. M., Agrawal, M., et al.: Neonatal gastrointestinal perforation. *J. Pediatr. Surg.* 1989, 24:888–892.

Shock

Strodel, W. E., Callahan, M., Weintraub, W. H., and Coran, A. G.: The effect of various resuscitative regimens on hemorrhagic shock in puppies. *J. Pediatr. Surg.* 1977, 12:809.
Paxson, C. L., Jr.: Neonatal shock in the first postnatal day. *Am. J. Dis. Child.* 1978, 132:509.
Pearson, H. A.: Post-hemorrhagic anemia in the newborn. *Pediatr. Rev.* 1982, 4:40–43.
Lees, M. H., and King, D. H.: Cardiogenic shock in the neonate. *Pediatr. Rev.* 1988, 9:258–266.
Molteni, R. A.: Perinatal blood loss. *Pediatr. Rev.* 1990, 12:47–54.
Shankaran, S., Elias, E., and Ilagan, N.: Subcapsular hemorrhage of the liver in the very low birth weight neonate. *Acta Paediatr. Scand.* 1991, 80:616–619.
Gill, A. B., and Weindling, A. M.: Echocardiographic assessment of cardiac function in shocked very low birth weight infants. *Arch. Dis. Child.* 1993, 68:17–21.

Extreme Cyanosis

Drummond, W. H., Gregory, G. A., Heymann, M. A., and Phibbs, R. H.: Independent effects of hyperventilation, tolazoline and dopamine on infants with persistent pulmonary hypertension. *J. Pediatr.* 1981, 98:603–611.
Lees, M. H., and King, D. H.: Cyanosis in the newborn. *Pediatr. Rev.* 1987, 9:36–42.

Cardiopulmonary Arrest

Lees, M. H.: Perinatal asphyxia and the myocardium (Editorial). *J. Pediatr.* 1980, 96:675.
Phillips, G. W. L., and Zeideman, D. A.: Relation of infant heart to sternum: Its significance in cardiopulmonary resuscitation. *Lancet* 1988, i:1024–1025.
Sinkin, R. A., and Davis, J. M.: Cardiopulmonary resuscitation of the newborn. *Pediatr. Rev.* 1990, 12:136–141.

Dysrhythmia

Bisset, G. S. III, Gaum, W., and Kaplan, S.: The ice bag: A new technique for interruption of supraventricular tachycardia. *J. Pediatr.* 1980, 97:593–595.
Southall, D. P., Johnson, A. M., Shinebourne, E. A., et al.: Frequency and outcome of disorders of cardiac rhythm and conduction in a population of newborn infants. *Pediatrics* 1981, 68:58–66.
Green, A. P., and Giattina, K. H.: Adenosine administration for neonatal SVT. *Neonat. Network* 1993, 12:15–18.

Bleeding

Hathaway, W. E.: The bleeding newborn. *Sem. Hematol.* 1975, 12:175.
Editorial: Bleeding in the newborn. *B.M.J.* 1977, 2:915.
Editorial: XIII, a lucky number? *Lancet* 1980, i:522.
Gross, S. J., Filston, H. C., and Anderson, J. C.: Controlled study of treatment for disseminated intravascular coagulation in the neonate. *J. Pediatr.* 1982, 100:445–448.
Schmidt, B. K., Vegh, P., Andrew, M., and Johnston, M.: Coagulation screening tests in high risk neonates: A prospective cohort study. *Arch. Dis. Child* 1992, 67:1196–1197.

Convulsions

Leay, A. R., and Bray, P. F.: Significance of seizures in infants weighing less than 2,500 grams. *Arch. Neurol.* 1977, 34:381.
Scher, M. S., Aso, K., Beggasly, M. E., et al.: Electrographic seizures in preterm and fullterm neonates: Clinical correlates, associated brain lesions, and risk for neurologic sequelae. *Pediatrics* 1993, 91:128–134.

Scrotal Swelling

Watson, R. A.: Torsion of spermatic cord in neonate. *Urology* 1975, 5:439.

Congenital Abnormalities

Cockington, R. A., and Vonwiller, J. B.: Acute emergencies in the newborn. *Med. J. Aust.* 1977, 24:900.
Lister, J.: Surgical emergencies in the newborn. *Br. J. Anaesth.* 1977, 49:43.
White, P., and Lebowitz, R. L.: Exstrophy of the bladder. *Radiol. Clin. North Am.* 1977, 15:93.
Ein, S. H., and Shandling, B.: A new non-operative treatment of large omphaloceles with a polymer membrane. *J. Pediatr. Surg.* 1978, 13:255.
Mollit, D. L., Ballantine, T. V. N., Grosfeld, J. L., and Quinter, P.: A critical assessment of fluid requirements in gastroschisis. *J. Pediatr. Surg.* 1978, 13:217.

COLOR DISORDERS

YELLOW-ORANGE (JAUNDICE)

Because multiple reasons for hyperbilirubinemia (clinically manifest by jaundice) exist, it is important to understand the accepted normal limits and the most common causes of jaundice in the first few days. The easiest approach is to consider the causes of clinically apparent jaundice by day of onset.

FIRST DAY

1. Hemolytic disease of the newborn: Rh incompatibility; ABO incompatibility; other incompatibility
2. Sepsis (bacterial infection)

SECOND DAY

1. Infection: bacterial, viral, or protozoal
2. Hemolytic disease of the newborn
3. Defects of red blood cell, usually enzyme deficiency
4. Enclosed hemorrhage

THIRD AND FOURTH DAYS

1. Physiologic jaundice (oxytocin induction may contribute)
2. Defects of red blood cells: morphologic abnormality (e.g., spherocytosis), enzyme defects (e.g., glucose-6-phosphate dehydrogenase deficiency), and hemoglobin abnormality
3. Infection (sepsis)
4. Enclosed hemorrhage (e.g., cephalhematoma)
5. Transient familial (Lucey-Driscoll) syndrome

FIFTH TO SEVENTH DAYS

1. Infection (sepsis)
2. Breast-milk jaundice (enzyme-inhibiting substances)

3. Defects of red blood cells: usually hemoglobin abnormality
4. Crigler-Najjar syndrome (congenital deficiency of glucuronyl transferase)
5. Galactosemia (check urine for reducing substance)
6. Hypothyroidism
7. Intestinal tract obstruction

The problems encountered at the end of the first week may be encountered in the second week, but the usual difficulty with jaundice presenting in the second week is differentiating between congenital biliary atresia and giant cell hepatitis. There is an increasing conviction that these two disorders are not separate entities but form parts of a continuum. In other words, hepatitis develops into biliary atresia, and the timing of diagnostic tests and therapeutic intervention may be critical. More recently, it has been recognized that a deficiency of α_1-antitrypsin may account for a large number of cases of "hepatitis." Increased use of parenteral alimentation has also been associated with an increase in cholestasis (see also Chapter 10).

Jaundice appearing within 48 hours always merits investigation. Physiologic jaundice may be the explanation for unconjugated bilirubin levels up to 12 mg/dl in formula-fed term infants and up to 15 mg/dl in premature infants and breast-fed term infants. Levels above this require investigation. Current practice usually attempts to limit the rise of bilirubin in most premature infants to keep it below 15 mg/dl or even lower in extreme prematurity (see Chapter 10).

WHITE (PALLOR)

Babies appear pale for many reasons; the normal term infant appears pale pink when sleeping quietly. In premature infants and aroused term infants who are pale, the following possibilities should come to mind: (1) cold, (2) acidosis (may also be hypoxemia), (3) hypovolemia, (4) shock, (5) cardiac anomaly or dysfunction, and (6) anemia.

The first four problems result in vasoconstriction of peripheral blood vessels, and the fifth results in decreased cardiac output. Attention should be directed to the environmental temperature, blood pressure, hemoglobin and/or hematocrit values, acid-base status, and any evidence of bleeding (e.g., intracranial hemorrhage) (see also Chapter 24, Neonatal Emergencies).

RED; RED-PURPLE (PLETHORA)

Most babies have a bright red skin color on the second day of life, particularly when aroused. Very premature infants are usually a similar bright red color in the first hours after delivery.

Other conditions to be considered are (1) overheated incubator (red), (2) hyperoxemia (red)—very high paO_2, hypervolemia (red-purple), and high hematocrit value (red-purple).

The environmental temperature and hematocrit value can be checked quickly, and when a baby is in an increased environmental oxygen concentration, the arterial pO_2 should be determined.

BLUE; BLUE-PURPLE (CYANOSIS)
(see also p. 285)

The first question to be asked is: Is the cyanosis peripheral or central? Peripheral cyanosis is frequently seen in the first few hours of life, with blueness of the hands and feet. It is caused by cooling and consequently is termed acrocyanosis. Central cyanosis involves blueness of mucous membranes but may be preceded by circumoral cyanosis.

The following disorders should be considered:

1. Cyanotic congenital heart disease
2. Hyperviscosity (high hematocrit) syndrome (see Chapter 20)
3. Cyanotic attacks associated with apnea (see Chapter 26)
4. Intrinsic pulmonary disease (e.g., respiratory distress syndrome, pneumonia)
5. Extrinsic pulmonary disease (e.g., pneumothorax, diaphragmatic hernia)
6. Persistent pulmonary hypertension—persistent fetal circulation (see pp. 122 to 124)
7. Metabolic disorders (e.g., hypoglycemia, producing convulsive equivalents)
8. Intracranial hemorrhage (see also pp. 233 to 236)
9. Methemoglobinemia

Rapid differentiation is not always possible, but initial evaluations of blood glucose (test tape) and hematocrit value, followed by pH and blood gas evaluations, may be revealing. A hyperoxia test (see Chapter 35) may strongly suggest cyanotic congenital heart disease if the paO_2 remains below 50 mm Hg. A significant rise in paO_2 (perhaps stimulated by continuous positive airway pressure) would suggest intrinsic pulmonary disease. Chest x-ray studies may quickly provide the answer but might be preceded by transillumination of the chest for pneumothorax. Lumbar puncture may eliminate meningitis or subarachnoid or intraventricular hemorrhage. Methemoglobinemia may be detected by hemoglobin electrophoresis or changes in spectral absorption patterns.

Remember that cyanosis results from a certain amount of reduced hemoglobin (about 3 to 4 g/dl in the newborn). Thus, severe desaturation is needed before cyanosis is seen in the anemic infant, whereas comparatively high saturation may be associated with cyanosis with a high hematocrit value.

GRAY

A combination of pallor and cyanosis may produce a grayish hue. The combination of shock and hypoxia is the most likely explanation. Congenital heart disease should always be considered, as well as sepsis, pneumothorax, and intracranial hemorrhage.

Rare causes are subcapsular hemorrhage (hematoma) of the liver and the gray baby syndrome that results from chloramphenicol toxicity (overdosage).

GREEN

The baby born through meconium-stained amniotic fluid may appear quite green on arrival in the nursery, but much of this color can be washed off. More lasting green staining is usually noted in extremely postmature (postterm) babies, particularly involving the umbilical cord, the head, and the nails of both fingers and toes.

Babies with very high levels of bilirubin may also have a greenish hue on top of the yellow-orange color (probably caused by biliverdin).

BRONZE

The bronze baby syndrome is occasionally seen when babies with elevated direct bilirubin levels receive phototherapy. The bronze color is a gray-green hue over the whole body. It may be related to disordered porphyrin metabolism.

TANNING

Phototherapy may also produce an increase in pigmentation of the skin, which later fades. This tanning seems to be more prominent in those who are destined to be heavily pigmented later.

BIBLIOGRAPHY

Yellow-Orange

Weldon, A. P., and Danks, D. M.: Congenital hypothyroidism and neonatal jaundice. *Arch. Dis. Child.* 1972, 47:469.

Bernstein, J., Chang, C. H., Brough, A. J., and Heidelberger, K. P.: Conjugated hyperbilirubinemia in infancy associated with parenteral alimentation. *J. Pediatr.* 1977, 90:361.

Morse, J. O.: Alpha-1-antitrypsin deficiency. *N. Engl. J. Med.* 1978, 299:1099.

Tan, K. L.: Glucose-6-phosphate dehydrogenase status and neonatal jaundice. *Arch. Dis. Child.* 1981, 56:874–877.

Lange, A. P., Secher, M. J., Westergaard, J. G., and Skovgard, I.: Neonatal jaundice after labour induced or stimulated by prostaglandin E_2 or oxytocin. *Lancet* 1982, i:991–994.

Maisels, M. J.: Jaundice in the newborn. *Pediatr. Rev.* 1982, 3:305–319.

Maisels, M. J. (ed.): Neonatal Jaundice. *Clin. Perinatol.* 1990, 17:245–511.

Red-Purple

Berggvist, G., and Zetterstrom, R.: Blood viscosity and peripheral circulation in newborn infants. *Acta Paediatr.* 1974, 63:865.

Saigal, S., and Usher, R.: Symptomatic neonatal plethora. *Biol. Neonate* 1977, 32:62.

Blue-Purple

Macintosh, T. F., and Walker, C. H. M.: Blood viscosity in the newborn. *Arch. Dis. Child.* 1973, 48:547.
Rao, P. S., Marino, B. L., and Robertson, A. F., III: Usefulness of CPAP in differential diagnosis of cardiac from pulmonary cyanosis in newborn infants. *Arch. Dis. Child.* 1978, 53:456.
Kitterman, J. A.: Cyanosis in the newborn infant. *Pediatr. Rev.* 1982, 4:13–23.

Green

Clifford, S. H.: Postmaturity—With placental dysfunction: Clinical syndrome and pathologic findings. *J. Pediatr.* 1954, 44:1.

Bronze

Tan, K. L., and Jacob, E.: The bronze baby syndrome. *Acta Paediatr.* 1982, 71:409–414.
Rubaltelli, F. F., Jori, G., and Reddi, E.: Bronze baby syndrome: A new porphyrin-related disorder. *Pediatr. Res.* 1983, 17:327–330.

Tanning

Woody, N. C., and Brodkey, M. J.: Tanning from phototherapy for neonatal jaundice. *J. Pediatr.* 1973, 82:1042.

26
RESPIRATORY SIGNS

APNEA

Although it is not entirely clear what constitutes clinically significant apnea, for practical purposes, infants with prolonged apnea require careful evaluation and appropriate management. A task force has defined prolonged apnea as ". . . cessation of breathing for 20 seconds or longer, or as a briefer episode associated with bradycardia, cyanosis or pallor." Bradycardia is usually defined as a heart rate of less than 100/min (or possibly 80/min) in this context. Broken apnea (intermittent respiratory movements in a prolonged apneic spell) and disorganized breathing, or obstructive apnea (in which chest wall movement continues without airflow), may be equally or more important in decreasing pO_2 levels. Apneic spells may accompany:

1. Intrinsic pulmonary disease—especially group B streptococcal pneumonia and severe respiratory distress syndrome
2. Sepsis and/or meningitis
3. Hypoglycemia
4. Intracranial hemorrhage or ischemia
5. Changing incubator temperature
6. Prematurity
7. Cardiac disease
8. Convulsions (seizures)
9. Anemia
10. Rapid eye movement sleep
11. Drug depression or withdrawal
12. Necrotizing enterocolitis
13. Obstruction of airway (from vomitus, mucus, and so on)
14. Gastroesophageal reflux
15. Hyperammonemia

To diagnose or eliminate many of these possible reasons for apnea, the following should be determined or obtained:

1. Temperature of baby and incubator
2. Blood pressure
3. Hematocrit value
4. Blood glucose (Dextrostix)
5. Chest radiograph

6. pH and blood gases

7. Sepsis workup, including lumbar puncture

8. Other studies (e.g., stool for blood, serum bilirubin level, electrocardiogram, electroencephalogram, serum ammonia level, cephalic ultrasonographic study).

It is unclear whether isolated hypocalcemia is directly responsible for apnea or whether circumstances predisposing to hypocalcemia also predispose to apnea.

Prematurity may remain as the only explanation for apnea, and this problem seems to be primarily caused by immaturity of the respiratory center. A common cause of apnea in small premature babies is the passage of a bowel movement (equivalent to straining at stool). This is usually easily documented, but apnea may precede a hard stool. A portion of a glycerin suppository may alleviate the problem.

Apnea at the end of the neonatal period may be caused by infection with respiratory syncytial virus. The author has also seen several babies with inguinal hernia whose apnea ceased after surgical correction.

Extremely premature infants (less than 32 weeks' gestation) are most prone to develop apnea because of immaturity of the respiratory center but may induce airway obstruction either by changes in position (producing neck flexion) or by changes in sleep state. The treatment regimen should start with tactile stimulation and may be followed by (1) increased inspired oxygen concentration, but this measure requires caution (limit to 5% increase), (2) 2 to 4 cm H_2O of continuous positive airway pressure (by use of nasal prongs), or (3) xanthine (aminophylline or caffeine) treatment.

Another treatment associated with a decrease in apneic spells is the oscillating water bed, but more recent evidence seems to refute this association. Doxapram therapy may also be successful in infants unresponsive to methylxanthines.

DYSPNEA (RESPIRATORY DISTRESS; BREATHING DIFFICULTY)

The major features of dyspnea are grunting, retractions (sternal and intercostal), and flaring of the nostrils (alae nasi). Chest and abdominal movements may be asynchronous or even paradoxical. Frequently, there is accompanying cyanosis (see Chapter 25) unless increased concentration of oxygen is used.

It is apparent that an enormous number of problems may result in respiratory distress. Although primary pulmonary disease accounts for most cases (see Chapter 9), disorders of the central nervous system and cardiovascular system should not be forgotten. Abdominal distension may limit diaphragmatic excursion, and certain metabolic problems may result in apnea or dyspnea.

The following classification may allow a reasoned approach to the problem.

RESPIRATORY SYSTEM

Primary Pulmonary Disease

1. Respiratory distress syndrome (hyaline membrane disease)
2. Pneumonia

3. Pulmonary hemorrhage
4. Chronic lung disease (bronchopulmonary dysplasia and Wilson-Mikity syndrome)
5. Congenital cystic disorders
6. Retained lung fluid syndrome (respiratory distress syndrome type II)
7. Atelectasis
8. Pulmonary interstitial emphysema
9. Immotile cilia syndrome

Intraluminal Obstruction

1. Atresia or stenosis (choanal, laryngeal)
2. Aspiration syndromes (meconium, blood, milk)
3. Upper airway (Pierre Robin syndrome, macroglossia, and so on)
4. Congenital lobar emphysema

Extrapulmonary Compression

1. Diaphragm problems (hernia, eventration, paralysis)
2. Pneumothorax, pneumomediastinum
3. Mediastinal tumors (including goiter)
4. Vascular ring or aberrant vessel
5. Pleural effusions (includes chylothorax)
6. Congenital dilation of pulmonary lymphatics

CENTRAL NERVOUS SYSTEM

1. Infection
2. Hemorrhage
3. Drugs
4. Anomalies
5. Phrenic nerve palsy

CARDIOVASCULAR SYSTEM

1. Congenital heart disease
2. Anemia
3. High hematocrit (hyperviscosity) syndrome
4. Hypotension (shock)

ABDOMINAL DISTENSION

1. Erythroblastosis fetalis
2. Obstructive uropathy

METABOLIC

1. Acidosis (infection, cooling, organic aciduria, and so on)
2. Hyperammonemia

Despite this formidable list, considerable differentiation can be achieved using clinical examination (including temperature), chest radiography, white blood count and differential, hematocrit value, and blood gas analysis. If none of these tests is revealing, a blood ammonia analysis may be helpful.

TACHYPNEA

Rapid respirations may accompany respiratory distress but may be observed as an isolated feature. Tachypnea is present when the respiratory rate exceeds 60/min. It may be a benign problem (transient tachypnea) or may prove to be the first sign of serious illness (congenital heart disease).

The following disorders should be considered when tachypnea alone is seen:

1. Metabolic acidosis: stimulating the blowing off of carbon dioxide in an attempt to compensate for it
2. Transient tachypnea of the newborn: retained lung fluid syndrome, detectable on x-ray study
3. Congenital heart disease: usually an early sign of congestive heart failure
4. Anemia
5. High hematocrit value
6. High environmental (incubator) temperature
7. Central nervous system irritation, such as meningitis or hemorrhage

STRIDOR

Stridor may be continuous or intermittent. Continuous stridor usually requires immediate investigation. It may be inspiratory, or expiratory, or both. Intermittent and inspiratory stridor is usually more benign. Stridor results from an intrinsic or extrinsic blockage of the upper airway (usually the trachea). A high-pitched noise is more likely the result of obstruction at the laryngeal level, whereas a low-pitched noise is more likely to be associated with tracheal problems. The following disorders should be considered.

LARYNX

1. Laryngeal web
2. Laryngeal stenosis
3. Vocal cord paralysis
4. Laryngeal cysts
5. Laryngeal tumors (e.g., hemangioma, papilloma)
6. Laryngeal edema (after extubation)

TRACHEA

1. Tracheal stenosis (hypoplasia)
2. Tracheal compression: vascular ring or aberrant vessels, enlarged thyroid (goiter), mediastinal tumors
3. Subglottic stenosis (following endotracheal intubation)

COMBINED

1. Simple (benign) congenital (laryngeal) stridor

Investigation will probably be directed toward the same items as those for apnea (see p. 298).

Disorders of the larynx can usually be ascertained by direct laryngoscopy. Lateral radiographs of the neck and chest with or without contrast material in the esophagus may demonstrate many tracheal problems, but more complicated procedures may be needed (e.g., arteriography), although ultrasonography is sometimes revealing.

Congenital laryngeal stridor has also been termed laryngomalacia. Because the epiglottis may also be large and floppy (omega epiglottis) and the trachea may be involved, chondromalacia is another alternative term. Although parents and personnel are disturbed, the baby is usually not bothered by it at all. It is usually heard with inspiration and disappears within 6 to 12 months.

PERSISTENT STUFFY AND RUNNY NOSE

The baby who has persistent rhinitis or nasal obstruction should be evaluated with the following possibilities in mind:

1. Reserpine or methyldopa administered to the mother
2. Pyogenic (bacterial) infection
3. Congenital syphilis (so-called snuffles)
4. Hypothyroidism
5. Choanal atresia (usually acute distress, but may be unilateral)
6. Nasal septal deviation (fracture)

SNEEZING

Because the neonate is an obligate nasal breather (although this is not *always* true), any minor obstruction is likely to trigger the sneeze reflex. This is a normal activity in most term babies, and parents should be reassured that the baby does not have the common cold (unless there is other evidence to the contrary).

COUGHING

Unlike sneezing, coughing is unusual in the neonate but has been associated with numerous infections seen later in the neonatal period. Chlamydial pneumonia and infection with either respiratory syncytial virus or adenoviruses, as well as pertussis, are infections to consider strongly.

Aspiration for any reason may predispose to coughing, so gastroesophageal reflux and H-type tracheoesophageal fistula may need to be considered.

BIBLIOGRAPHY

Apnea

Kattwinkel, J.: Apnea in the neonatal period. *Pediatr. Rev.* 1980, 2:115–120.
Philip, A. G. S.: Neonatal inguinal hernia and recurrent apnea. *Hosp. Pract.* 1980, 15(Aug): 21–24.
Rigatto, H.: Apnea. *Pediatr. Clin. North Am.* 1982, 29:1105–1116.
Avery, M. E., and Frantz, I. D. III: To breathe or not to breathe: What have we learned about apneic spells and sudden infant death? (Editorial) *N. Engl. J. Med.* 1983, 309:107–108.
Dransfield, D. A., Spitzer, A. R., and Fox, W. W.: Episodic airway obstruction in premature infants. *Am. J. Dis. Child.* 1983, 137:441–443.
Henderson-Smart, D. J., Pettigrew, A. G., and Campbell, D. J.: Clinical apnea and brainstem neural function in preterm infants. *N. Engl. J. Med.* 1983, 308:353–357.
Van Someren, V., and Stothers, J. K.: A critical dissection of obstructive apnea in the human infant. *Pediatrics* 1983, 71:721–725.
Paton, J. Y., Nanayakkara, C. S., and Simpson, H.: Observations on gastro-oesophageal reflux, central apnoea and heart rate in infants. *Eur. J. Pediatr.* 1990, 149:608–612.
Kumita, H., Mizuno, S., Shinohara, M., et al.: Low-dose doxapram therapy in premature infants and its CSF and serum concentrations. *Acta Paediatr. Scand.* 1991, 80:786–791.
Upton, C. J., Milner, A. D., and Stokes, G. M.: Apnoea, bradycardia, and oxygen saturation in preterm infants. *Arch. Dis. Child.* 1991, 66:381–385.
Scanlon, J. E. M., Chin, K. C., Morgan, M. E. I., et al.: Caffeine or theophylline for neonatal apnoea. *Arch. Dis. Child.* 1992, 67:425–428.

Dyspnea

Avery, M. E., Fletcher, B. D., and Williams, R. G.: *The Lung and Its Disorders in the Newborn Infant,* 4th ed. W. B. Saunders, Philadelphia, 1981, pp. 127–328.
Whitelaw, A., Evans, A., and Corrin, B.: Immotile cilia syndrome: A new cause of neonatal respiratory distress. *Arch. Dis. Child.* 1981, 56:432–435.
Schreiner, R. L., and Bradburn, N. C.: Newborns with acute respiratory distress: Diagnosis and management. *Pediatr. Rev.* 1988, 9:279–285.

Stridor

Arthurton, M. W.: Stridor in a paediatric department. *Proc. R. Soc. Med.* 1970, 63:712.
McSwiney, P. F., Cavanagh, N. P. C., and Languth, P.: Outcome in congenital stridor (laryngomalacia). *Arch. Dis. Child.* 1977, 52:215.
Burch, M., Balaji, S., Deanfield, J. E., and Sullivan, I. D.: Investigation of vascular compression of the trachea: The complementary roles of barium swallow and echocardiography. *Arch. Dis. Child.* 1993, 68:171–176.

Stuffy Nose

Silverman, S. H., and Liebow, S. G.: Dislocation of the triangular cartilage of the nasal septum. *J. Pediatr.* 1975, 87:456.

Coughing

Hammerschlag, M. R.: Chlamydial pneumonia in infants. *N. Engl. J. Med.* 1978, 298:1083–1084.

Hall, C. B., Kopelman, A. E., Douglas, R. G., et al.: Neonatal respiratory syncytial virus infection. *N. Engl. J. Med.* 1979, 300:393–396.

27
CARDIAC SIGNS

CARDIAC MURMUR

A comprehensive review of all the causes of murmurs heard in the neonatal period is beyond the scope of this book (see Chapter 8). Nevertheless, certain points are worth remembering.

1. A murmur heard on the first day of life is most likely to be benign (usually associated with flow through the ductus arteriosus); murmurs discovered later usually require investigation but are also frequently benign.

2. Absence of a murmur on the first day (and subsequently) by no means excludes the diagnosis of congenital heart disease.

3. The louder and more widely transmitted the murmur, the more likely it is to be significant, but small defects can create a lot of turbulence.

4. Location of the maximal intensity is not reliable in differentiation; for example, a patent ductus arteriosus murmur may be heard at the left lower sternal edge, whereas a ventricular septal defect murmur may be heard at the second left interspace.

5. Premature infants who have pulmonary disease followed by a murmur have a patent ductus arteriosus until proven otherwise.

6. The murmur of patent ductus arteriosus is usually only systolic in timing to begin with. The typical "machinery" murmur occurs much later.

Investigations include hemoglobin and hematocrit determination (for anemia or hyperviscosity), chest x-ray study, and electrocardiograph. When two-dimensional echocardiography is available, this noninvasive technique may quickly detect structural abnormalities of the heart. If all of these results are within normal limits, the parents should be reassured that the murmur is of no real significance. However, careful evaluation should be carried out at follow-up visits, and signs of cardiac failure should be kept in mind.

BRADYCARDIA

A heart rate below 100/min may be normal in some babies, especially in the latter part of the neonatal period. More commonly, however, another explanation exists. Bradycardia is a common accompaniment of prolonged apnea and seems to accompany hypoxia. Congenital heart block, with or without associated cardiac abnormalities, is the most likely explanation, particularly if the heart rate is very slow. Congenital complete heart block may be associated with maternal systemic lupus erythematosus. An occasional cause of heart block (acquired) is severe hypocalcemia, and the author has seen several babies respond dramatically to slow infusion of calcium gluconate when low serum calcium level has been documented. Bradycardia has been reported in term babies who develop pulmonary interstitial emphysema (for Cardiopulmonary Arrest, see p. 285).

TACHYCARDIA

The most common causes of slightly increased heart rate are overheating (fever), crying, and early cardiac failure. Methylxanthine overdosage, when used in the treatment of apnea, may induce tachycardia of moderate degree.

When very fast rates are encountered (over 200 to 300 beats/min), some form of atrial tachycardia is usually present. This phenomenon may be documented on the electrocardiograph, and treatment should be started as soon as the diagnosis is made. Oxygen, intravenous fluids, and digoxin form the basis of treatment (see Chapter 24, Neonatal Emergencies).

HEART SOUNDS HEARD BEST ON THE RIGHT SIDE

Four diagnoses require careful consideration when heart sounds are heard best on the right side of the chest: (1) true dextrocardia, (2) pneumothorax (tension on left), (3) diaphragmatic hernia, and (4) atelectasis of a major portion of the right lung.

True dextrocardia may or may not be accompanied by situs inversus of the abdominal organs. If the liver and other organs appear to be in their usual location, a high risk of intrinsic cardiac abnormality exists. With total situs inversus, congenital heart disease is unlikely.

Both left-sided tension pneumothorax and diaphragmatic hernia (which most frequently occurs on the left side) produce an apparent dextrocardia, which can be excluded on chest x-ray study. Pneumothorax might be ruled out by transillumination of the chest.

Atelectasis of the right lung is perhaps the least likely of the four diagnoses to cause significant mediastinal shift but may be the result of aspirated blood or meconium, inspissated mucus blocking the right main stem bronchus, or hyperinflation of the left lung, such as occurs in unilateral pulmonary interstitial emphysema. In the somewhat older baby, postextubation atelectasis, following the use of assisted ventilation, needs to be considered.

MUFFLED HEART SOUNDS

Heart sounds that initially are easily heard but that later become muffled may be caused by pneumomediastinum or pericardial effusion. The former is detected on chest x-ray study (usually easier on the lateral) or by transillumination, whereas the latter may be confirmed by echocardiography.

LARGE HEART ON CHEST RADIOGRAPH

In the presence of other cardiac symptoms, a large heart usually accompanies congestive heart failure or pericardial effusion. An apparently large heart may merely be a large cardiothymic shadow during expiration. Other causes of an enlarged heart without a cardiac murmur are (1) myocarditis, (2) endocardial fibroelastosis, (3) glycogen storage disease, and (4) other rare causes such as rhabdomyoma or aberrant left coronary artery. Hypoglycemia may also result in cardiac enlargement (see Chapter 17).

HYPERTENSION

The incidence of elevated blood pressure in the neonatal period appears to be increasing, but this may be the result of more careful observations (for normal values see Appendix 6). It has been linked closely to renovascular problems and activation of the renin-angiotensin syndrome. Thrombi related to high placement of umbilical artery catheters (tip above renal arteries) and patent ductus arteriosus have been described. Considerable day-to-day fluctuations of systolic and diastolic blood pressures have been observed. Diagnosis may depend on angiographic and radionuclide evaluation. The renal scan (using radioactive technetium) provides valuable information regarding the function of each kidney.

Endocrine causes of hypertension are rare. Somewhat more likely is obstructive uropathy (documented with intravenous pyelogram or ultrasonography). An aggressive medical approach with antihypertensive agents may be necessary, but the natural history of hypertension presenting in the newborn period is not clear. Occasionally, a rapid rate of increase in blood pressure produces hypertensive encephalopathy. Surgery for unilateral renal disease may be needed.

When hypertension is limited to the upper extremities (especially the right arm), coarctation of the aorta is likely to be the cause. Another cause to keep in mind is the use of phenylephrine eye drops for pupillary dilation, which can cause transient hypertension.

HYPOTENSION

Most newborn infants have blood pressures that seem low to the uninitiated. However, when blood pressure falls below defined levels (see Appendix 6), the cause must be investigated. Although there is not always a direct relationship between blood pressure and blood volume, a low blood pressure immediately suggests hypovolemia. If peripheral perfusion is adequate, no action may be necessary, but if perfusion is poor, steps to support blood volume should be taken. Initially, one may use albumin, followed by whole blood, fresh-frozen plasma, packed red blood cells, or a combination of the last two. Pressor agents may also be needed, particularly when echocardiography indicates poor cardiac contractility.

The possibility that hemorrhage may have occurred or that metabolic acidosis and/or infection has resulted in decreased blood pressure should initiate a search for the source and institution of appropriate measures (see Shock section in Chapter 24). Air leaks should also be considered.

For Dysrhythmia (arrhythmia), see pp. 286 to 287.

BIBLIOGRAPHY

Barr, P. A., Bailey, P. E., Sumners, J., and Cassady, G.: Relation between arterial blood pressure and blood volume and effect of infused albumin in sick preterm infants. *Pediatrics* 1977, 60:282.

Brazy, J. E., and Blackmon, L. R.: Hypotension and bradycardia associated with airblock in the neonate. Preliminary report. *J. Pediatr.* 1977, 90:796.

Chameides, L., Truex, R. C., Vetter, V., et al.: Association of maternal systemic lupus erythematosus with congenital complete heart block. *N. Engl. J. Med.* 1977, 297:1204.

Evans, D. J., Silverman, M., and Bowley, N. B.: Congenital hypertension due to unilateral renal vein thrombosis. *Arch. Dis. Child.* 1981, 56:306–308.

Lees, B. J., and Cabal, L. A.: Increased blood pressure following pupillary dilation with 2.5% phenylephrine hydrochloride in preterm infants. *Pediatrics* 1981, 68:231–234.

Editorial: Delayed closure of the ductus. *Lancet* 1983, ii:436–437.

Sheftel, D. N., Hustead, V., and Friedman, A.: Hypertension screening in the follow-up of premature infants. *Pediatrics* 1983, 71:763–766.

Emery, E. F., Greenough, A., and Gamsu, H. R.: Randomised controlled trial of colloid infusions in hypotensive preterm infants. *Arch. Dis. Child.* 1992, 67:1185–1188.

Hodgman, J. E., Hoppenbrouwers, T., and Cabal L. A.: Episodes of bradycardia during early infancy in the term-born and preterm infant. *Am. J. Dis. Child.* 1993, 147:960–964.

See also Chapter 8.

ABDOMINAL SIGNS

28

SINGLE UMBILICAL ARTERY

Single umbilical artery is seen in approximately 1% of all live births. It is more common in twins and in infants with chromosomal defects. There are several associated abnormalities, primarily involving the cardiovascular, gastro-intestinal, and renal systems. Although at one time, single umbilical artery was considered to be a useful marker for other abnormalities, it now seems unlikely that any undetected abnormalities will be revealed by investigation if single umbilical artery is the only obvious abnormality. Nevertheless, discovery of single umbilical artery should alert the examiner to other possible abnormalities. If any minor abnormalities are found, it may be valuable to evaluate the kidneys with ultrasonography (i.e., a noninvasive technique).

VOMITING

Many babies vomit occasionally for no apparent reason. When vomiting occurs with some regularity, consideration should be given to both medical and surgical conditions. Bile-stained vomitus is almost invariably caused by a problem requiring surgery (intestinal obstruction), but regurgitation of yellow-tinged mucus is not uncommon in the first 24 hours after birth.

MEDICAL REASONS

1. Sucking and swallowing difficulties
2. Swallowed air
3. Sepsis and/or meningitis
4. Urinary tract infection or abnormality (hydronephrosis)
5. Necrotizing enterocolitis (may be surgical)
6. Hiatus hernia
7. Drug withdrawal
8. Congenital adrenal hyperplasia (adrenogenital syndrome)
9. Kernicterus
10. Gastroesophageal reflux

SURGICAL REASONS

1. Esophageal atresia (early)
2. Vascular ring (involving esophagus)
3. Congenital hypertrophic pyloric stenosis (late, usually postneonatal)
4. Duodenal obstruction (atresia, stenosis, annular pancreas, and so on)
5. Intestinal atresia
6. Malrotation
7. Volvulus
8. Duplication of bowel
9. Hirschsprung's disease (congenital megacolon)

Differentiation of the various medical causes is aided by knowledge of the maternal history, observation of the baby feeding, presence of abdominal distension (see later) or evidence of infection (see Chapter 15), and laboratory investigations. Hiatus hernia (congenital short esophagus) seems to be uncommon in the United States but quite common in Great Britain. Esophagitis may result in blood-flecked vomitus. Similar features may occur when marked gastroesophageal reflux is present, although the significance of reflux is still debated. It has been shown that the prone position, particularly with the child inclined and head up, is superior to the sitting position for the prevention of reflux. Thickening the feedings may be beneficial. Preliminary work suggests that metoclopramide may also decrease symptomatic reflux.

Disorders that require surgical intervention can be roughly classified into those without abdominal distension and those with abdominal distension. The former are usually upper intestinal problems. Esophageal atresia (with or without tracheoesophageal fistula) is associated with excessive amounts of mucus on the first day of life. Vascular ring usually has accompanying stridor. Pyloric stenosis occasionally presents problems late in the neonatal period, with forceful to projectile vomiting of feedings without bile. The other disorders usually have accompanying abdominal distension, and a barium enema and upper gastrointestinal tract series may be needed to differentiate among them.

BLOODY VOMITUS

Vomiting of milk with small amounts of blood in it may be the result of cracked nipples (as well as hiatus hernia) in the breast-fed baby. Larger quantities of blood may be vomited in the early neonatal period, making it difficult to know whether it is swallowed maternal blood or whether it is from the baby (because peptic ulcer is not rare in the newborn period). If the blood is red, it may be distinguished by using the Apt test (see p. 380), which shows persistence of pink supernatant after addition of sodium hydroxide in the presence of fetal hemoglobin (baby's blood), as opposed to a yellow-brown color seen in adult hemoglobin (maternal blood). If the blood is already altered ("coffee-grounds" material), the Apt test cannot be applied (it is no longer apt).

DIARRHEA

Loss of large amounts of fluid and electrolytes into the bowel constitutes diarrhea. Many breast-fed babies have loose yellow stools that are not considered to be diarrhea. Diarrheal stools are usually green in the neonatal period, indicating decreased transit time. Phototherapy for hyperbilirubinemia may also result in decreased transit time and increased fluid loss in the stool, which is not true diarrhea. Loose, green, frequent, small stools may result from gross deficiency of food intake.

The following classification of diarrhea in the newborn may be helpful.

FALSE DIARRHEA

Breast-milk stools
"Phototherapy stools"
"Starvation stools"

DIARRHEA WITHOUT BLOOD

Systemic infection
Enteral infection: viral, bacterial
Disaccharidase deficiency (may be induced by phototherapy)
Monosaccharidase deficiency (rare)

DIARRHEA WITH BLOOD

Enteral infection: *Salmonella* (rare); *Shigella;* pathogenic *Escherichia coli*
Necrotizing enterocolitis
Hypersensitivity to cow's milk (rare)

Stool cultures are indicated in most cases. Some strains of *E. coli* may not be considered enteropathogenic until an epidemic occurs and extensive serogrouping is performed (see Enteritis section in Chapter 15).

If diarrhea disappears with parenteral feeding but reappears with reintroduction of disaccharide in the diet, a disaccharidase deficiency should be considered.

BLOOD IN THE STOOL

In addition to disorders listed earlier in association with diarrhea, the following may cause difficulty:

1. Swallowed maternal blood
2. Hemorrhagic disease of the newborn: preventable with vitamin K, usually appears on the second day

3. Rectal perforation (via rectal thermometer)
4. Mesenteric thrombosis
5. Bleeding gastric ulcer (due to stress)
6. False-positive result caused by povidone-iodine

When the stool is streaked with blood, the most likely explanation is an anal fissure.

DELAYED PASSAGE OF MECONIUM

The first meconium stool is passed within 24 hours in 90% of babies. Some babies seem to have delay secondary to a meconium plug. Many times, relief of such a plug results in no further difficulties. However, approximately 10% of babies who have delay in passage of the first stool for 24 hours have a bilirubin level (maximum) of greater than 15 mg/dl. Meconium plug is somewhat more common in infants with intrauterine growth retardation in our experience. It may be one end of a spectrum extending through meconium ileus to meconium peritonitis, and cystic fibrosis (mucoviscidosis) should always be considered. Delay in the passage of meconium until after 36 to 48 hours in the term baby should raise the possibility of intestinal atresia or obstruction, Hirschsprung's disease (congenital megacolon due to aganglionosis), cystic fibrosis of the pancreas, hypermagnesemia, or hypothyroidism.

Some premature infants have considerable delay in the passage of meconium, partly because of lack of feeding by mouth, partly because of ileus (caused by infection, hypoxia, and so on), and probably also because of immaturity of the nervous system.

CONSTIPATION

In addition to delay of passage of the first meconium stool, the baby may have continued difficulty in passing bowel movements, which may necessitate a search for the following problems: Hirschsprung's disease (aganglionosis of the colon); anterior placement of the anus; retroperitoneal or other masses, causing extrinsic compression; or hypothyroidism (later in the newborn period).

ABDOMINAL DISTENSION

Although it is apparent that obstruction of the lower part of the intestine is likely to result in obvious abdominal distension (Fig. 28–1), there are many other reasons for this finding. In particular, the premature infant who has a distended abdomen may be suffering from sepsis or meningitis; necrotizing enterocolitis; ileus caused by hypoxia or hypermagnesemia; perforation of a viscus, such as the stomach; swallowed air after a feeding or if the baby is being treated with continuous positive airway pressure by nasal prongs; or eye occlusion during phototherapy.

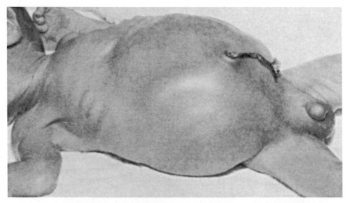

FIGURE 28–1. Gross abdominal distension with intestinal loops seen through the abdominal wall in a small premature infant suspected of having neonatal sepsis.

These conditions are generally associated with increased amounts of air in the abdomen. Distension may also be caused by enlarged solid organs, such as

1. Liver: subcapsular hematoma; TORCH complex; cardiac failure
2. Kidney: hydronephrosis, polycystic kidneys, nephroblastoma (Wilms' tumor), congenital mesoblastic nephroma
3. Adrenal: neuroblastoma, hemorrhage
4. Spleen: TORCH complex (especially toxoplasmosis)
5. Ovary: large cysts are occasionally encountered but usually resolve spontaneously.

Another broad category is distension caused by fluid in the abdomen, which comes under the heading of ascites. Some causes of ascites are hydrops fetalis (usually Rh incompatibility, but also α-thalassemia and congenital syphilis), obstructive uropathy, peritonitis (including meconium peritonitis), congenital nephrosis, or chylous and biliary ascites (rare). Investigation may be directed to the appropriate area by consideration of whether the distension is caused by solid, liquid, or gas.

SCAPHOID ABDOMEN

The abdomens of all babies are relatively flat until swallowed air has distended the intestines. A flat or scaphoid abdomen after a few hours is most likely the result of (1) diaphragmatic hernia or other diaphragmatic problem (eventration or paralysis); (2) absence of viscera, e.g., renal agenesis (Potter's syndrome); or (3) a "gasless" abdomen secondary to failure to swallow gas, such as that caused by a central nervous system defect, paralysis, or moribund state.

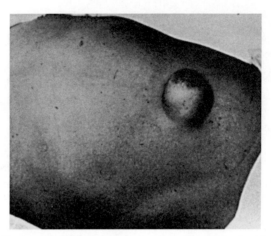

FIGURE 28–2. Umbilical hernia. This condition is more common in the black population.

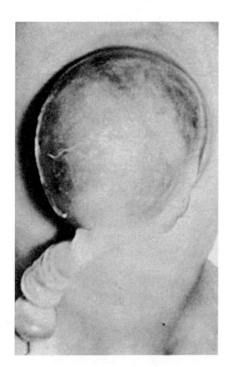

FIGURE 28–3. Large omphalocele (exomphalos), showing the umbilical cord emerging from the enclosing sac.

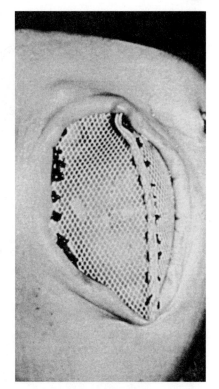

FIGURE 28–4. Postoperative photograph of the baby in Figure 28–3, showing a prosthesis minimizing tension of the abdominal wall.

DEFECTS OF THE ABDOMINAL WALL

Minor defects at the umbilical ring may result in protrusion of intestine into an umbilical hernia (Fig. 28–2). Although rather unsightly, no specific therapy is required. It is more common in blacks and premature infants.

Three disorders usually require surgical consultation and deserve a word of explanation. When the abdominal contents protrude into the umbilical cord, the condition is called omphalocele (exomphalos) (Figs. 28–3 and 28–4). When this protrusion is large, the covering of the intestine may be so thinned out that the covering layer ruptures. Intestines may be exposed. When this occurs, it may be difficult to distinguish from gastroschisis (Fig. 28–5). This disorder is the result of a defect in the abdominal wall lateral to the umbilicus, almost invariably on the right side. Again, the bowel is exposed, but the umbilical cord is present lateral to the bowel (see also Chapter 24, Neonatal Emergencies).

Another defect of the abdominal wall is called prune-belly syndrome, in which there is absence of abdominal musculature (Fig. 28–6). This condition is unlikely to be confused with omphalocele or gastroschisis but must be distinguished from ascites. There may be associated renal anomalies.

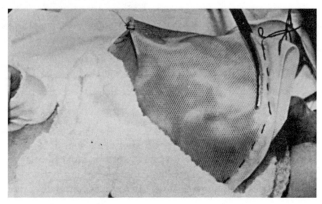

FIGURE 28–5. Postoperative photograph of a baby with gastroschisis, showing prosthesis covering the exteriorized intestines. Slow replacement of intestine into the abdominal cavity can be achieved with this technique.

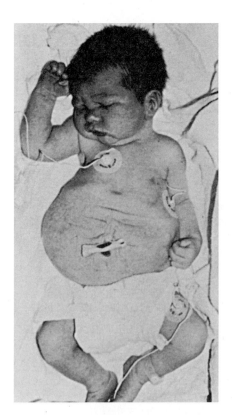

FIGURE 28–6. Prune-belly syndrome, showing abdominal distension and wrinkled skin.

DRAINAGE FROM THE UMBILICUS

After the umbilical cord drops off (between 4 and 10 days after birth) some drainage may be noted from the umbilical stump. Most frequently, this drainage is caused by exudation from excessive granulation tissue, but if it is grossly yellow, it may be caused by staphylococcal infection. If fluid rapidly reaccumulates after the umbilicus is wiped, two other disorders should be considered: (1) persistent (patent) omphalomesenteric duct, communicating with the gut, and (2) patent urachus, communicating with the bladder.

BIBLIOGRAPHY

Single Umbilical Artery

Cogswell, J. J.: The single umbilical artery. *Dev. Med. Child. Neurol.* 1974, 16:79.
Heifetz, S. A.: Single umbilical artery: A statistical analysis of 237 autopsy cases and review of the literature. *Perspect. Pediatr. Pathol.* 1984, 8:345–378.
Leung, A. K. C., and Robson, W. L. M.: Single umbilical artery: A report of 159 cases. *Arch. Dis. Child.* 1989, 143:108–111.
Bourke, W. G., Clarke, T. A., Mathews, T. G., et al.: Isolated single umbilical artery—The case for routine renal screening. *Arch. Dis. Child.* 1993, 68:600–601.

Vomiting

Balistreri, W. F., and Farrell, M. K.: Gastroesophageal reflux in infants. *N. Engl. J. Med.* 1983, 309:790–792.
Lilien, L. D., Srinivasan, G., Pyati, S. P., et al.: Green vomiting in the first 72 hours in normal infants. *Am. J. Dis. Child.* 1986, 140:662–664.
Bailey, P. V., Tracy, T. F., Jr., Connors, R. H., et al.: Congenital duodenal obstruction: A 32-year review. *J. Pediatr. Surg.* 1993, 28:92–95.

Bloody Vomitus

Johnson, D., L'Heureux, P., and Thompson, T.: Peptic ulcer disease in early infancy: Clinical presentation and roentgenographic features. *Acta Paediatr.* 1980, 69:753–760.

Diarrhea

Lester, R.: "Diarrhea" and malabsorption in the newborn (Editorial). *N. Engl. J. Med.* 1977, 297:505.
Editorial: Colitis in term babies. *Lancet* 1983, i:1083.

Blood in the Stool

Hait, W. N., Snepar, R., and Rothmen, C.: False-positive Hematest due to povidone-iodine (Letter). *N. Engl. J. Med.* 1977, 297:1350.

Delayed Passage of Meconium

Clark, D. A.: Times of first void and first stools in 500 newborns. *Pediatrics* 1977, 60:457.
Editorial: Meconium ileus. *Lancet* 1982, i:1000.
Olsen, M. M., Luck, S. R., Lloyd-Still, J., and Raffensperger, J. G.: The spectrum of meconium disease in infancy. *J. Pediatr. Surg.* 1982, 17:479–481.
Fakhoury, K., Durie, P. R., Levison, H., and Canny, G. J.: Meconium ileus in the absence of cystic fibrosis. *Arch. Dis. Child.* 1992, 67:1204–1206.

Weaver, L. T., and Lucas, A.: Development of bowel habit in preterm infants. *Arch. Dis. Child.* 1993, 68:317–320.

Constipation

Hendren, W. H.: Constipation caused by anterior location of the anus and its surgical correction. *J. Pediatr. Surg.* 1978, 13:505.

Malangoni, M. A., Grosfeld, J. L., Ballantine, T. V. N., and Kleiman, M.: Congenital rectal stenosis: A sign of a presacral pathologic condition. *Pediatrics* 1978, 62:584.

Abdominal Distension

Griscom, N. T., Colodny, A. H., Rosenberg, H. K., et al.: Diagnostic aspects of neonatal ascites: Report of 27 cases. *Am. J. Roentgenol.* 1977, 128:961.

Henderson, K. C., and Torch, E. M.: Differential diagnosis of abdominal masses in the neonate. *Pediatr. Clin. North Am.* 1977, 24:557.

Preis, O., and Rudolph, N.: Abdominal distension in newborn infants on phototherapy—role of eye occlusion. *J. Pediatr.* 1979, 94:816.

Gerber, A., Gold, J. H., Bustamante, S., et al.: Congenital mesoblastic nephroma. *J. Pediatr. Surg.* 1981, 16:758–759.

Cohen, M. D., Schreiner, R., and Lemons, J.: Neonatal pneumoperitoneum without significant adventitious pulmonary air: Use of metrizamide to rule out perforation of the bowel. *Pediatrics* 1982, 69:587–589.

Gale, G. B., D'Angio, G. J., Uri, A., et al.: Cancer in neonates: The experience at the Children's Hospital of Philadelphia. *Pediatrics* 1982, 70:409–413.

Wilson, D. A.: Ultrasound screening for abdominal masses in the neonatal period. *Am. J. Dis. Child.* 1982, 136:147–151.

Johnson, J. F., and Robinson, L. H.: Localized bowel distension in the newborn: A review of the plain film analysis and differential diagnosis. *Pediatrics* 1984, 73:206–215.

Schwartz, M. Z., and Shaul, D. B.: Abdominal masses in the newborn. *Pediatr. Rev.* 1989, 11:172–179.

Campbell, B. A., Garg, R. S., Garg, K., et al.: Perinatal ovarian cyst: A non-surgical approach. *J. Pediatr. Surg.* 1992, 27:1618–1619.

Duffy, L. F.: Malformations of the gut. *Pediatr. Rev.* 1992, 13:50–54.

Defects of Abdominal Wall

Seashore, J. H.: Congenital abdominal wall defects. *Clin. Perinatol.* 1978, 5:61.

Woodhouse, C. R. J., Ransley, P., and Innes-Williams, D.: Prune belly syndrome—Report of 47 cases. *Arch. Dis. Child.* 1982, 57:856–859.

Kirk, E. P., and Wah, R. M.: Obstetric management of the fetus with omphalocele or gastroschisis: A review and report of one hundred twelve cases. *Am. J. Obstet. Gynecol.* 1983, 146:512–518.

Nakayama, D. K., Harrison, M. R., Gross, B. H., et al.: Management of the fetus with an abdominal wall defect. *J. Pediatr. Surg.* 1984, 19:408–413.

Tucci, M., and Bard, H.: The associated anomalies that determine prognosis in congenital omphaloceles. *Am. J. Obstet. Gynecol.* 1990, 163:1646–1649.

Stringer, M. D., Brereton, R. J., and Wright, V. M.: Controversies in the management of gastroschisis: A study of 40 patients. *Arch. Dis. Child.* 1991, 66:34–36.

Loder, R. T., Guiboux, J-P., Bloom, D. A., and Hensinger, R. N.: Musculo-skeletal aspects of prune-belly syndrome: Description and pathogenesis. *Am. J. Dis. Child.* 1992, 146:1224–1229.

Drainage from the Umbilicus

Geneiser, N. B., Becker, M. H., Grosfeld, J., and Kaufman, H.: Draining umbilicus in infants. *N. Y. State J. Med.* 1974, 74:182.

29

NEUROLOGIC SIGNS

JITTERINESS

Infants may be jittery or tremulous for benign reasons in some cases, and in others the reasons are ominous. Most causes of jitteriness may also result in convulsions (see the following section). One method of evaluation may be helpful in distinguishing whether or not jitteriness is benign. If the tremors of the limbs are of low amplitude and high frequency (rapid, fine movements), it is likely that the condition will prove to be benign (usually metabolic in origin). If the tremors are of high amplitude and low frequency (slow, coarse movements), it is more likely to be ominous (resulting from a problem of the central nervous system).

Many newborn infants become quite jittery just before a feeding (eager anticipation) without demonstrating low blood glucose values. Infants of diabetic mothers frequently demonstrate unexplained jitteriness, even though they are more prone to develop the metabolic problems associated with jitteriness.

Causes of jitteriness are classified in Table 29–1.

Placing a baby on its abdomen or giving it a feeding may abolish jitteriness. If not, one should direct attention toward the prenatal course or events during labor and delivery, blood glucose level, and hematocrit value. If these are normal, further investigation may be necessary.

CONVULSIONS (SEIZURES; FITS)

Typical generalized tonic-clonic convulsive activity noted in older children and adults is seen only rarely in newborns. More frequently, intermittent hypertonicity occurs with deviation of the eyes, and there may be jerking of one limb or twitching of only the fingers and toes. Unilaterality cannot be used as a localizing sign. Conversely, bilateral convulsions do not rule out a focus on one side (e.g., subdural hematoma). However, focal seizures will frequently yield a focal injury when cephalic ultrasonography, electroencephalography, and radionuclide scanning results are combined.

An unusual presentation of convulsions on the fifth day of life has been described as a possibly distinct entity; the cause is uncertain, but zinc deficiency has been suggested, although the problem seems to have disappeared after 1985. There are certain so-called convulsive equivalents (or subtle seizures) that are

TABLE 29–1. CAUSES OF NEONATAL JITTERINESS

Metabolic Disorders
  Hypoglycemia
  Hypocalcemia
  Hypomagnesemia

CNS Disorders
  Hemorrhage
  Hypoxia
  Congenital abnormality
  Hyperviscosity (high hematocrit) syndrome

Drug Withdrawal
  Heroin
  Methadone
  Barbiturates

Idiopathic
  Prefeeding
  Others

CNS = central nervous system.

frequently seen in the neonate. The most common are apnea, circumoral cyanosis (seen more frequently with metabolic problems), eye blinking, and repetitive sucking or chewing (mouthing) movements (more common with central nervous system problems). Small premature infants frequently have sudden jerking movements that are of brief duration and not repetitive. A distinguishing feature of clonic movements of a limb is that they cannot be stopped by flexing the limb (other jerks or jitteriness can).

The same kind of classification can be used for convulsions as for jitteriness, and although convulsions are less common, the list is longer (Table 29–2).

Unfortunately, hypoxic-ischemic encephalopathy secondary to perinatal asphyxia remains the most common cause of convulsions. This diagnosis is not easily confirmed, although increased levels of creatine kinase brain-type isoenzyme (CK-BB) or hypoxanthine may be helpful. The electroencephalogram is almost invariably deranged but may not be diagnostic of hypoxic injury. Hemorrhage can be detected with cephalic ultrasonography or computed tomographic scan, and blood glucose and serum calcium levels are easily determined. Hematocrit value determination with a white blood count and differential can be performed quickly and easily; this information may suggest hyperviscosity or infection.

Treatment is usually initiated with phenobarbital, but other pharmacologic agents may be needed (see pp. 289 to 290). Prognosis varies with the cause, but if the clinical examination and electroencephalographic results are normal 1 week after the seizure, the long-term outlook is good.

LETHARGY

Surprisingly, almost all the disorders that may produce convulsions (listed earlier) can also produce lethargy, particularly infection and hypoxia. In addi-

TABLE 29–2. CAUSES OF NEONATAL CONVULSIONS

Metabolic Disorders
  Hypoglycemia*
  Hypocalcemia*
  Hypomagnesemia
  Hyponatremia or hypernatremia
  Pyridoxine deficiency or dependency
  Aminoacidopathies (e.g., hyperglycinemia)

CNS Disorders
  Congenital abnormality
  Intracranial hemorrhage*
  Hypoxic-ischemic encephalopathy*
  Cerebral edema
  Infection (meningitis or encephalitis)
  Kernicterus
  Hyperviscosity (high hematocrit) syndrome

Narcotic Withdrawal
  Heroin
  Methadone

*Most common.
CNS = central nervous system.

tion, hypothermia (cooling) may induce lethargy, and babies with congenital hypothyroidism exhibit lethargy as one manifestation of that disorder. Lethargy may also be seen with organic acidurias, such as methylmalonic or propionic aciduria.

HYPOTONIA (FLOPPY BABY)

Almost all premature infants display some degree of hypotonia. The less mature the baby, the greater the degree of hypotonia. In the term baby on admission to the nursery, hypotonia (Fig. 29–1) may reflect (1) maternal anesthesia or analgesia, (2) *hypermagnesemia* after magnesium sulfate is given to the mother, or (3) fetal or neonatal hypoxia. If hypotonia persists after perinatal asphyxia, the prognosis is not as good as with progression to either extensor or flexor tone. If none of these diagnoses seems likely, congenital abnormalities should be sought. Hypotonia is an almost universal feature of Down's syndrome (mongolism). It is also a feature of the Prader-Willi syndrome (HHHO syndrome: hypotonia, hypomentia, hypogonadism, and obesity), which may be suspected in the newborn period.

Most babies appear much more hypotonic immediately after being fed than at other times. It is therefore important to take this into consideration when assessing tone.

A baby who seems alert but has extreme flaccidity of the arms and legs probably has suffered a high spinal cord injury, presumably as the result of obstetric trauma.

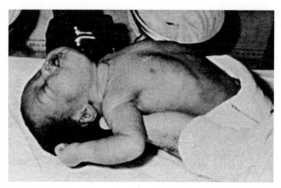

FIGURE 29–1. Demonstration of generalized hypotonia (floppy baby).

As with other neurologic manifestations, infection is an important cause of hypotonia, either as sepsis, meningitis, or encephalitis. In addition, infant botulism has extreme weakness as the most prominent feature. Intracranial hemorrhage must always be considered.

Less common problems that may require special studies for differentiation are Werdnig-Hoffmann disease (progressive spinal muscle atrophy), myasthenia gravis, congenital myotonic dystrophy, Pompe's (cardioskeletal) form of glycogen storage disease, Ehlers-Danlos syndrome (cutis hyperelastica), congenital muscular dystrophy, and congenital benign hypotonia.

Muscle biopsy, electromyography, serum enzyme determinations, and nerve conduction velocity studies may be helpful in distinguishing these disorders. Myasthenia gravis may be diagnosed by administering neostigmine. Consultation with a pediatric neurologist is usually required.

DISORDERS OF CRY

The baby with a rather weak, shrill, high-pitched cry frequently is suffering from intracranial pathology (meningitis or hemorrhage). Such a cry is referred to as a "cerebral cry" in Britain. Infants with brain abnormalities may also have a delay in crying after a stimulus when compared with normal infants.

This type of cry needs to be distinguished from the rather harsh, "angry cat" cry associated with the chromosomal disorder involving the short arm of chromosome 5, referred to as cri-du-chat syndrome. There are usually associated physical abnormalities (microcephaly, anti-mongoloid slant of eyes, and low-set ears).

A hoarse cry in a child with large fontanels (or coarse features, large tongue, lethargy, and constipation) may be associated with congenital hypothyroidism. More frequently, it is likely to be encountered in a baby in the period immediately after removal of an endotracheal tube. It may also be seen in association with conditions of the larynx that produce stridor.

BIBLIOGRAPHY

Convulsions

Herzlinger, R. A., Kandall, S. R., and Vaughan, H. G.: Neonatal seizures associated with narcotic withdrawal. *J. Pediatr.* 1977, 91:638.

Goldberg, H. J., and Sheeny, E. M.: Fifth day fits: An acute zinc deficiency syndrome? *Arch. Dis. Child.* 1982, 57:633–635.

Walsh, P., Jedeikin, R., Ellis, G., et al.: Assessment of neurologic outcome in asphyxiated term infants by use of serial CK-BB isoenzyme measurement. *J. Pediatr.* 1982, 101:988–992.

Lipp-Zwahlen, E. A., Tuchschmid, P., Silberschmidt, M., and Duc, G.: Arterial cord blood hypoxanthine: A measure of intrauterine hypoxia? *Biol. Neonate* 1983, 44:193–202.

Myers, G. J., and Cassady, G.: Neonatal seizures. *Pediatr. Rev.* 1983, 5:67–72.

Ellison, P. H.: Management of seizures in the high-risk infant. *Clin. Perinatol.* 1984, 11:175–188.

Volpe, J. J.: Commentary on duration of anticonvulsant therapy. In *1984 Year Book of Pediatrics.* Oski, F. A., and Stockman, J. A. III (eds.). Year Book Medical Publishers, Chicago, 1984, pp. 363–365.

Legido, A., Clancy, R. R., and Berman, P. H.: Neurologic outcome after electroencephalographically proven neonatal seizures. *Pediatrics* 1991, 88:583–596.

Hypotonia

Brown, J. K., Purvis, R. J., Forfar, J. O., and Cockburn, F.: Neurological aspects of perinatal asphyxia. *Dev. Med. Child Neurol.* 1974, 16:567–580.

Stephenson, J. B. P.: Prader-Willi syndrome: Neonatal presentation and later development. *Dev. Med. Child Neurol.* 1980, 22:792–799.

Dubowitz, V.: Evaluation and differential diagnosis of the hypotonic infant. *Pediatr. Rev.* 1985, 6:237–243.

Rais-Bahrami, K., McDonald, M. G., Eng, G. D., and Rosenbaum, K. N.: Persistent pulmonary hypertension in newborn infants with congenital myotonic dystrophy. *J. Pediatr.* 1994, 124:634–635.

Disorders of Cry

Wasz-Hockert, O., Lind, J., Vuorenkoski, V., et al.: *The Infant Cry: A Spectrographic and Auditory Analysis. Clin. Dev. Med.* No. 29. SIMP, Lavenham Press, Suffolk, England, 1968.

30
ABNORMALITIES OF THE HEAD AND NECK

LARGE HEAD

The infant with intrauterine growth retardation may appear to have a large head but is usually found to have a head circumference below the 50th percentile. There are three major reasons for a large head without other apparent abnormalities: hydrocephalus, hydranencephaly, or familial. Another rare disorder is megalocephalus or macrocephaly (associated with mental retardation).

Hydranencephaly may be distinguished by transillumination (see Figs. 8–21 and 8–22), but hydrocephalus may require more sophisticated studies, such as cephalic ultrasound or computed tomographic scan.

SMALL HEAD

In contrast to infants who are small for gestational age, infants of diabetic mothers often appear to have a small head when compared with the rest of the body, but the head circumference falls within normal limits.

True microcephaly may be familial and not necessarily associated with mental retardation. However, microcephaly may be secondary to (1) high-dose intrauterine radiation, such as atomic; (2) cytomegalovirus infection (Fig. 30–1); (3) toxoplasmosis; (4) chromosomal abnormalities; or (5) generalized intrauterine growth retardation of uncertain cause.

ODD-SHAPED SKULL

Various types of premature closure of cranial sutures (craniostenosis, craniosynostosis) may produce unusually shaped skulls. One of the more frequently seen abnormalities is acrocephaly (or oxycephaly), in which the head is high and rounded. It may be associated with syndactyly, as in Apert's syndrome. Narrowing from front to back is called brachycephaly, narrowing from side to side is scaphocephaly, and asymmetric synostoses produce plagiocephaly.

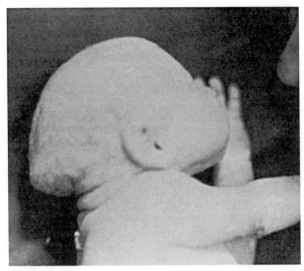

FIGURE 30–1. Microcephaly in a baby with intrauterine cytomegalovirus infection.

Plagiocephaly may also be seen as part of the "molded baby syndrome," in association with limited hip abduction and torticollis.

SWELLING ON THE HEAD

The only confusion that seems to arise is between cephalhematoma and caput succedaneum. There should be no confusion, because a caput is usually present at delivery, is situated in the occipital area, crosses suture lines, and quickly gets smaller. Conversely, a cephalhematoma usually takes several hours to develop, is bounded by suture lines, is most frequently seen in the parietal region, and may persist for weeks to months. As it resolves, it may liquefy in the center and may occasionally give the impression of a depressed fracture. However, it is uncommon to have any kind of fracture underlying a cephalhematoma, although linear fractures have been reported in up to 25% of cases. More commonly, it becomes quite firm (rubbery) and may become calcified. Certain areas of the head and neck may be subject to pressure during the delivery process, which later gives rise to localized swelling caused by subcutaneous fat necrosis (Fig. 30–2). Swellings over the base of the skull or in the region of the posterior fontanel, that is, in the midline, most likely are caused by an encephalocele. Diffuse swelling not limited by suture lines may be the result of subgaleal (subaponeurotic) hemorrhage.

ABNORMAL HAIR PATTERNS

It was originally suggested that abnormally placed hair whorls could indicate defective brain morphogenesis. More recently, it has been suggested that

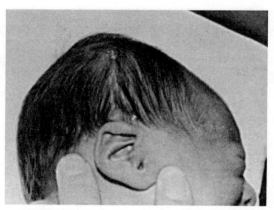

FIGURE 30–2. An area of excoriation (caused by forceps) overlies a swelling on the scalp that has a rubbery consistency and represents subcutaneous fat necrosis.

similar problems may be indicated by hair that does not lie flat during the neonatal period (unruly hair). Both of these findings should serve as stimuli to careful evaluation of the central nervous system both in the neonatal period and during the first year of life.

LARGE FONTANEL

There is a wide range of size of the anterior fontanel in most term babies, but the posterior fontanel is rarely palpable. If both fontanels appear to be large, the possibility of congenital hypothyroidism should be considered. In infants with intrauterine growth retardation, the anterior fontanel may be large (Fig. 30–3), and this phenomenon correlates with the retardation of epiphyseal ossification at the knee in term infants, which can be seen radiographically.

Rubella syndrome and chromosomal abnormalities may produce intrauterine growth retardation with large fontanels. In addition, a recent survey suggests that black term infants have somewhat larger fontanels than whites.

INCREASED TENSION OF ANTERIOR FONTANEL

The most common disorders that produce increased tension of the anterior fontanel are meningitis, intracranial hemorrhage, cerebral edema (secondary to hypoxia), congestive heart failure, and hydrocephalus.

"SQUASHED" FACIES

The classic features of Potter's facies associated with bilateral renal agenesis are a squashed appearance with flattening of the nose, deep folds below the

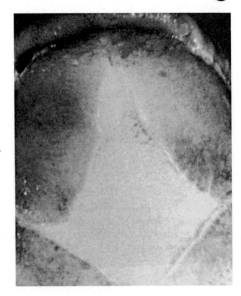

FIGURE 30–3. Postmortem photograph, showing very large anterior fontanel.

eyes, and large, floppy ears ("elephant ears"), which may be low set (Fig. 30–4). The same features have been observed after prolonged leakage of amniotic fluid, resulting in oligohydramnios, and may point to pulmonary hypoplasia.

ASYMMETRY OF FACIAL MOVEMENTS

The usual reason for asymmetric facial movements is facial palsy (Fig. 30–5). Facial palsy is most likely to result from pressure on the facial nerve (probably by the sacral promontory), but it may be a congenital abnormality. A transient palsy has been observed in association with otitis media. It is not obvious in repose but becomes apparent during crying. Another cause is congenital hypoplasia of the depressor anguli oris muscle. The importance of distinguishing this problem from facial palsy is its association with other malformations, particularly congenital heart disease.

DEFECTS OF SKULL BONES

Two problems should be considered when softness of the bones of the skull is encountered. The first is the condition called craniotabes, in which a localized area of softness is encountered, usually in the occipitoparietal region secondary to prolonged engagement of the fetal head. This area often pops in and out (like compressing a soft Ping-Pong ball) under the palpating finger. The other condition is osteogenesis imperfecta (fragilitas ossium), which in its severest form has "islands of bone floating in a sea of membrane." Fractures of the long bones are likely to be seen, together with very blue sclerae.

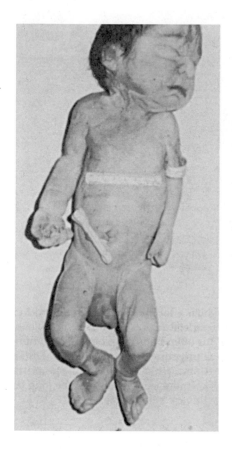

FIGURE 30–4. Baby with bilateral renal agenesis and Potter's facies, showing compression abnormalities, low-set ears, and redundant skin.

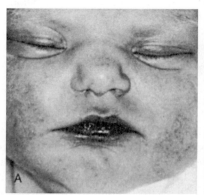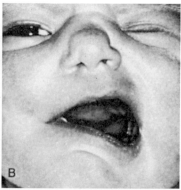

FIGURE 30–5. Right facial nerve palsy. *A,* During sleep, the right nasolabial fold is flattened. *B,* During crying, the right eye is open, and the mouth is pulled to the left.

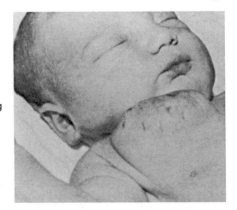

FIGURE 30–6. Large hemangioma involving the right neck and upper chest.

SWELLING OF THE NECK

A central swelling is most likely to be caused by congenital goiter (enlargement of the thyroid gland). This condition may be caused by maternal antithyroid treatment, maternal ingestion of iodides (in certain cough medicines) or goitrogens (kale), maternal deficiency of iodine intake, or defects in thyroxine metabolism (inborn errors).

A lateral swelling is most likely to be a hemangioma (Fig. 30–6), or lymphangioma (when large it is called cystic hygroma). A palpable nodule in the lateral neck is most frequently a sternomastoid hematoma ("tumor").

A swelling over the back of the neck may communicate with the central nervous system and is an encephalocele (Figs. 30–7 and 30–8).

HEAD TILTED OR TWISTED

The most common reason for a tilted or twisted head is an abnormal position adopted in utero, which is the preferred position after birth. Sometimes,

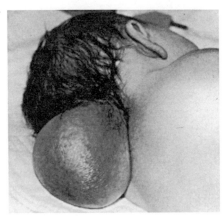

FIGURE 30–7. An encephalocele over the back of the neck.

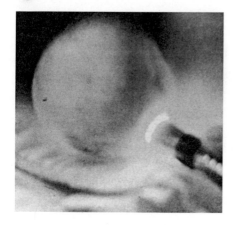

FIGURE 30–8. Same baby as in Figure 30–7: transillumination of the encephalocele shows the neural elements outlined.

the problem persists because of congenital muscular torticollis. It is interesting to note that torticollis is associated with hip dislocation in approximately 20% of cases and may be related to breech presentation.

BIBLIOGRAPHY

Small Head

Miller, R. W., and Blot, W. J.: Small head size after in-utero exposure to atomic radiation. *Lancet* 1972, ii:784.
Haslam, R. H. A., and Smith, D. W.: Autosomal dominant microcephaly. *J. Pediatr.* 1979, 95:701.

Odd-Shaped Skull

Hanson, J. W., Sayers, M. P., Knopp, L. M., et al.: Subtotal neonatal calvariectomy for severe craniosynostosis. *J. Pediatr.* 1977, 91:257.

Swelling on the Head

Zelson, C., Lee, S. J., and Pearl, M.: Incidence of skull fractures underlying cephalhematomas in newborn infants. *J. Pediatr.* 1974, 85:371.

Abnormal Hair Patterns

Smith, D. W., and Greely, M. J.: Unruly scalp hair in infancy: Its nature and relevance to problems of brain morphogenesis. *Pediatrics* 1978, 61:783.

Large Fontanel

Tan, K. I.: Wide sutures and large fontanels in the newborn. *Am. J. Dis. Child.* 1976, 130:386.
Philip, A. G. S.: Fetal growth retardation: Femurs, fontanels, and follow-up. *Pediatrics* 1978, 93:150.
Faix, R. G.: Fontanelle size in black and white term newborn infants. *J. Pediatr.* 1983, 100:304–306.

"Squashed" Facies

Perlman, M., Williams, J., and Hirsch, M.: Neonatal pulmonary hypoplasia after prolonged
leakage of amniotic fluid. *Arch. Dis. Child.* 1976, 51:349.

Asymmetry of Facial Movements

Alexion, D., Manolidis, C., Papaevangellou, G., et al.: Frequency of other malformations
in congenital hypoplasia of depressor anguli oris muscle syndrome. *Arch. Dis. Child.*
1976, 51:891.
Monreal, F. J.: Asymmetric crying facies: An alternative interpretation. *Pediatrics* 1980,
65:146.

Defects of Skull Bones

Graham, J. M., and Smith, D. W. Parietal craniotabes in the neonate—Its origin and
significance. *J. Pediatr.* 1979, 95:114.

Swelling of Neck

Streeto, J. M.: Drugs and congenital goiter. *Lancet* 1970, ii:212.
Fonkalsrud, E. W.: Surgical management of congenital malformations of the lymphatic
system. *Am. J. Surg.* 1974, 128:152.
Chervenak, F. A., Isaacson, G., Blakemore, K. J., et al.: Fetal cystic hygroma: Cause and
natural history. *N. Engl. J. Med.* 1983, 309:822–825.

31

ABNORMAL EYE EXAMINATION

EYES WIDE APART (HYPERTELORISM)

The distance between the eyes may be increased in several syndromes. The following distances are useful for the physician who is deciding whether or not hypertelorism exists:

Interpupillary distance (range) = 3.5 – 4.5 cm (term infant)
Inner canthal distance (range) = 1.5 – 2.5 cm (term infant)

CLOUDY CORNEA

Several reasons for haziness of the cornea exist. Most frequently, these are rupture of Descemet's membrane (unilateral, secondary to trauma during forceps delivery) (Fig. 31–1), congenital glaucoma (increased tension in eyeball), or congenital rubella infection.

CATARACT (OPACITY OF THE LENS)

Cataract may be subdivided into three major causes: (1) familial (hereditary; dominant), (2) congenital rubella infection (usually other features) (Fig. 31–2), or (3) galactosemia (not present at birth). Although the most common established cause is hereditary, this accounts for only 25% of the cases. More than 50% are of unknown cause.

MEMBRANOUS LESION BEHIND THE PUPIL

A membranous lesion behind the pupil may be the remnant of the hyaloid membrane seen early in gestation. In premature infants, the gradual disappearance of the anterior vascular capsule of the lens may cause confusion, but it is useful in assessing gestational age (see Chapter 6).

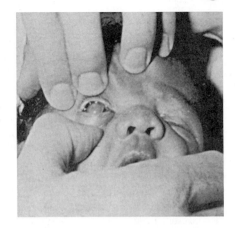

FIGURE 31-1. Cloudy cornea caused by rupture of Descemet's membrane secondary to forceps delivery.

DISCHARGE FROM THE EYES

This problem can be simplified by the statement that discharge (drainage) from the eyes in the first 24 hours is caused by chemical conjunctivitis in most cases (secondary to silver nitrate instillation, although it is now used infrequently). Discharge at a later time is most likely bacterial or chlamydial (see p. 190).

When the lacrimal duct is partly blocked (congenital lacrimal stenosis), there may be a slight swelling below the eye. Pressure over the swelling may produce pus at the inner canthus of the eye. Conjunctivitis is usually absent.

CONJUNCTIVAL HEMORRHAGE

Conjunctival (or subconjunctival) hemorrhage is seen quite frequently. It seems to be more common after prolonged labor (when the mother may also have subconjunctival hemorrhage) or after precipitate delivery. It may reflect

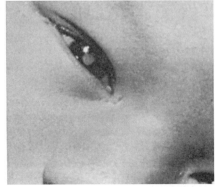

FIGURE 31-2. Cataract in a baby with congenital rubella syndrome.

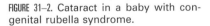

hemorrhage of the retina but, like most retinal hemorrhages, subsides quickly. The importance of conjunctival hemorrhage is the parental concern that it may generate. Parents should be reassured that it will quickly subside.

DEFECT OF THE IRIS

A defect of the iris is called a coloboma and may be an isolated defect or part of a more extensive failure of development of the face. Deafness is sometimes associated. Coloboma is also part of the CHARGE association, which includes coloboma, heart disease, atresia choanae, retarded growth and development, genital anomalies, and ear anomalies. When the iris is completely absent, a condition called aniridia, the possibility of Wilms' tumor should be considered (it is present in one third of the cases).

PROMINENT IRIS VESSELS

In preterm infants, the finding of prominent iris vessels may indicate active proliferation of retinal vessels associated with retinopathy of prematurity. When the retina is examined, this usually correlates with the presence of "plus" disease. The possibility of treatment with cryotherapy or laser therapy should be considered.

LARGE-APPEARING IRIS

When the iris appears to fill most of the orbit or appears considerably larger than usual, one should suspect congenital glaucoma (buphthalmos), and early ophthalmologic consultation is needed.

PUPIL SIZE AND RESPONSE

The pupillary light reflex is absent in all infants younger than 30 weeks' gestational age and consequently cannot be used to assess neurologic status in very preterm infants. The reflex is reliably present after 35 weeks' gestation. Until the reflex is established, the pupil appears somewhat large.

PALE OPTIC DISC

Examination of the normal newborn fundus may be confusing. The optic disc appears pale and may suggest optic atrophy. This is a normal finding.

WHITE AREAS ON THE RETINA

White areas on the retina may be the result of scarring caused by retrolental fibroplasia (retinopathy of prematurity). They are most likely to be found on the temporal side of the retina in a preterm infant whose birth weight was less than 1200 g. Prolonged exposure to oxygen (or more particularly to high levels of paO_2) has been implicated but is by no means the only explanation. This condition is seen late in the neonatal period.

Chorioretinitis due to toxoplasmosis or cytomegalovirus infection might also need to be considered.

BIBLIOGRAPHY

Baum, J. D., and Bulpitt, C. J.: Retinal and conjunctival hemorrhage in the newborn. *Arch. Dis. Child.* 1970, 45:344.

Haddad, H. M.: Birth trauma of the eye. *Pediatr. Digest* 1970, April:29.

Feingold, M., and Bossert, W. H.: Normal values for selected physical parameters. *Birth Defects Orig. Artic. Ser. X* 1974, (13):7. National Foundation March of Dimes.

Williams, H.: Congenital cataracts. *Dev. Med. Child. Neurol.* 1976, 18:806.

Yasunaga, S., and Kean, E. H.: Effect of three ophthalmic solutions on chemical conjunctivitis in neonate. *Am. J. Dis. Child.* 1977, 131:159.

Angell, L. K., Robb, R. M., and Berson, F. G.: Visual prognosis in patients with ruptures in Descemet's membrane due to forceps injuries. *Arch. Ophthalmol.* 1981, 99:2137–2139.

Beller, R., Hoyt, C. S., Marg, E., and Odom, J. V.: Good visual function after neonatal surgery for congenital monocular cataracts. *Am. J. Ophthalmol.* 1981, 91:559–565.

Broughton, W. L., and Parks, M. M.: An analysis of treatment of congenital glaucoma by goniotomy. *Am. J. Ophthalmol.* 1981, 91:566–572.

Egge, K., Lyng, G., and Maltau, J. M.: Effect of instrumental delivery on the frequency and severity of retinal hemorrhages in the newborn. *Acta Obstet. Gynecol. Scand.* 1981, 60:153–155.

Fryns, J. P., Beirinckx, J., DeSutter, E., et al.: Aniridia-Wilms' tumor association and 11p interstitial deletion. *Eur. J. Pediatr.* 1981, 136:91–92.

Lucey, J. F., and Dangman, B.: A re-examination of the role of oxygen in retrolental fibroplasia. *Pediatrics* 1984, 73:82–96.

Committee Report: An international classification of retinopathy of prematurity. *Pediatrics* 1984, 74:127–133.

Palmer, E. A., and Phelps, D.: Multicenter trial of cryotherapy for retinopathy of prematurity. *Pediatrics* 1986, 77:428–429.

Calhoun, J. H.: Cataracts in infancy. *Pediatr. Rev.* 1988, 9:227–233.

Robinson, J., and Fielder, A. R.: Pupillary diameter and reaction to light in preterm neonates. *Arch. Dis. Child.* 1990, 65:35–38.

Kutiyanawala, M., Wyse, R. K. H., Brereton, R. J., et al.: CHARGE and esophageal atresia. *J. Pediatr. Surg.* 1992, 27:558–560.

32
SKIN CHANGES

In addition to the abnormalities of color noted in Chapter 25, numerous other changes are seen rather frequently in the newborn infant.

ERYTHEMA TOXICUM NEONATORUM

Erythema toxicum neonatorum is a common blotchy erythematous eruption that may appear anywhere on the body but is most typically seen over the trunk and back. Occasionally, the center of an erythematous patch looks almost pustular, although more frequently, vesicular lesions contain clear (or whitish) fluid. The characteristic progression is for these erythematous areas to appear prominently on one area of the body and to be almost completely different in distribution only a few hours later. Perhaps the easiest way to think of it is as transient urticaria of the newborn (Fig. 32–1).

Confusion may arise with the pustular form, most frequently when such lesions are on the abdomen. If fluid expressed from one of the pustules is examined under the microscope, eosinophils are prominent and are virtually diagnostic.

HARLEQUIN PHENOMENON

Harlequin phenomenon is not rare, but it is not nearly as common as erythema toxicum. The baby has markedly different coloring of the two sides of the body, with a sharp line of demarcation at the midline (Fig. 32–2). The dependent half is bright red, whereas the upper half is very pale. The explanation offered is "vascular instability."

When the body position is changed, the marked difference quickly disappears, although the sides may be reversed if the baby is turned to the opposite side. It may be seen more commonly in babies under phototherapy lights.

PHOTOTHERAPY RASH

Frequently, a baby being treated with phototherapy develops a rather fine blotchy erythematous rash. This condition is probably a variant of erythema

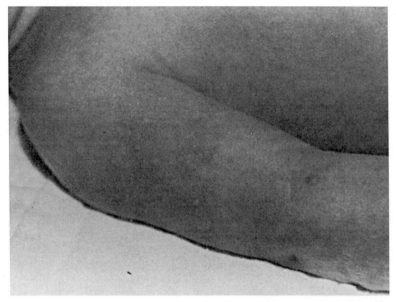

FIGURE 32–1. Baby with an erythematous eruption over the upper arm with superimposed vesiculopustular lesions (indistinctly seen). A more pustular lesion is seen in the antecubital fossa. Four hours later, this lesion had disappeared, which is typical of pustular erythema toxicum.

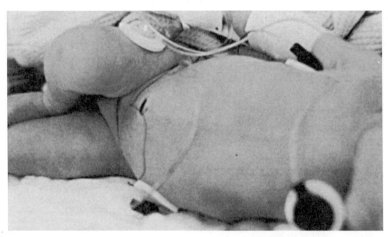

FIGURE 32–2. Harlequin phenomenon, showing a sharp line of demarcation at the midline between the pallor of the elevated part of the body and the erythema of the dependent part.

toxicum because blood flow through the skin is increased during phototherapy. Almost invariably, it disappears when treatment is discontinued.

NEVI (BIRTHMARKS)

Three major groups of nevi exist: (1) vascular, (2) pigmented, and (3) sebaceous. Capillary hemangiomas, which are very common, are most commonly seen over the eyelids, on the forehead between the eyes, and at the nape of the neck. The color is pink or red. Such a birthmark is called a nevus flammeus. It is usual for these to fade almost completely within a few months, but they may be apparent in later years at times when peripheral vasodilation occurs. More permanent lesions, whose color is dark red or purple, are referred to as port-wine stains and may be extensive. This type of nevus may be amenable to treatment using pulsed dye laser therapy. They may be associated with lesions within the skull and may produce convulsions (Sturge-Weber syndrome).

Strawberry nevi are also hemangiomas, which may be barely detectable at birth, but often have a pale "halo" around them and become more prominent in the first few weeks of life. They remain prominent for several months and then usually involute over 1 or 2 years. Some very large lesions (apparently quite deforming) have undergone complete spontaneous resolution.

The third major type of vascular nevus is the cavernous hemangioma, which is akin to an iceberg. The portion that is visible above the skin represents only a small part of the whole. In contrast to the other two types, the edge is very ill-defined. This type is more important because of the greater likelihood of complications. These include hemihypertrophy when a limb is involved, consumptive coagulopathy secondary to thrombosis, and ulceration.

Pigmented nevi are frequently covered with hair and are mostly situated over the lower trunk and back. This is sometimes referred to as a "bathing trunk" nevus (Fig. 32–3), but much smaller (or larger) areas can be involved. A minor variant is the bluish discoloration called a Mongolian blue spot seen

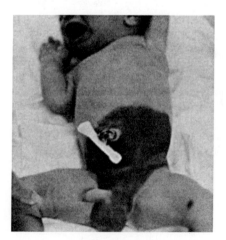

FIGURE 32–3. Pigmented nevus with a "bathing trunk" distribution.

frequently over the lower back and buttocks of the pigmented races (they are not bruises).

The sebaceous nevus is infrequently seen, but it can be quite misleading to the uninitiated (Fig. 32–4). This lesion is a slightly raised area usually on the scalp, particularly encroaching on the forehead. The color is usually a yellow-orange or salmon and the surface is somewhat irregular. It is potentially malignant, and a dermatologist should be consulted within the first few weeks after birth.

PUSTULES

Staphylococcal skin lesions produce pustules that may be present as early as the fourth day, but more typically they occur between 10 and 14 days of age. They are most frequently seen around the umbilicus or where two skin surfaces come into contact—the groin, axillae, and neck folds (Fig. 32–5). Pustular erythema toxicum is more likely to occur in the first 3 or 4 days, with a back and trunk distribution. Occasionally, the pustules are not limited in size and become bullae (pemphigus). Rarely, a desquamating (exfoliative) process occurs (Ritter's disease). In black infants, vesicopustules present at birth may be seen with pustular melanosis. This disorder may also be seen in white infants and has been called pustulosis; when pustular lesions are present on the hands and feet, this appearance is almost pathognomonic. The condition is benign.

VESICLES

Some infants have multiple, superficial, easily ruptured, clear vesicles without inflammation. This condition is called miliaria crystallina and results from subcorneal retention of fluid from the sweat glands. The vesicles are not usually present at birth but appear within a few days. Less common causes of vesicles are Herpesvirus hominis (simplex) infection, varicella-zoster infection (neonatal

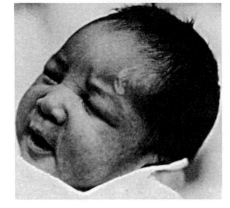

FIGURE 32–4. Sebaceous nevus on the scalp and forehead.

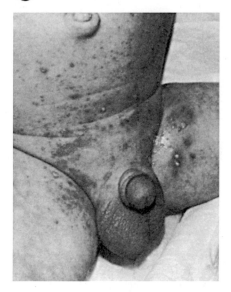

FIGURE 32–5. A 10-day-old baby (note the absence of an umbilical cord) with pustules in the groin, which proved to be staphylococcal in origin (compare with Figure 32–1).

chickenpox), incontinentia pigmenti, urticaria pigmentosa, and pustular melanosis—vesicles may be on palms and soles. Additional causes of vesicopustular lesions are congenital cutaneous candidiasis and congenital tuberculosis.

BLISTERS

Somewhat similar to vesicles but frequently more linear, fluid-filled blisters may be seen on the upper extremity, usually on the radial side in babies born at term. These seem to be the result of vigorous sucking on the extremity before delivery ("sucking blisters"). No treatment is necessary.

The skin may also blister in some preterm infants after the removal of adhesive tape.

SCALP DEFECTS

Absence of skin can occur in any location, but this rare disorder (cutis aplasia) is most frequently encountered on the scalp in the midline in the region of the crown of the head (Fig. 32–6). The appearance is one of a sharply demarcated ulcer without erythema or drainage. These defects may be seen with trisomy 13, whereas more generalized defects have been associated with a twin that fails to develop (fetus papyraceus).

PEELING SKIN

By far the most common cause of peeling (desquamation) noted at birth is dysmaturity (intrauterine growth retardation or postmaturity). Peeling of the

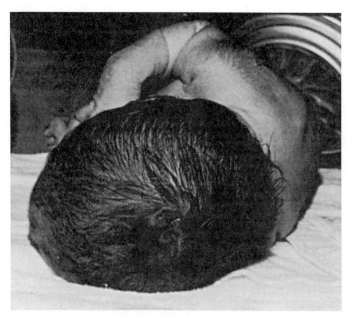

FIGURE 32–6. Two scalp defects (cutis aplasia) can be seen indistinctly at the crown of the head. An erythematous ulcerated area is present, from which no hair is growing.

hands and feet may be seen with congenital syphilis and peeling of the whole baby in the different types of congenital ichthyosis (Fig. 32–7). More localized, but large, areas of peeling may be seen in epidermolysis bullosa. This last condition usually involves more than the superficial layers (so that normal skin is not seen beneath) and therefore may be life threatening in its severest form.

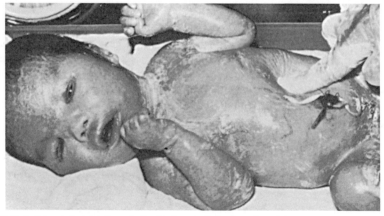

FIGURE 32–7. Congenital ichthyosis (collodion baby), showing thickened, cracked, parchment-like skin over the whole body.

The same is true of the exfoliative form of staphylococcal skin infection (otherwise known as the staphylococcal scalded-skin syndrome).

PETECHIAE AND PURPURA

Petechia and purpura refer to bleeding into the skin, so that blanching does not occur with pressure. Pinpoint lesions are referred to as petechiae, and larger lesions are called purpura. The causes are numerous and are summarized below:

1. *Mechanical:* trauma at the time of delivery, including precipitate delivery.
2. *Capillary fragility:* secondary to hypoxia or infection.
3. *Thrombocytopenia*
   a. Immune-type: maternal thrombocytopenia, antibody transfer to fetus.
   b. Infection: bacterial sepsis, TORCH complex.
   c. Blood disorders: hemolytic disease of the newborn, congenital leukemia.
   d. Toxic effects: maternal hypertension, maternal drug ingestion, such as quinine.
   e. Consumptive: disseminated intravascular coagulation, and so on.

If petechiae are confined to the head and neck, it is usually unnecessary to investigate the situation further. Petechiae over the back or trunk and on the limbs usually require investigation, which would begin with a platelet count and might include a white blood cell count and differential, blood group and Coombs test, sepsis workup, and tests for agents in the toxoplasmosis, rubella, cytomegalovirus, and herpes simplex complex.

If the mother has thrombocytopenia, possible diagnoses are idiopathic, lupus, drug-induced, or inherited. When maternal platelets are normal, the physical examination may provide further clues. Hepatosplenomegaly suggests infection or congenital leukemia. Limb abnormalities may suggest a trisomy syndrome or Fanconi's anemia. Absence of the radius is a specific associated abnormality (TAR baby—thrombocytopenia with absent radius). (For treatment, see p. 287).

If widespread purpuric spots are present, the appearance may be characterized as a "blueberry muffin baby," which has been associated with rubella, cytomegalovirus, and toxoplasmosis infections (see Chapter 15). When these spots have a slightly nodular texture, one may need to consider congenital leukemia, congenital self-healing reticulohistiocytoma, and cutaneous erythropoiesis secondary to twin-twin transfusion (in the anemic twin).

BRUISING

Quite extensive bleeding into the skin may be categorized as bruising. This is common in the extremely preterm infant soon after delivery. Such extravasation of blood may contribute to hypovolemia immediately and hyperbilirubinemia later.

Another form of "bruising" in the extremely low-birth-weight infant may be the result of hemorrhagic necrosis of the dermis secondary to alcohol absorption.

Therefore, alcohol should be used cautiously in extremely low-birth-weight infants.

FIRM (INDURATED) SKIN

Certain infants develop a hardness of the skin and subcutaneous tissues, which has a firm, waxy texture. This most commonly affects the extremities but can affect any area of the body. The probable cause of this hardness is sclerema neonatorum. Sclerema may result from decreased blood flow at the periphery, resulting in cooling of the subcutaneous tissues and a change in the physical properties of subcutaneous fat. This is most frequently associated with severe forms of neonatal sepsis but can be seen in association with poor cardiac output (e.g., secondary to congenital heart disease or hypovolemia) or prolonged metabolic acidosis. It is also seen in neonatal cold injury. Correction of the underlying disorder is the primary form of treatment. Corticosteroids or adrenocorticotropic hormone were recommended in the past; more recently, exchange transfusion has been used in infants with sepsis.

Sclerema is distinguished from edema by lack of pitting with compression. Occasionally, there seems to be a combination of the two, called scleredema.

The areas of firmness may be more localized and situated in areas more likely to be subjected to pressure in utero or to trauma at delivery. In such cases, a diagnosis of subcutaneous fat necrosis may be made.

SWEATING

Sweating is uncommon in the newborn infant, especially the preterm infant. The most important cause is cardiac failure associated with underlying congenital heart disease (especially with too much pulmonary blood flow). Sweating is sometimes seen when the incubator temperature has been set too high (with a large baby) and in the infant of a diabetic mother. Other possibilities are cerebral cortex irritation and narcotic withdrawal. Palmar sweating (emotional sweating) may be documented during painful procedures.

MOTTLING (CUTIS MARMORATA)

When the skin of a baby shows generalized mottling (appearing somewhat like marble) there are several possibilities. The most likely possibility is that the baby is cold, which results in decreased perfusion at the periphery. The same mechanism accounts for mottling seen with acidosis. Both of these problems are more likely with prematurity, but the premature infant may be mottled for no apparent reason. An exaggeration of this benign condition is seen with congenital cutis marmorata. Hypothyroidism should also be considered, and hypertension should be sought, with the possibility of renal pathology. (For localized mottling, see Fig. 35–9.)

BIBLIOGRAPHY

Hodgman, J. E., Freedman, R. I., and Levan, N. E.: Neonatal dermatology. *Pediatr. Clin. North Am.* 1971, 18:713.
Solomon, L. M., and Esterly, N. B.: *Neonatal Dermatology.* W. B. Saunders, Philadelphia, 1973.
Hurwitz, S.: A visual guide to neonatal skin eruptions. *Contemp. Pediatr.* 1985, 2(Sept):82–92.

Nevi

Holmes, L. B.: The practical significance of birthmarks. *Pediatrics* 1976, 58:150.
Illingworth, R. S.: Thoughts on treatment of strawberry naevi. *Arch. Dis. Child.* 1976, 51:38.
Alper, J., Holmes, L. B., and Mihm, M. C., Jr.: Birthmarks with serious medical significance: Nevocellular nevi, sebaceous nevi and multiple café au lait spots. *J. Pediatr.* 1979, 95:696.
Strauss, R. P., and Resnick, S. D.: Pulsed dye laser therapy for port-wine stains in children: Psychosocial and ethical issues. *J. Pediatr.* 1993, 122:505–510.

Pustules

Merlob, P., Metzker, A., and Reisner, S. H.: Transient neonatal pustular melanosis. *Am. J. Dis. Child.* 1982, 136:521–522.

Skin Defects

Kosnik, E. J., and Sayers, M. P.: Congenital scalp defects: Aplasia cutis congenita. *J. Neurosurg.* 1975, 42:32.
Mannino, F. L., Jones, K. L., and Benirschke, K.: Congenital skin defects and fetus papyraceus. *J. Pediatr.* 1977, 91:958.

Peeling Skin

Melish, M. E., and Glasgow, L. A.: Staphylococcal scalded skin syndrome. The expanded clinical syndrome. *J. Pediatr.* 1971, 78:958.

Petechiae and Purpura

Handin, R. I.: Neonatal immune thrombocytopenia—the doctor's dilemma. *N. Engl. J. Med.* 1981, 305:951–953.
Cines, D. B., Dusak, B., Tomaski, A., et al.: Immune thrombocytopenic purpura and pregnancy. *N. Engl. J. Med.* 1982, 306:826–830.
Oski, F. A., and Naiman, J. L.: Thrombocytopenia in the newborn. In *Hematologic Problems in the Newborn,* 3rd ed. W. B. Saunders, Philadelphia, 1982, pp. 175–222.
Schwartz, J. L., Maniscalco, W. M., Lane, A. T., and Currao, W. J.: Twin transfusion syndrome causing cutaneous erythropoiesis. *Pediatrics* 1984, 74:527–529.
Ornvold, K., Jacobsen, S. V., and Neilsen, M. H.: Congenital self-healing reticulohistiocytoma: A clinical histological and ultrastructural study. *Acta Paediatr.* 1985, 74:143–147.

Bruising

Harpin, V. A., and Rutter, N.: Percutaneous alcohol absorption and skin necrosis in a preterm infant. *Arch. Dis. Child.* 1982, 57:477–479.

Firm Skin

Solomon, L. M., and Esterly, N. B.: Diseases of the subcutaneous tissues. In *Neonatal Dermatology.* W. B. Saunders, Philadelphia, 1973, pp. 203–207.
Xanthou, M., Xypolyta, A., Anagnostakis, D., et al.: Exchange transfusion in severe neonatal infection with sclerema. *Arch. Dis. Child.* 1975, 50:901.

Vonk, J., Janssens, P. M. W., Demacker, P. N. M., and Folkers E.: Sub-cutaneous fat necrosis in a neonate in association with aberrant plasma lipid and lipoprotein values. *J. Pediatr.* 1993, 123:462–464.

Sweating

Harpin, V. A., and Rutter, N.: Sweating in premature babies. *J. Pediatr.* 1982, 100:614–619.
Rutter, N.: The evaporimeter and emotional sweating in the neonate. *Clin. Perinatol.* 1985, 12:63–77.

Mottling

South, D. A., and Jacobs, A. H.: Cutis marmorata telangiectatica congenita (congenital generalized phlebectasia). *J. Pediatr.* 1978, 93:944.
Adelman, R. D.: Neonatal hypertension. *Pediatr. Clin. North Am.* 1978, 25:99–110.

33

MISCELLANEOUS PRESENTING SIGNS

MALFORMED NAILS

The nails of the fingers and toes are usually not very prominent (although present) in most very premature infants. Absence (or severe hypoplasia) may occur in certain forms of ectodermal dysplasia (Fig. 33–1) and the nail-patella syndrome and after maternal phenytoin ingestion.

Staining (yellow-green) of the nails is most commonly associated with postmaturity.

EDEMA

Most very premature infants are somewhat edematous. Infants of diabetic mothers were once considered to be edematous, but it is now recognized that the increase in tissue is primarily fat.

The following conditions are worthy of consideration when the history is appropriate:

1. *Rh incompatibility and other causes of hydrops fetalis* (Fig. 33–2): this is a generalized problem, and this type of massive edema has multiple causes (see next section).

2. *Late edema of prematurity:* seems to occur at approximately 35 to 36 weeks' maturity in infants born before 32 weeks' gestation.

3. *Turner's syndrome:* hands and feet; female infant.

4. *Congestive cardiac failure:* a late sign.

5. *Congenital lymphedema* (Milroy's disease): particularly if unilateral or asymmetric.

6. *Excessive fluid administration:* may have associated renal problems.

7. *Increased capillary permeability:* leakage across "sick" blood vessels, such as after profound hypoxia or cold injury.

8. *With vitamin E deficiency* (associated with hemolytic anemia).

9. During paralysis with *pancuronium bromide* (Pavulon).

10. *Zinc deficiency* in low-birth-weight infants.

11. *Myotonic dystrophy* (history of polyhydramnios).

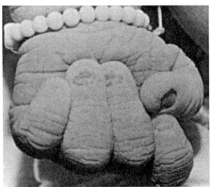

FIGURE 33–1. Ectodermal dysplasia, showing poorly formed nails and a wrinkled appearance of the skin of the hand.

HYDROPS

Hydrops fetalis secondary to Rh incompatibility is discussed in Chapter 10. However, this is now a relatively unusual cause of hydrops; a nonimmunologic problem is much more likely to be the cause. Many disorders may produce nonimmunologic hydrops fetalis, some of which are outlined in Table 33–1. Investigations may be directed toward the most likely causes, with incorporation of physical findings into such decisions (e.g., features of Down's syndrome suggest that chromosome analysis be performed).

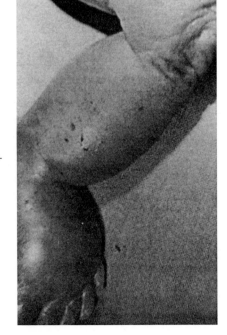

FIGURE 33–2. Severe edema of the lower extremity.

TABLE 33–1. SOME CONDITIONS ASSOCIATED WITH NONIMMUNOLOGIC HYDROPS FETALIS

Cardiovascular	Cardiac malformations
	Fetal arrhythmias
	Arteriovenous shunts
Chromosomal	Turner's syndrome
	Trisomies 21 and 18
	Triploidy
Hematologic	Twin-twin transfusion
	Fetomaternal hemorrhage
	Homozygous α-thalassemia
Infection (intrauterine)	Parvovirus B19
	Syphilis
	Toxoplasmosis
	Cytomegalovirus
Placental	Chorioangioma
Pulmonary	Diaphragmatic hernia
	Cystic adenomatoid malformation
	Lymphangiectasia
Renal	Congenital nephrosis
	Wilms' tumor
	Genitourinary obstruction
Miscellaneous	Maternal diabetes mellitus
	Achondroplasia
	Liver dysfunction
Idiopathic	

Initial investigations include a complete blood count and chest radiography. With anemia in the baby, the mother's blood should be evaluated for fetal red blood cells with the Kleihauer-Betke test, and the infant's blood should be evaluated with hemoglobin electrophoresis.

AMBIGUOUS GENITALIA

There may be great difficulty in some cases in determining whether a baby is a boy or a girl. The difficulty arises most often in congenital adrenal hyperplasia because of masculinization of the female, with a scrotal appearance of fused labia being difficult to distinguish from the male with a perineal hypospadias and cryptorchidism (Figs. 33–3 through 33–5).

The problem cannot be ignored and will not go away, so the parents must be told of the concern, and a recommendation should be made to defer naming the child or to choose a name suitable for a boy or a girl. Investigations must be started at once.

The history should include whether or not progestative hormones or other drugs were taken during pregnancy. It should also include questions about any similar cases of sexual ambiguity or instances of sudden unexplained neonatal death in the family. If a family history is positive, congenital adrenal hyperplasia (adrenogenital syndrome) is likely to be the diagnosis.

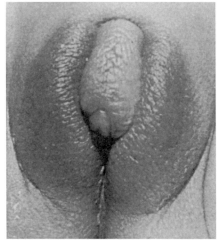

FIGURE 33–3. Ambiguous genitalia in a baby with congenital adrenal hyperplasia (adrenogenital syndrome). The "phallus" lies between the labia majora rather than arising above this region.

The following investigations should be performed: (1) buccal smear for sex chromatin (not reliable until third day); (2) 24-hour urine specimen for 17-ketosteroids and pregnanetriol; (3) serum sodium and potassium levels and acid-base status; and (4) radiographic studies: urethrovaginography, intravenous pyelography (or renal ultrasonography), and perhaps bone age assessment. Chromosome studies may also be necessary.

The baby should be carefully observed for the following complications related to adrenal insufficiency: salt-losing crisis, dehydration, and failure to gain weight.

In approximately 90% of the cases, the diagnosis is female sex with congenital adrenal hyperplasia. In the remaining 10%, the diagnosis is among the following: (1) other forms of female pseudohermaphroditism, (2) true hermaph-

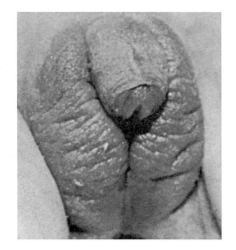

FIGURE 33–4. Another example of ambiguous genitalia secondary to congenital adrenal hyperplasia. In this baby the labia are scrotalized and are partly fused together.

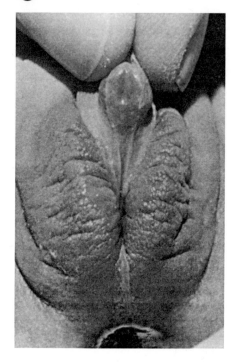

FIGURE 33–5. Same baby as in Figure 33–4, showing the "phallus" to be a clitoris and the vaginal introitus lying beneath.

roditism, or (3) male sex with hypospadias, perineal urethra, and bifid scrotum (particularly when the testes are absent).

When the diagnosis is congenital adrenal hyperplasia, the child should be raised in accordance with the genetic and gonadal sex. In other cases, the primary consideration in sex assignment is the serviceability of the external genitalia.

SWELLING OF SCROTUM

Scrotal swelling is common in the first few days of life. The differential diagnosis is primarily between hydrocele (which transilluminates, cannot easily be reduced in size, and is the most likely diagnosis) and inguinal hernia (which does not transilluminate easily and may be reducible) (Figs. 33–6 and 33–7). It may be part of generalized edema or, with discoloration, may indicate torsion of the testes.

Another reason for blueness of the scrotum is intraperitoneal bleeding, which may communicate with the scrotum.

UNDESCENDED TESTES (CRYPTORCHIDISM)

The testes may be undescended in 3% of full-term boys. Of these, about 50% descend within a month. When both testes are undescended, several prob-

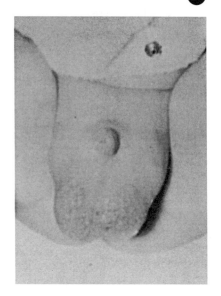

FIGURE 33–6. Bilateral swelling of the upper scrotum that was caused by inguinal hernias.

lems need to be considered. In the presence of hypotonia, particularly if there are dysmorphic facial features, the Prader-Willi syndrome (hypotonia, hypomentia, hypogonadism, and obesity syndrome) should be considered. If there is hypospadias and a small phallus, the "scrotum" may be scrotalized labia in the adrenogenital syndrome. Cryptorchidism is also seen with Klinefelter's syndrome and other complex disorders of sex chromosomes.

NONSPECIFIC SYMPTOMS AND SIGNS

In addition to jitteriness, lethargy, apnea, and circumoral cyanosis, which are rather nonspecific, at least two other symptoms are frequently reported by the nursing staff. These are poor feeding and "baby doesn't look good."

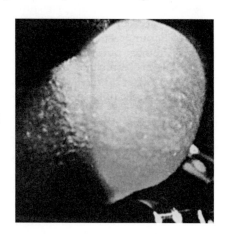

FIGURE 33–7. Transillumination of a left-sided hydrocele of the scrotum.

The baby who appears unwell to the intuitive nursing staff always deserves a second look. Four major groups of disorder should be considered: (1) *metabolic:* hypoglycemia, hypocalcemia, and so on; (2) *infection:* bacterial, viral, or protozoal; (3) *central nervous system hemorrhage or abnormality;* and (4) *toxic manifestation:* drug withdrawal. The following investigations are suggested in cases in which doubt exists:

1. Check maternal record: for diabetes mellitus, drug ingestion, and so on.
2. Obtain a complete blood count: consider high hematocrit syndrome and infection.
3. Use glucose test tapes (and/or blood glucose).
4. Obtain serum calcium and phosphorus levels, but can use Q_0T_c via electrocardiography to screen.
5. Obtain blood culture (and other cultures, e.g., urine, cerebrospinal fluid).
6. Determine serum electrolytes.
7. Perform lumbar puncture, for infection or hemorrhage.
8. Perform transillumination of skull (via Chun gun or similar device).
9. Perform amino acid screen.
10. Perform cephalic ultrasonography, for hemorrhage (consider computed tomographic scan and subdural taps).

ABNORMAL TEMPERATURE

Details of the normal range of temperature and the reasons for derangement are discussed in Chapter 5, Thermoregulation. To summarize, fever is most likely to be caused by increased environmental temperature (incubator) and may be caused by infection, dehydration, intracranial hemorrhage, or drug withdrawal. Fever later in the newborn period may also be caused by bundling in warm climates and is frequently encountered in infants with bronchopulmonary dysplasia (usually without explanation); it may also occur immediately after delivery in which maternal epidural anesthesia was used. Low temperature is most likely the result of inability to prevent heat loss, such as when the baby is out of the warmer while procedures are being performed, but it may also be caused by infection (sepsis) and possibly hypothyroidism.

SMALL-FOR-GESTATIONAL AGE

When a baby of low birth weight (< 2500 g) is found to be below the 10th percentile for gestational age, several possible explanations exist. With many infants, there is little that can be done, but some may require specific investigations. With any small for gestational age (intrauterine growth retardation) baby, the following questions should be asked (see also pp. 208 to 212):

1. Is there any maternal or placental problem that might have contributed (e.g., maternal cardiorespiratory disease or placental infarction)?
2. Is there evidence of chromosomal abnormality?
3. Is there evidence of other congenital abnormality?

4. Could this baby have had chronic intrauterine infection (TORCH complex)?

LARGE-FOR-GESTATIONAL AGE

By far, the most significant cause of largeness for gestational age is diabetes in the mother (see pp. 204 to 207). Other causes of largeness for gestational age are (1) *familial;* (2) *Beckwith's syndrome:* macroglossia, omphalocele, visceromegaly, and hypoglycemia (Fig. 33–8); (3) *postmaturity* with continued growth; and (4) *hydrops fetalis:* because of excessive accumulation of water. For further information see Chapters 6 and 16.

DWARFISM

Infants who are disproportionately short for their gestational age are considered to have dwarfism. The most common form of dwarfism is achondroplasia, which is characterized by shortening of the proximal portions of the extremities. The upper to lower body segment ratio is usually greater than 2 to 1. A less severe form is called hypochondroplasia.

Shortening of the distal extremities is seen with chondroectodermal dysplasia (Ellis–van Creveld syndrome) and mesomelic dwarfism. There are many

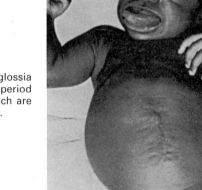

FIGURE 33–8. This infant with macroglossia was operated on in the neonatal period for an omphalocele, both of which are features of Beckwith's syndrome.

other forms of dwarfism, some of which are lethal. Two forms associated with a narrow chest are asphyxiating thoracic dystrophy and thanatophoric dwarfism. Polydactyly is associated with chondroectodermal dysplasia and asphyxiating thoracic dystrophy. Fractures may be associated with osteogenesis imperfecta congenita.

Achondroplasia is autosomal dominant, but most cases are new mutations. Most other forms of dwarfism have different forms of inheritance, and genetics consultation and counseling are recommended.

DELAYED PASSAGE OF URINE

Many babies pass urine in the delivery room, and the information is not transmitted to the nursery. Most babies (over 90%) pass urine within 24 hours, and almost 100% pass urine within 48 hours. Failure to pass urine within 2 days may be the result of (1) insufficient fluid intake, (2) bilateral renal agenesis (Potter's syndrome), (3) urethral obstruction (should have palpable bladder), (4) neurogenic bladder (with meningomyelocele), (5) tubular or cortical necrosis (secondary to shock and/or hypoxia), or (6) anticonvulsant drugs taken by the mother (possibly).

HEMATURIA (BLOODY URINE)

When hematuria is obvious to the naked eye (gross hematuria), it can be quite alarming. Perhaps the most common cause today is a generalized hemorrhagic problem (see Bleeding in Chapter 24, Neonatal Emergencies). Many rare causes of hematuria exist, the most important of which are renal venous thrombosis (usually treated conservatively), polycystic disease of the kidney, and obstructive uropathy. In some infants, the cause is never found. Pink urine may also be caused by urates.

When hematuria is detected only by test tapes or under the microscope (microscopic hematuria), the most likely antecedent is any stress to the baby, particularly asphyxia and infection. It may also follow a suprapubic bladder tap. Care should be exercised in obtaining urine specimens to make sure that iodinated preparations do not contaminate the specimen. The povidone-iodine preparations can produce a false-positive result for blood with test tapes.

OLIGURIA (DECREASED URINE OUTPUT)

Oliguria is most likely to follow hypoxia (or asphyxia), hypotension, or shock (caused by infection or blood loss). In other words, it is the result of "prerenal" renal failure. Particularly with asphyxia and meningitis, the syndrome of inappropriate antidiuretic hormone response should be considered. Decreased urine output may occur after administration of indomethacin. Another unusual cause is urate nephropathy, but other intrinsic renal anomalies (e.g., polycystic kidneys, renal dysgenesis or agenesis, obstructive uropathy) should be considered. Fluid restriction may be necessary (especially with inappropriate antidiuretic hormone response).

Renal failure may be distinguished from prerenal oliguria by use of fractional excretion of sodium (> 2.5) or a renal failure index (> 4), where

$$\text{Renal failure index} = \frac{\text{urinary sodium (mEq/L)}}{\text{urine/serum creatinine}}$$

ABNORMAL SMELL

Babies who are born after prolonged rupture of the membranes may have an unpleasant (foul-smelling) odor related to bacteria, which may have produced an amnionitis.

When an abnormal smell occurs after several days, it is most likely the result of an inborn error of metabolism involving amino acids. In phenylketonuria, there is a musty or "mousy" smell; with isovalericacidemia, there is a smell of sweaty feet; and a maple syrup smell may be detected with maple syrup urine disease (the name comes from the color rather than the smell).

PAIN ON MOVEMENT OF A LIMB

There are two major considerations in pain on limb movement: fracture and osteomyelitis. At present, fracture of bones other than the clavicle is very uncommon in term infants but could produce pain in the first few days after birth. Because of increased survival of extremely low-birth-weight infants (<1000 g), rickets of prematurity (or osteopenia) is seen more frequently and has been associated with fractures of long bones, usually after several weeks. The more likely explanation for pain is osteomyelitis, which is unlikely in the first few days after delivery.

BIBLIOGRAPHY

Edema

Lewy, J. E., and Moel, D. I.: Pathogenesis and management of edema in the newborn. *Clin. Perinatol.* 1975, 2:117.
Editorial: Anasarca in the newborn. *Lancet* 1979, ii:729.
Pearse, R. G., and Höweler, C. J.: Neonatal form of dystrophia myotonica: Five cases in preterm babies and review of earlier reports. *Arch. Dis. Child.* 1979, 54:331–338.
Kumar, S. P., and Anday, E. K.: Edema, hypoproteinemia and zinc deficiency in low-birth-weight infants. *Pediatrics* 1984, 73:327–329.

Hydrops

Hutchison, M., Drew, J. H., Yu, V. Y. H., et al.: Nonimmunologic hydrops fetalis: A review of 61 cases. *Obstet. Gynecol.* 1982, 59:347–352.
Carlton, D. P., McGillivray, B. C., and Schreiber, M. D.: Non-immune hydrops fetalis: A multidisciplinary approach. *Clin. Perinatol.* 1989, 16:839–851.

Ambiguous Genitalia

Donahoe, P. L. K., and Hendren, W. H.: Evaluation of the newborn with ambiguous genitalia. *Pediatr. Clin. North Am.* 1976, 23:361.
Kottmeier, P. K., and Velcek, F. T.: Ambiguous genitalia in the neonate. *Clin. Perinatol.* 1978, 5:163.

Swelling of Scrotum

Watson, R. A.: Torsion of spermatic cord in neonate. *Urology* 1975, 5:439.

Undescended Testes

Aughton, D. J., and Cassidy, S. B.: Physical features of Prader-Willi syndrome in neonates. *Am. J. Dis. Child.* 1990, 144:1251–1254.
Ansell, P. E., Bennet, V., Bull, D., et al.: Cryptorchidism: A prospective study of 7500 consecutive male births, 1984–8. *Arch. Dis. Child.* 1992, 67:892–899.

Small-for-Gestational Age

Andrews, B. (ed.): The small-for-date infant. *Pediatr. Clin. North Am.* 1970, 17:1–229.
Lang, J. M., Cohen, A., and Lieberman, E.: Risk factors for small-for-gestational-age birth in a preterm population. *Am. J. Obstet. Gynecol.* 1992, 166:1374–1378.

Large-for-Gestational Age

Iffy, L., Chatterton, R. T., and Jakobovitz, A.: The "high weight for dates" fetus. *Am. J. Obstet. Gynecol.* 1973, 115:238.
Lubchenco, L. O.: The infant who is large for gestational age. In *The High Risk Infant.* W. B. Saunders, Philadelphia, 1976, pp. 165–180.

Dwarfism

Clark, R. N.: Congenital dysplasias and dwarfism. *Pediatr. Rev.* 1990, 12:149–159.

Delayed Passage of Urine

Moore, E. S., and Galvez, M. B.: Delayed micturition in newborn period. *J. Pediatr.* 1972, 80:867.
Robson, W. J., and Davies, R. H.: Transient retention of urine in the neonatal period. *J. Pediatr. Surg.* 1974, 9:863.
Clark, D. A.: Times of first void and first stool in 500 newborns. *Pediatrics* 1977, 60:457.
Levene, M. I.: Retention of urine in the neonate, possibly due to anticonvulsant drugs. *Arch. Dis. Child.* 1977, 52:975.

Hematuria

Emanuel, B., and Aronson, N.: Neonatal hematuria. *Am. J. Dis. Child.* 1974, 128:204.
Hait, W. N., Snepar, R., and Rothman, C.: False-positive hematest due to povidone-iodine (Letter). *N. Engl. J. Med.* 1977, 297:1350.
Brem, A. S.: Neonatal hematuria and proteinuria. *Clin. Perinatol.* 1981, 8:321–332.
Oliver, W. J., and Kelsch, R. C.: Renal venous thrombosis in infancy. *Pediatr. Rev.* 1982, 4:61–66.

Oliguria

Ahmadian, Y., and Lewy, P. R.: Possible urate nephropathy of the newborn infant as a cause of transient renal insufficiency. *J. Pediatr.* 1977, 91:96.
Mathew, O. P., Jones, A. S., James, E., et al.: Neonatal renal failure: Usefulness of diagnostic indices. *Pediatrics* 1980, 65:57.
Springate, J. E., Fildes, R. D., and Feld, L. G.: Assessment of renal function in newborn infants. *Pediatr. Rev.* 1987, 9:51–56.
Karlowicz, M. G., and Adelman, R. D.: Acute renal failure in the neonate. *Clin. Perinatol.* 1992, 19:139–158.

34

INTERPRETING LABORATORY TESTS AND X-RAY STUDIES

INTERPRETING SOME COMMON LABORATORY TESTS

HEMATOCRIT

1. The normal range of cord blood values is 40 to 60%.
2. Heel-stick values (especially if unwarmed) may give falsely elevated values. Equilibration occurs in the first 3 to 4 hours, at which time the hematocrit value is likely to be at a maximum.
3. Despite considerable depletion of blood volume, the hematocrit value may remain stable as a result of vasoconstriction.
4. In the absence of a history of maternal bleeding or blood group incompatibility, a low hematocrit value at birth suggests fetomaternal hemorrhage.

NUCLEATED RED BLOOD CELLS

1. The preterm infant usually has a slight increase in the number of circulating nucleated red blood cells, which are rarely present in term infants.
2. Hemolysis is likely to produce an increase in the reticulocyte count and number of nucleated red blood cells.
3. In the absence of hemolysis, an increased number of nucleated red blood cells may indicate exposure to infection or hypoxia (asphyxia). This latter condition seems to be common in babies with severe intrauterine growth retardation, in which there is presumably chronic hypoxemia (see Chapter 16).

WHITE BLOOD COUNT

1. A wide range of total leukocyte counts exists, especially in the first 24 hours after birth. Values vary with age, but the usual range is 5000 to 30,000/mm^3 (5.0 to 30.0 $\times$ 10^9/L). Initial values below 7500 are suspicious, as are values above 20,000 after the first week.
2. Usually, an increase in total leukocytes and absolute neutrophils occurs

by 8 to 12 hours after delivery, with a gradual fall after this. A falling leukocyte or neutrophil count in the first few hours suggests infection.

3. Lower leukocyte counts are seen in preterm infants.

4. The immature to total neutrophil ratio is not influenced by gestational age. Values over 0.2, especially over 0.3, raise the possibility of infection, but asphyxial insult should be sought.

5. A total leukocyte count of less than 5000/mm^3 together with an immature total neutrophil ratio of greater than 0.2 strongly suggests infection.

6. Decreased neutrophils (neutropenia) may follow maternal hypertension, but profound neutropenia (< 1000/mm^3) suggests bacterial infection. Viral infection can also produce neutropenia.

7. Increased numbers of eosinophils are seen with chlamydial infection and in infants growing while receiving parenteral nutrition.

8. A very high immature to total neutrophil ratio (> 0.8) suggests depletion of neutrophil storage pool in bone marrow.

9. A leukemoid response can be seen during recovery from infection and has also been seen in some infants with Down's syndrome.

PLATELETS

1. Normal values are above 150,000/mm^3 (150 $\times$ 10^9/L) and below 400,000/mm^3 (400 $\times$ 10^9/L).

2. Thrombocytopenia may be seen after maternal hypertension.

3. Values below 30,000/mm^3 usually require platelet transfusion (see also Chapter 24, Neonatal Emergencies, p. 287).

4. Increased platelet counts (thrombocytosis) may be encountered in some infants recovering from infection.

BLOOD GASES AND pH

1. Respiratory acidosis is documented when pH decreases with an increased pCO$_2$. This indicates inadequate ventilation and suggests that ventilatory assistance may be needed. If ventilation is being assisted, some method of improving minute ventilation is needed (see Appendix 7).

2. Metabolic acidosis is documented when pH decreases but pCO$_2$ remains normal. Compensated metabolic acidosis exists when pH is normal but pCO$_2$ is decreased. Metabolic acidosis may be caused by hypoxemia (if pO$_2$ is low) but suggests that administration of base (usually sodium bicarbonate) is required (see also pp. 218 to 220).

3. Heel-stick (capillary) blood gases usually show a significant discrepancy of pO$_2$ versus arterial pO$_2$, but capillary values of 35 to 50 mm Hg usually equate with arterial values of 50 to 100 mm Hg. Although capillary values above 50 mm Hg may reflect arterial values below 100 mm Hg, frequently they are above this level. Heelstick pCO$_2$ and especially pH are fairly accurate.

4. A sudden increase in pH and pCO$_2$ is probably the result of contamina-

tion of an arterial sample by bicarbonate in the line. The sample should be repeated, and care should be taken to clear the line.

GLUCOSE

1. Falsely low values may be seen when glucose oxidase test tapes (e.g., Dextrostix) are used. This is the result of exposure to oxygen when the bottle has been opened for some time.

2. Although very-low-birth-weight infants (particularly < 1000 g) may not tolerate normal amounts of glucose, transient elevations of glucose may follow resuscitation procedures as a result of exogenous or endogenous catecholamines (see also pp. 214 to 216).

ELECTROLYTES
(see also pp. 221 to 222)

1. The most common reason for decreased sodium and potassium levels is sampling error. This problem is usually associated with umbilical artery (or other central) catheters, with dilution of the sample by infusion fluid.

2. Anion gap can be calculated from: $Na - (Cl + CO_2)$, which should be 12 ± 2 mEq/L. If acidosis is associated with a normal anion gap, gastrointestinal or renal loss of bicarbonate is likely. When acidosis is associated with an increased anion gap, increased acid production or failure to excrete acid is likely to be present, and an inborn error of metabolism may be present.

3. Increased potassium levels may follow excessive squeezing of the heel for heel-stick samples, or they may be seen with hemolyzed samples.

4. Decreased potassium levels may be associated with alkalemia (usually secondary to hyperventilation).

BILIRUBIN

1. Age at sampling is the most important consideration. Elevated levels in the first 24 and possibly 48 hours (over 10 and 12 mg/dl, respectively) suggest that a pathologic explanation be sought.

2. Accuracy of determinations is suspect, and levels within 1 mg/dl should probably be considered the same.

TOTAL PROTEIN

1. Levels increase with advancing gestational age, with a mean of about 3.5 g/dl at 28 weeks' gestation to 6.0 g/dl at term.

2. Albumin level can be estimated as at least 60% of total protein.

COAGULATION STUDIES

1. Most coagulation-related times (prothrombin, partial thromboplastin, bleeding, and so on) are somewhat prolonged, particularly in the preterm infant. Occasionally, there is a hypercoagulable state.
2. Increased partial thromboplastin time may be the result of a heparin effect. This results from failure to clear the residual fluid in the infusion line after small amounts of heparin have been added to the infusate. This effect can be overcome by a reptilase test.

LIVER ENZYMES

1. It is usual to have some increase in the liver enzyme levels during the neonatal period. "Normal adult" levels may indicate liver failure and suggest that blood ammonia be checked.
2. Marked increases in aspartate aminotransferase and alanine aminotransferase levels suggest parenchymal damage, secondary either to asphyxia or infection.
3. A marked increase in gamma glutamyl transpeptidase level suggests cholestatic injury, which may follow use of parenteral nutrition for 2 weeks or more.
4. An increased serum alkaline phosphatase level may indicate incipient neonatal rickets (sometimes called osteopenia). Long bone x-ray studies are indicated.

INTERPRETING SOME COMMON X-RAY FINDINGS

CHEST

Shift of the Mediastinum

1. There are two reasons for true mediastinal shift:
   a. Something pulling: usually atelectasis (collapse of lung).
   b. Something pushing: either tension pneumothorax, diaphragmatic hernia, or hyperinflated lung (for some reason). Opacity on one side or the other suggests fluid, either pleural effusion or chylothorax.
2. Remember that the mediastinum may appear to be shifted if the chest is partially rotated.

Reticulogranular Appearance

Reticulogranular appearance is usually the result of alternating areas of inflation and atelectasis. The two most common reasons for this finding are respiratory distress syndrome (hyaline membrane disease) and pneumonia (caused by group B streptococci and other organisms). When seen in the first 24 hours in a preterm infant, it may be impossible to distinguish between the two. If it appears after an apparently normal chest x-ray study in the first 24 hours, pneumonia is likely. When it is seen in the first 12 hours after acute antepartum hemorrhage, it is most likely respiratory distress syndrome.

Linear Marking Over Lateral Chest

Although the possibility of a small pneumothorax should always be kept in mind, a confusing finding is commonly associated with skin folds. The presence of a skin fold is usually confirmed by the ability to follow the line beyond the limits of the thorax, whereas a pneumothorax is obviously confined to the thoracic cavity.

Diffuse Haziness in Both Lung Fields

1. Retained lung fluid is the most likely explanation and is a normal finding in many babies evaluated within the first hours after delivery.
2. When diaphragms are high, diffuse atelectasis is probable.
3. When diaphragms are in a normal position, pulmonary edema and the exudative phase of bronchopulmonary dysplasia should be considered.

Rapid Improvement

Rapid improvement in aeration of the chest is usually the result of absorption of retained lung fluid or resolution of atelectasis after the use of mechanical ventilation. However, in some small babies, there may be apparent radiographic improvement, although other findings suggest deterioration. This finding is most likely caused by pulmonary interstitial emphysema, with interstitial air producing apparently improved aeration. This appearance can be confusing to the uninitiated.

Thin Ribs

When the chest radiograph of an infant with respiratory difficulty is evaluated, the ribs may appear extremely thin. This finding is usually associated with some neuromuscular disorders, such as congenital myotonic dystrophy.

Large Heart (see p. 307)

ABDOMEN

Gasless Abdomen

1. There are two basic reasons for the appearance of a gasless abdomen: either air is unable to enter the bowel, or it is being eliminated more rapidly than it enters.
2. The possibility of esophageal atresia without a communicating tracheo-

esophageal fistula should be considered if it occurs early, especially if the baby has a great deal of mucus.

3. The most common reasons include sickness, a neurologic problem, or paralysis. Under all of these circumstances, swallowing of air may not occur; thus, air does not pass into the intestine.

"Frothy" Appearance of Bowel

1. The most likely explanation is the presence of loose stool with air bubbles within the lumen of the intestine.

2. When it is present in the right-lower quadrant, one should consider the possibility of meconium ileus (when the problem is within the bowel) or necrotizing enterocolitis, in which the intramural air may produce bubbles rather than the more classic "railroad-track" appearance.

3. Both meconium ileus and necrotizing enterocolitis can produce changes elsewhere in the bowel; therefore, the location is not crucial.

Dilated Loops of Bowel

1. The rule of thumb is: compare bowel loops with width of vertebral body (L-1); pathology is likely if 90 to 95% of bowel loops are wider than L-1.

2. In the term baby, the most likely explanations are intestinal obstruction (for one of several reasons) or ileus caused by asphyxia or sepsis.

3. In the preterm baby, ileus as a result of asphyxia or sepsis is still a strong possibility, but one should always consider necrotizing enterocolitis. Intestinal obstruction is less likely.

BIBLIOGRAPHY

Osborne, J. P., Murphy, E. G., and Hill, A.: Thin ribs on chest x-ray: A useful sign in the differential diagnosis of the floppy newborn. *Dev. Med. Child. Neurol.* 1983, 3:343–345.

Procedures

35

DIAGNOSTIC TECHNIQUES

MONITORING

HEART RATE

To measure heart rate, a simple rate recorder (cardiotachometer) is usually used with electrodes attached to the chest wall and leg or abdomen, but it may have an electrocardiograph readout with a cardioscope (Fig. 35–1). However, it is important to be aware that seizures, tremulousness, or hiccups may produce artifacts. Occasionally, beat-to-beat variability is used.

RESPIRATION AND APNEA

Impedance monitoring records electrical activity across the chest, usually with electrodes placed on the lateral chest wall, but electrical activity can be detected with arm leads. This method has the advantage of being able to detect heart rate at the same time. *Pneumatic* monitoring records chest wall movement by transmission of an air-filled mattress. Displacement of air in the mattress is detected in a central sensing device (Fig. 35–2). This device has the advantage of using no leads (electrodes) on the baby. These monitors are rarely used at this time.

With either of these methods, dangerous exceptions ("broken" apnea, upper airway obstruction, or "disorganized breathing") may not be recorded, but hypoxemia will occur. Although devices to detect nasal air flow are available, they have not been used frequently in clinical practice. Because the major concern is hypoxemia, oxygen saturation monitors (pulse oximetry) and transcutaneous oxygen tension monitors have been used extensively (see later in this chapter).

TEMPERATURE

Temperature is usually recorded continuously whenever an infant servocontrol mechanism is being used with either an incubator or a radiant heat warmer. Baby's temperature is recorded with a thermistor probe attached to the upper abdomen, overlying the liver, or between the scapulae. Manual monitoring

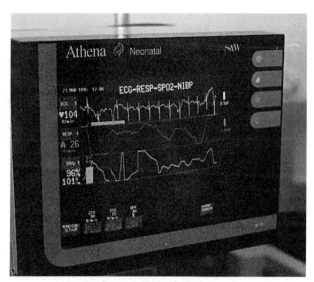

FIGURE 35–1. This monitor records heart rate, respiration rate, and oxygen saturation. It can also be used to record arterial and venous blood pressures.

usually involves taking an axillary temperature (Fig. 35–3) (see Chapter 5). More recently, infrared thermometers have been introduced, which may provide a rapid measurement from the tympanic membrane. Possible hazards (such as overheating and increased fluid loss) with the use of infant radiant warmers should be understood (see Bibliography).

BLOOD PRESSURE

Blood pressure should be measured in the following groups of babies: (1) those who require prolonged resuscitation in the delivery room, (2) those who have more than mild respiratory difficulty, (3) those who look pale or mottled, and (4) those who are cyanotic, especially without respiratory distress (i.e., congenital heart disease). The technique for measuring blood pressure varies

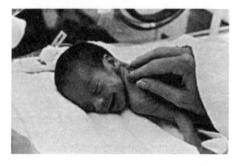

FIGURE 35–2. A premature infant lying on the lower part of a pneumatic apnea monitor. The individual units of this air mattress are connected to a single sensor, so that any chest wall movement transmits the movement of air past the sensor.

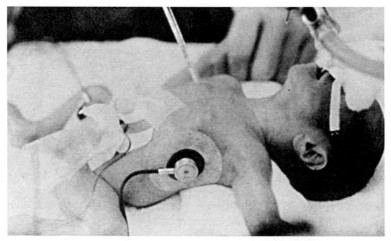

FIGURE 35–3. Temperature being recorded in the axilla in a premature infant monitored on a ventilator.

with the availability of the equipment and the clinical management used (for normal values see Appendix 6).

Direct Method

When an arterial catheter (usually umbilical) is in place, intraarterial pressures may be detected by using a transducer. This method also allows a continuous recording to be obtained.

Indirect Method

OSCILLOMETRY. Several devices are now available that measure blood pressure noninvasively and automatically. The blood pressure cuff is self-inflating; oscillations in blood pressure are used to determine the systolic and diastolic values. Mean arterial pressure as well as heart rate can also be determined. Continuous (or, strictly speaking, very frequent intermittent) measurements that seem to correlate closely with direct measurements can be performed.

ULTRASONOGRAPHIC TECHNIQUE. This method employs a cuff and external transducer and detects vessel movement, giving systolic and diastolic measurements.

DOPPLER TECHNIQUE. This method employs a cuff and external transducer to detect blood flow and is therefore reliable only for systolic measurement.

FLUSH TECHNIQUE. Always available, this method uses a cuff and tourniquet technique to produce pallor in the limb, with flushing as pressure is lowered slowly to systolic pressure.

INFECTION DETECTION

GASTRIC ASPIRATE SMEAR

A smear of gastric aspirate should be stained, either with Wright's stain to detect polymorphonuclear leukocytes (pus cells), with more than 5 per high-power field being significant, or with Gram's stain to detect organisms, especially β-hemolytic streptococcus group B. The number of pus cells is more an indication of amnionitis than infection of the neonate (and the cells are maternal in origin). A single bacterial organism, especially in large numbers, suggests exposure to a specific infection.

BLOOD CULTURES

A culture is usually obtained from peripheral veins after the skin is cleaned with an iodinated preparation. The safest vessel is the antecubital vein, but it may be necessary to use the external jugular or femoral vein. It may be possible (with suitable precautions) to use blood from heel-stick samples. Umbilical artery catheter samples seem to be reliable when obtained within 8 to 12 hours of delivery, and they probably remain reliable for several days after this. As little as 0.5 to 1.0 ml of blood may be enough, although larger samples may increase the yield.

URINE CULTURE

Culture samples taken by the bag technique are notoriously unreliable in the neonate. The most reliable sample method is suprapubic bladder aspiration (bladder tap). When the bladder is palpable, the skin is cleaned with an iodinated preparation. The baby's legs should be held down by an assistant. It may be necessary to try to prevent inadvertent passage of urine by gently squeezing the penis in the male or placing a finger in the rectum of the female. A 1½-inch 21-gauge needle is inserted just above the symphysis pubis at about 10° from the perpendicular, with slight traction on the plunger of the syringe. With a full bladder, urine should be aspirated after ½ to ¾ inch of the needle is inserted. Microscopic and chemical examination may also be carried out.

CAUTION: It is probably best not to perform this procedure in the presence of marked abdominal distension because of the risk of bowel perforation. It may be possible to use transillumination or ultrasonography to detect a full bladder.

CEREBROSPINAL FLUID CULTURE

After the skin is cleaned with an iodinated preparation, a lumbar puncture should be performed using a needle with a stylet. Although frequently performed with scalp vein needles, this method carries the risk of introducing a small piece of skin, which may result in a spinal tumor. Fluid specimens are usually examined microscopically and chemically.

Great care should be taken in positioning the baby to avoid excessive flexion of the trunk or neck (with resultant hypoxemia). The number of white blood cells in cerebrospinal fluid may not always be increased with meningitis; thus, the fluid should always be sent for culture.

WHITE BLOOD CELL COUNT AND DIFFERENTIAL

An abnormally high or low count with a change in the distribution of cells may be very helpful. In the author's experience, low values are more helpful than high values. A total white blood cell count of less than $5000/mm^3$, and particularly less than $4000/mm^3$, suggests the presence of infection. An increased number of immature forms (bands) of greater than $2000/mm^3$ or an increased band to total neutrophil ratio (≥ 0.2) suggests infection (see Chap. 15).

"MINI"-SEDIMENTATION RATE

Older methods for determining erythrocyte sedimentation rate usually required large amounts of blood. The microhematocrit tube method is simple to perform and seems to be reliable. The microhematocrit tube (with internal diameter of 1.1 mm) is filled completely with blood (from a heel-stick sample). One end is closed with sealant, and the other (open) end is wiped free of superfluous blood. The tube is placed in a vertical position for 1 hour, and the distance from the meniscus to the column of blood is read. Values are usually 1 to 4 mm. Values above 10 mm may support a diagnosis of infection, but values above 15 mm are even more indicative. Increased values have been observed in ABO incompatibility, so blood groups should be checked.

OTHER NONSPECIFIC TESTS (see discussion in Chapter 15)

With the advent of rapid, quantitative determinations of acute-phase proteins (using nephelometric techniques), C-reactive protein and α_1-acid glycoprotein values seem to provide supporting evidence for infection. A buffy-coat smear for organisms engulfed by white cells is sometimes helpful, but the nitroblue tetrazolium test seems to have limited application. Changes in platelet counts and immunoglobulin M occur late. Interleukin-6 is the most promising of the newer tests.

NEUROLOGIC EVALUATION

LUMBAR PUNCTURE (SPINAL TAP)

Lumbar puncture is performed in the same manner as cerebrospinal fluid culture (see previous discussion). In this case, microscopic or gross examination for blood is usually indicated. In some cases of intraventricular hemorrhage, the fluid is initially clear and then becomes blood tinged ("blood in the third tube"). This situation usually contrasts with a traumatic tap, which starts out bloody but clears with manipulation of the needle ("clearing of the third tube").

SUBDURAL TAP

A subdural tap should be considered in the presence of a bulging fontanel, after traumatic delivery, or if convulsions or other gross neurologic abnormalities are not explained by other investigations. In many centers, it should be possible to document a subdural collection of fluid with computed tomography and sometimes with ultrasonography.

Short-beveled ½-inch needles with a stylet are available for this procedure. The head is usually shaved if hair is prominent, and the scalp is cleaned with an iodinated preparation. The needle is inserted away from the midline at the lateral angle of the anterior fontanel. A sharp pop is experienced as the dura (which is quite tough) is perforated. More than 0.5 to 1.0 ml of fluid is considered abnormal.

TRANSILLUMINATION OF THE SKULL

Standardization of this technique has been accomplished in recent years by using the Chun gun device, which permits a high-intensity light to be applied to the baby's head while dissipating heat. In hydranencephaly, the whole skull lights up (see Fig. 8–22). In premature babies, there is usually a greater zone of

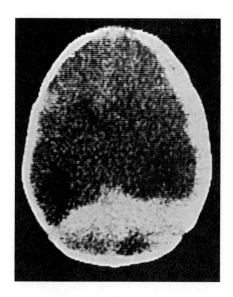

FIGURE 35–4. Computed tomograph of a term baby with subdural hemorrhage, demonstrated by the white area seen posteriorly (courtesy of W. C. Allan).

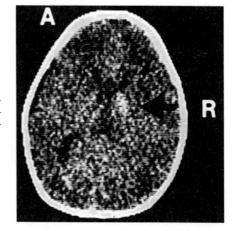

FIGURE 35–5. Computed tomograph showing a right-sided germinal matrix hemorrhage (arrow) (courtesy of W. C. Allan).

transillumination over the frontal bones. The cheek may be used as a reference standard, but normal values are now available. Other transillumination devices can also be used.

COMPUTED TOMOGRAPHY

Computed tomography (Figs. 35–4 to 35–6) radically changed our way of thinking about the frequency and extent of intraventricular hemorrhage in very-low-birth-weight infants, but it has now been replaced almost completely for this purpose by cephalic ultrasonography. Nevertheless, it remains extremely valuable for detection of subarachnoid and subdural hemorrhage as well as for examination of the posterior fossa. In term infants, the development of areas of

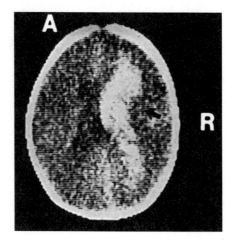

FIGURE 35–6. Computed tomograph showing intraventricular hemorrhage (arrow). The right lateral ventricle is filled with blood (courtesy of W. C. Allan).

hypodensity after asphyxia suggests a poor prognosis. Hypodensities in preterm infants are more difficult to interpret.

CEPHALIC ULTRASONOGRAPHY

Since it was first reported on in 1979, cephalic ultrasonography has revolutionized our understanding of neonatal intracranial pathology. The major advantage of this technique over computed tomography is that it can be performed at the bedside without having to disturb the baby; a second advantage is that it does not involve ionizing radiation. In most cases, the information can be obtained within about 5 minutes. Intraventricular or periventricular hemorrhage is easily detected (Fig. 35–7), and increased ventricular size can also be recognized and followed (Fig. 35–8). Initially, linear-array devices were used, but now a sector scan is more typically used.

MAGNETIC RESONANCE IMAGING

Magnetic resonance imaging was earlier called nuclear magnetic resonance imaging but is frequently abbreviated now to MRI. Introduced in the early 1980s, it is now an established imaging technique that does not use ionizing radiation. Unfortunately, like computed tomography, magnetic resonance imaging requires that the baby be moved to the machine, and certain technical difficulties make this difficult to accomplish in the sickest infants. It is important to eliminate any ferrous metals from the baby's environment. Otherwise, needles and other objects can become high-velocity projectiles when the magnets are turned on. The particular advantage of this technique is that it can demonstrate effects on myelination.

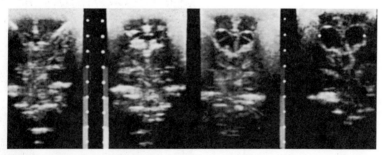

FIGURE 35–7. Ultrasound demonstration of intraventricular hemorrhage and posthemorrhagic hydrocephalus. These coronal views were taken over the course of 2 weeks by use of a linear-array scan and show (left to right) germinal matrix hemorrhage, intraventricular hemorrhage, intraventricular hemorrhage and ventricular dilation, and further ventricular dilation (courtesy of J. D. Horbar).

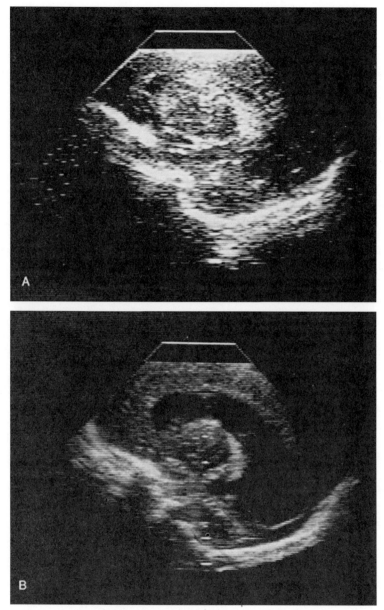

FIGURE 35–8. Ultrasound demonstration of intraventricular hemorrhage and posthemor-rhagic hydrocephalus. These sagittal views were taken with a sector scan and show blood in the ventricle *(A)* followed by marked ventricular dilation *(B)*.

INTRACRANIAL PRESSURE MONITORING

Intracranial pressure monitoring is another noninvasive technique, and it may prove valuable in the treatment of infants who are of low birth weight or who suffered asphyxia at birth. Pressure can be measured by placing a sensor over the anterior fontanel. Difficulties with reliable application of the sensor have limited the practical usefulness of this technique.

RESPIRATORY EVALUATION

BLOOD GASES

Three major sources for measuring pH, pO_2, and pCO_2 exist:

1. *Umbilical artery catheters:* usually intermittent sampling, but occasionally continuous pO_2 recording
2. *Radial or temporal artery:* intermittent needle sampling or continuous catheter (but contraindicated for temporal)
3. *Warmed heel (or finger):* blood obtained by stylet prick (sometimes referred to as capillary or arterialized blood gases)

Umbilical Artery Catheters

Umbilical artery catheters can also be used for infusion of fluid and may allow easy blood sampling for other studies. Many risks are inherent in this technique that require close attention. *Hemorrhage* is the most important complication, and great care should be taken to ensure that all connections are as firm as possible. Other problems are *spasm of an artery,* producing blanching of a limb (Fig. 35–9) (reflex vasodilatation by warming the opposite limb may resolve the problem), and *thromboembolic phenomena,* which may be minimized by using 1 unit of heparin per milliliter of infusion fluid or silicone catheters. *Hypertension* may follow high placement in the aorta. The techniques for placement, sampling, and removal of umbilical artery catheters are contained in Appendix 1.

Radial or Temporal Arteries

These arteries are the preferred sites for sampling in some centers. The risk of hemorrhage is more transient but may require 15 minutes of firm pressure after needle puncture. Arterial samples from these sites may more accurately reflect the pO_2 in arteries supplying the retina than samples taken from the lower end of the aorta (postductal samples). The possibility of producing cerebral ischemia exists with catheter placement in the temporal artery. Transillumination may help in catheterizing the radial artery.

Warmed Heel

Samples from a warmed heel are fairly reliable for pH and pCO_2 but need to be interpreted cautiously for pO_2. We try to maintain capillary pO_2 between

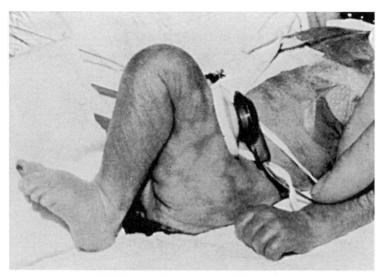

FIGURE 35–9. Severe blanching of the foot and mottling of the thigh suggest arterial spasm or a thromboembolic phenomenon. A few minutes later, the umbilical artery catheter was removed, and normal color returned to the limb, suggesting spasm.

35 and 50 mm Hg, which corresponds to arterial pO_2 levels of approximately 50 to 100 mm Hg.

PULSE OXIMETRY

In the mid-1980s, oxygen saturation monitors were introduced into neonatology and became accepted rapidly. These devices are also called pulse oximeters and use a light source and detector to measure oxygenated hemoglobin. Because they do not involve heat, they can be left in place for relatively prolonged periods of time. However, the site should be changed from time to time. It is important to remember that erroneous values will be observed if the pulse is not being detected. The rate for the pulse oximeter should be the same as for the heart rate monitor. When the extremity to which the sensor is applied is moving, the oxygen saturation measurement may be inaccurate.

Different devices may also give different ranges of oxygen saturation. It is generally difficult to accurately predict arterial oxygen tension (PaO_2) when the oxygen saturation (SpO_2) is above 95 or 96%, because the oxygen dissociation curve is flat in its upper portion. By use of the Nellcor oximeter, hypoxemia and hyperoxemia were avoided by keeping SpO_2 values between 92 and 96%, but lower comparable levels have been seen with the Ohmeda device.

TRANSCUTANEOUS OXYGEN TENSION ($tcpO_2$)

Transcutaneous oxygen tension measurement was developed in West Germany and depends on the fact that oxygen passes across the skin when a small area is heated a few degrees above body temperature. An oxygen electrode placed on the skin provides a continuous recording that closely reflects the arterial pO_2 in most clinical situations. These devices are now standard features of most intensive care nurseries and are particularly helpful when changes are made in settings for respiratory assistance because there is a rapid response time, which quickly reflects the baby's status. In addition, nursing care can be improved by careful attention to continuous $tcpO_2$ reading. When two electrodes are used (double-site monitoring), changes in blood flow through the ductus can be documented, when shunting is right to left.

TRANSCUTANEOUS CARBON DIOXIDE TENSION (tcpCO₂)

Shortly after the introduction of transcutaneous oxygen monitoring, devices to measure carbon dioxide were constructed. In recent years, combined $tcpO_2/tcpCO_2$ electrodes have been available. It is not as necessary to have a heated electrode for $tcpCO_2$ monitoring as it is for $tcpO_2$ monitoring, because carbon dioxide diffuses more easily than oxygen. Continuous $tcpCO_2$ recording is helpful in assessing ventilation strategies.

HYPEROXIA TEST

The hyperoxia test has been used to differentiate between pulmonary and cardiac disease. The pO_2 is measured with arterial blood gases or a $tcpO_2$ electrode, and the baby is placed in 100% oxygen for 15 to 20 minutes. A paO_2 of over 100 mm Hg (especially > 150 mm Hg) makes lung disease probable and cyanotic congenital heart disease unlikely. A further refinement of this technique is to add continuous positive airway pressure. With transcutaneous monitoring, the response may be observed in as little as 5 minutes.

RESPIROGRAPHY

In addition to the respiration rate and apnea monitor mentioned earlier, it may be valuable to examine the waveform of respirations. This provides a better assessment of respiratory activity and may demonstrate periods of hypoventilation or broken apnea. Such periods could result in bradycardia without triggering the apnea alarm. A nasal thermistor or other system (e.g., expired carbon dioxide) to measure air flow may be best.

TRANSILLUMINATION OF THE CHEST WALL

Detection of pneumothorax and pneumomediastinum has been greatly helped by use of a high-intensity light source on the chest wall (Figs. 35–10 and 35–11). It has also been possible to use a penlight, which may be easier to manipulate with a sick infant in an incubator. A wide area of transillumination

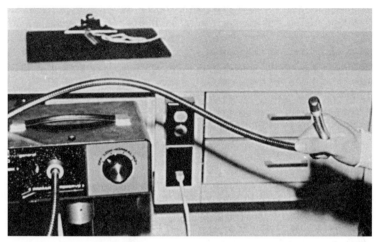

FIGURE 35–10. Transillumination device used to detect pneumothorax and pneumomedias-tinum.

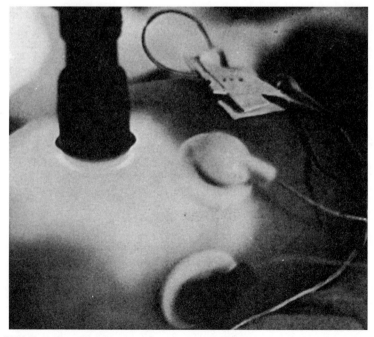

FIGURE 35–11. Transillumination of a pneumomediastinum using the Chun gun.

is virtually diagnostic of pneumothorax or pneumomediastinum. With experience, this technique eliminates the need for emergency chest x-ray study (see Figs. 9–5 and 9–6).

POSITION OF TUBES

The position of endotracheal tubes and umbilical artery catheters should always be checked by x-ray study. The tip of the endotracheal tube should lie just below the medial ends of the clavicles (approximately halfway between the vocal cords and the carina). There are theoretical advantages to low placement of umbilical artery catheters, with the tip at L3-4 (just above the bifurcation of the aorta), but many people prefer high placement (T6-10), particularly in very preterm infants, because of a higher frequency of mottling with low placement.

EVALUATION OF PHARYNGEAL ASPIRATE

Prediction of subsequent respiratory difficulty in the form of respiratory distress syndrome was initially performed on gastric aspirate specimens by use of the foam stability (shake) test. A simpler technique called bubble clicking has been used to predict and follow respiratory difficulty. When performed on pharyngeal secretions, it compared favorably with the lecithin-to-sphingomyelin ratio. The walls of the bubbles show rhythmic movements (clicking) under the microscope if they contain surfactant. These tests are used infrequently.

URINE EVALUATION

GLUCOSE

The presence of large amounts of glucose in urine may indicate that the baby is unable to tolerate the intravenous fluid prescribed. This problem occurs most frequently in very preterm infants. Most frequently, this requires reduction of the dextrose concentration from 10% to 5% to prevent an osmotic diuresis. In small for gestational age infants, the possibility of transient neonatal diabetes mellitus should be considered.

PROTEIN

Stressed newborns frequently have small amounts of protein in the urine. Large amounts of protein suggest congenital nephrotic syndrome.

SPECIFIC GRAVITY

A high or low specific gravity may indicate underhydration or overhydration, respectively. Fluid orders should be checked. (Some clinicians prefer the more accurate measure—osmolality.)

REDUCING SUBSTANCE

If results of glucose testing are negative, the presence of reducing substance in the urine could indicate galactosemia and is a useful screening test whenever this diagnosis is considered.

RED COLOR

A brick-red color may appear on the diaper because of the presence of urates and is sometimes confused with blood. Microscopic examination may be necessary.

BLOOD

See section on Hematuria in Chapter 33.

pH

Urine in small premature infants may be alkaline in the first days of life, especially in infants with respiratory distress syndrome, but in term infants, a pH of 7 or above raises the possibility of renal tubular acidosis.

STOOL EVALUATION

ALBUMIN

Various techniques have been used to detect albumin in the first meconium, which may indicate cystic fibrosis. Simple test strips are probably unreliable, giving both false-positive and false-negative results.

REDUCING SUBSTANCE

Large amounts (3+) of reducing substance in the stool of babies with either diarrhea or abdominal distension may provide an early indication of necrotizing enterocolitis, if the baby has been formula fed. Smaller amounts are common in breast-fed babies.

BLOOD

See section on Blood in the Stools in Chapter 28.

BONE MARROW EXAMINATION

Bone marrow examination is rarely performed in the newborn period. However, it may be a reliable source for rapid chromosome analysis and may be helpful in differentiating some cases of anemia. It may also be indicated in neonatal sepsis to document depletion of the neutrophil storage pool when granulocyte transfusion is considered. Preferred sites are the upper third of the tibia (anterior approach) and the iliac crest.

APT TEST

The Apt test is used to differentiate neonatal from maternal blood. (*This test is not applicable unless the blood is red.*)

1. Mix 1 volume of specimen (vomitus or stool) with 5 volumes of water. Centrifuge mixture and separate clear pink supernatant.
2. Add 1 part sodium hydroxide (0.25 N NaOH) to 4 parts supernatant. Mix and observe color change after 2 minutes.
3. Hemoglobin A (maternal blood) changes from pink to yellow-brown.
4. Hemoglobin F (neonatal blood) remains pink.

KLEIHAUER TECHNIQUE

The Kleihauer technique can be used to estimate fetomaternal hemorrhage (see also p. 244). To obtain the number of maternal cells, 5 fields are counted and divided by 5. The number of fetal cells is obtained by counting 30 fields and dividing by 30. One may then derive the percentage of fetal cells.

If the percentage of fetal cells is 1%, then approximately 50 ml of blood has been transferred from the fetus to the mother, assuming a maternal blood volume of 4500 ml.

TRANSCUTANEOUS BILIRUBINOMETRY

Determination of the degree of jaundice has been estimated with several simple devices (icterometers), but the most reliable technique seems to be a reflectance meter, in which a flash of light penetrates the skin and a fiberoptic bundle transmits the reflected light to a spectrophotometric module. Quite good correlations between the bilirubin index derived with the device and serum bilirubin measurements have been documented in term babies. How valuable this technique is in preterm infants is less clear. The device can be used to screen babies who should have a serum bilirubin determination. With earlier discharge of term infants and a more relaxed attitude toward moderate increases in bilirubin levels, transcutaneous bilirubinometry has been used less in the past few years.

RADIOLOGIC TECHNIQUES

In addition to routine x-ray examinations of the chest and abdomen, which are the most frequently ordered, other evaluations may be of considerable help. Bone x-ray studies and barium enemas are the most common of the less frequently ordered tests. Intravenous pyelographs are less frequently needed since the introduction of renal ultrasonography, but a voiding cystourethrogram may help to demonstrate outflow obstruction or ureteral reflux. One should remember that while the umbilical artery is patent, assessment of renal lesions may be greatly enhanced and bleeding gastric ulcer may be diagnosed by transumbilical aortography.

MISCELLANEOUS

Ultrasonography (other than cephalic ultrasonography), echocardiography, and radionuclide scans all have a place in neonatology, but space precludes further discussion of these valuable techniques.

Newer techniques are near-infrared spectroscopy and magnetic resonance spectroscopy to evaluate brain metabolism. Pulmonary function testing of the newborn has improved, and several other noninvasive techniques are currently being investigated and will probably be introduced into clinical practice in the next few years.

BIBLIOGRAPHY

Fletcher, M. A., MacDonald, M. G., and Avery, G. B. (eds.): *Atlas of Procedures in Neonatology*. J. B. Lippincott, Philadelphia, 1983.

Monitoring

Grausz, J. P.: Interscapular skin temperatures in the newborn infant. *J. Pediatr.* 1970, 76:752.
Peabody, J. L., Philip, A. G. S., and Lucey, J. F.: "Disorganized breathing"—An important form of apnea and cause of hypoxia (Abstract). *Pediatr. Res.* 1977, 11:540.
Stanger, P., Lister, G., Silverman, N. H., and Hoffman, J. I. E.: Electrocardiograph monitor artifacts in a neonatal intensive care unit. *Pediatrics* 1977, 60:689.
Warburton, D., Stark, A. R., and Taeusch, H. W.: Apnea monitor failure in infants with upper airway obstruction. *Pediatrics* 1977, 60:742.
Committee on Environmental Hazards, American Academy of Pediatrics: Infant radiant warmers. *Pediatrics* 1978, 61:113.
de Swiet, M., Fayers, P., and Shinebourne, E. A.: Systolic blood pressure in a population of infants in the first year of life: The Brompton Study. *Pediatrics* 1980, 65:1028–1035.
Versmold, H. T., Kitterman, J. A., Phibbs, R. H., et al.: Aortic blood pressure during the

first 12 hours of life in infants with birth weight 610 to 4,220 grams. *Pediatrics* 1981, 67:607–613.

Pellegrini-Caliumi, G., Agostino, R., Nodari, S., et al.: Evaluation of an automatic oscillometric method and of various cuffs for the measurement of arterial pressure in the neonate. *Acta Paediatr. Scand.* 1982, 71:791–797.

Darnall, R. A.: Non-invasive monitoring of blood pressure in the neonate. *Clin. Perinatol.* 1985, 12:31–49.

Johnson, K. J., Bhatia, P., and Bell, E. F.: Infrared thermometry of newborn infants. *Pediatrics* 1991, 87:34–38.

Infection Detection

Shaywitz, B. A.: Epidermoid spinal cord tumors and previous lumbar punctures. *J. Pediatr.* 1972, 80:638.

Adler, S. M., and Denton, R. L.: The erythrocyte sedimentation rate in the newborn period. *J. Pediatr.* 1975, 86:942.

Cowett, R. M., Peter, G., Hakanson, D. O., and Oh, W.: Reliability of bacterial culture of blood obtained from an umbilical artery catheter. *J. Pediatr.* 1976, 88:1035.

Vasan, U., Lim, D. M., Greenstein, R. M., and Raye, J. R.: Origin of gastric aspirate polymorphonuclear leukocytes in infants born after prolonged rupture of membranes. *J. Pediatr.* 1977, 91:69.

Manroe, B. L., Weinberger, A. G., Rosenfeld, C. R., and Browne, R.: The neonatal blood count in health and disease: I. Reference values for neutrophilic cells. *J. Pediatr.* 1979, 95:89–98.

Visser, V. E., and Hall, R. T.: Urine culture in the evaluation of suspected neonatal sepsis. *J. Pediatr.* 1979, 94:635–638.

Knudson, R. P., and Alden, E. R.: Neonatal heel-stick blood culture. *Pediatrics* 1980, 65:505–507.

Philip, A. G. S., and Hewitt, J. R.: Early diagnosis of neonatal sepsis. *Pediatrics* 1980, 65:1036.

Visser, V. E., and Hall, R. T.: Lumbar puncture in the evaluation of suspected neonatal sepsis. *J. Pediatr.* 1980, 96:1063–1067.

Weisman, L. E., Merenstein, G. B., and Steenbarger, J. R.: The effect of lumbar puncture position in sick neonates. *Am. J. Dis. Child.* 1983, 137:1077–1079.

Philip, A. G. S.: *Neonatal Sepsis and Meningitis.* G. K. Hall Publishing Company, Boston, 1985.

Neurologic Evaluation

Cheldelin, L. V., Davis, P. C., Jr., and Grant, W. W.: Normal values for transillumination of skull using a new light source. *J. Pediatr.* 1975, 87:937.

Swick, H. M., Cunningham, M. D., and Shields, L. K.: Transillumination of the skull in premature infants. *Pediatrics* 1976, 58:658.

Vyhmeister, N., Schneider, S., and Cha, C.: Cranial transillumination norms of the premature infant. *J. Pediatr.* 1977, 91:980.

Philip, A. G. S.: Non-invasive monitoring of intracranial pressure: A new approach for neonatal clinical pharmacology. *Clin. Perinatol* 1979, 6:123.

Fitzhardings, P. M., Flodmark, O., Fitz, C. R., and Ashby, S.: Prognostic value of computed tomography as an adjunct to assessment of the term infant with postasphyxial encephalopathy. *J. Pediatr.* 1981, 99:777–781.

Dubowitz, L. M. S., and Bydder, G. M.: Nuclear magnetic resonance imaging in the diagnosis and follow-up of neonatal cerebral injury. *Clin. Perinatol.* 1985, 12:243–260.

Byrne, P., Welch, R., Johnson, M. A., et al.: Serial magnetic resonance imaging in neonatal hypoxic-ischemic encephalopathy. *J. Pediatr.* 1990, 117:694–700.

Steinlin, M., Dirr, R., Martin, E., et al.: MRI following severe perinatal asphyxia: Preliminary experience. *Pediatr. Neurol.* 1991, 7:164–170.

Respiratory Evaluation

Jones, R. W. A., Baumer, J. H., Joseph, M. C., and Shinebourne, E. A.: Arterial oxygen tension and response to oxygen breathing in differential diagnosis of congenital heart disease in infancy. *Arch. Dis. Child.* 1976, 51:667.

Wyman, M. L., and Kuhns, L. R.: Accuracy of transillumination in the recognition of pneumothorax and pneumomediastinum in the neonate. *Clin. Pediatr.* 1977, 16:323–324.

Karna, P., and Poland, R. L.: Monitoring critically ill newborn infants with digital capillary blood samples: An alternative. *J. Pediatr.* 1978, 92:270.

Parkinson, C. E., Supramaniam, G., and Harvey, D.: Bubble clicking in pharyngeal aspirates compared with lecithin/sphingomyelin ratio. *Biol. Neonate* 1978, 131:71.

Pearse, R. G.: Percutaneous catheterization of the radial artery in newborn babies using transillumination. *Arch. Dis. Child.* 1978, 53:549.

Prian, G. W., Wright, G. B., Rumack, C. M., and O'Meara, O. P.: Apparent cerebral embolization after temporal artery catheterization. *J. Pediatr.* 1978, 93:115.

Blumenfeld, T. A., Turi, G. K., and Blanc, W. A.: Recommended site and depth of newborn heel skin punctures based on anatomical measurements and histopathology. *Lancet* 1979, i:230–233.

Gottschalk, S. K., and Schuth, C. R.: The use of a penlight as an aid in diagnosing pneumothorax (Note). *Clin. Pediatr.* 1980, 19:725.

Long, J. G., Philip, A. G. S., and Lucey, J. F.: Excessive handling as a cause of hypoxemia. *Pediatrics* 1980, 65:203.

O'Neill, J. A., Jr., and Neblett, W. W., III: Management of major thromboembolic complications of umbilical artery catheters. *J. Pediatr. Surg.* 1981, 16:972–978.

Garg, A. K., Houston, A. B., Laing, J. M., and Mackenzie, J. R.: Positioning of umbilical arterial catheters with ultrasound. *Arch. Dis. Child.* 1983, 58:1017–1018.

Pasnick, M., and Lucey, J. F.: Practical uses of continuous transcutaneous oxygen monitoring. *Pediatr. Rev.* 1983, 5:5–12.

Peabody, J. L., and Emery, J. R.: Non-invasive monitoring of blood gases in the newborn. *Clin. Perinatol.* 1985, 12:147–160.

Hay, W. W., Jr., Thilo, E., and Curlander, J. B.: Pulse oximetry in neonatal medicine. *Clin. Perinatol.* 1991, 18:441–472.

Blanchette, T., Dziodzio, J., and Harris, K.: Pulse oximetry and normoxemia in neonatal intensive care. *Respir. Care* 1991, 36:25–32.

Kempley, S. T., Bennett, S., Loftus, B. G., et al.: Randomized trial of umbilical artery catheter position: Clinical outcome. *Acta Paediatr. Int. J. Paediatr.* 1993, 82:173–176.

Thilo, E. H., Anderson, D., Wasserstein, M. L., Schmidt, J., and Luckey, D.: Saturation by pulse oximetry: Comparison of the results obtained by instruments of different brands. *J. Pediatr.* 1993, 122:620–626.

Stool Evaluation

Book, L. S., Herbst, J. J., and Jung, A. L.: Carbohydrate malabsorption in necrotizing enterocolitis. *Pediatrics* 1976, 57:201.

Desai, N., and Nousia-Arvanitakis, S.: False-negative meconium test results in screening for cystic fibrosis. *J. Pediatr.* 1977, 91:449.

Lacey, J. A., and Whisler, K. E.: Test strip meconium screening for cystic fibrosis. *Am. J. Dis. Child.* 1977, 131:71.

White, R. K., Homer, R., and Pennock, C. A.: Faecal excretion of oligosaccharides and other carbohydrates in normal neonates. *Arch. Dis. Child.* 1978, 53:913.

Bone Marrow Examination

Page, B. M., and Coulter, J. B. S.: Bone marrow aspiration for chromosome analysis in newborn. *B.M.J.* 1978, 1:1455.

Transcutaneous Bilirubinometry

Strange, M., and Cassady, G.: Neonatal transcutaneous bilirubinometry. *Clin. Perinatol.* 1985, 12:51–62.

Schumacher, R. E., Thornberg, J. M., and Gutcher, G. R.: Transcutaneous bilirubinometry: A comparison of old and new methods. *Pediatrics* 1985, 76:10–14.

Radiologic Techniques

Lang, E. K.: Contributions of arteriography in the assessment of renal lesions encountered in the neonatal period and infancy. *Radiology* 1974, 110:429.

Fliegel, C. P., Herzog, B., Signer, E., and Nars, P.: Bleeding gastric ulcer in a newborn infant diagnosed by transumbilical aortography. *J. Pediatr. Surg.* 1977, 12:589.

Miscellaneous

Philip, A. G. S.: Non-invasive diagnostic techniques in newborn infants. *Pediatr. Clin. North Am.* 1982, 29:1275–1298.

Philip, A. G. S. (ed.): Noninvasive neonatal diagnosis. *Clin. Perinatol.* 1985, 12:1–304.

Brans, Y. W. (ed.): Newer technologies and the neonate. *Clin. Perinatol.* 1991, 18:389–651.

36

THERAPEUTIC TECHNIQUES

BLOOD

SIMPLE TRANSFUSION

Newborn infants are given blood when hypovolemia (pathologic or iatrogenic), shock, infection, or anemia producing clinical difficulty occurs. The first three conditions probably require whole blood (or red cells reconstituted with plasma), whereas anemia usually requires packed cells.

The most common reason for whole blood transfusion is replacement of blood taken for sampling. The following guidelines should be adhered to:

1. Keep an accurate record of the volume of all blood samples withdrawn—preferably attached to the incubator or crib.

2. When approximately 10% of blood volume is removed (8 ml in 1-kg infant, 16 ml in 2-kg infant, and so on), replace with packed red blood cells (if this amount is removed within 3 or 4 days).

3. Do not depend on a falling hematocrit value to decide about blood transfusion, because babies frequently hemoconcentrate up to 10% depletion. However, if the hematocrit value is falling, blood volume may be 15% depleted (but intracranial hemorrhage should be considered).

4. Blood pressure should be measured frequently in babies having multiple blood samples withdrawn; if pressure is low (or dropping), packed red blood cells or albumin should be given (see blood pressure chart, Appendix 6).

5. The volume of blood to be given should be the same as the volume withdrawn, with an additional 2 to 5 ml, depending on the size of the baby. Blood transfusions for reasons other than blood sampling should be a maximum of 20 ml/kg of whole blood or 10 to 12 ml/kg of packed cells, except in unusual circumstances, such as continuous, profuse blood loss.

It is also important to remember that blood transfusion is not without risk. In particular, transmission of cytomegalovirus has been associated and may be avoided by screening blood for cytomegalovirus or using frozen (deglycerated) reconstituted red blood cells. Recently, the possibility of transmitting the virus of acquired immunodeficiency syndrome has been of great concern. It is possible to screen donors for the human immunodeficiency virus. Remember also that Jehovah's Witnesses do not accept blood products.

EXCHANGE TRANSFUSION

The major reason for performing exchange transfusion remains blood group (or type) incompatibility, in which there may be three considerations: (1) correction of anemia, (2) removal of sensitized red blood cells, and (3) reduction of hyperbilirubinemia.

Because of the possible toxic effects of high levels of bilirubin on the central nervous system, hyperbilirubinemia remains the main indication for exchange transfusion not associated with hemolytic disease of the newborn. Although evidence to support a more widespread use of exchange transfusion in improving oxygenation or preventing intraventricular hemorrhage was presented a few years ago, this finding has not been confirmed.

Exchange transfusion should be considered in the following situations:

1. With *Rh incompatibility* (or minor group incompatibility), a sensitized mother, and positive Coombs' test result on cord blood:
   a. Initial hemoglobin level of less than 10 g/dl
   b. Rate of rise in bilirubin level of greater than 1 mg/dl/hr (successive determinations 4 hours apart)
   c. Bilirubin level of greater than 10 mg/dl by 12 hours of age
   d. Bilirubin level of greater than 20 mg/dl at any age
2. *ABO incompatibility,* with positive direct or indirect Coombs' test result: indication c (above).
3. *Hyperbilirubinemia* from other causes (if no hemolysis, bilirubin level >25 mg/dl in term infant).
4. *Neonatal sepsis,* especially when associated with sclerema.
5. *Accumulation of toxic agents,* such as hyperammonemia, drug overdose.
6. Symptomatic *high hematocrit syndrome:* use partial exchange (see pp. 242 to 243).

As noted in Chapter 10, bilirubin toxicity is more likely to occur in preterm (premature) infants. Consequently, phototherapy should be used earlier and exchange transfusion considered at lower levels, such as 15 mg/dl, in sick premature infants.

For exchange transfusion technique, see Appendix 2.

OTHER BLOOD PRODUCTS

When bleeding or shock occurs, fresh-frozen plasma or albumin may be substituted for fresh whole blood until the latter is available. Occasionally other fractions, such as platelets, are required (see also Chapter 24, Neonatal Emergencies).

PHLEBOTOMY

Removal of approximately 15 ml/kg of blood with partial albumin or plasma replacement (5 ml/kg) is performed when hyperviscosity (high hematocrit) syndrome is present (see Chapter 20). An alternative is partial exchange transfusion of approximately 40 ml/kg of fresh-frozen plasma. The simplest technique is to proceed as if an exchange transfusion were to be performed. Obviously, if an umbilical artery catheter is in place, it can be used for this purpose.

RESPIRATORY SUPPORT

USE OF OXYGEN AND HEADBOX

Use of Oxygen

1. Environmental oxygen should always be measured by concentration (percent) and not by liter flow (except when nasal cannulae are used).

2. Any baby who develops generalized cyanosis should have the oxygen concentration level increased to a level at which cyanosis is relieved.

3. Whenever oxygen concentration needs to remain over 35 to 40% for several hours, measurement of arterial oxygen tension (PaO_2) is desirable. This is most easily accomplished via an umbilical artery catheter. Transcutaneous pO_2 (or oxygen saturation) measurements can be used, when available, to provide continuous measurements.

4. Attempts should be made in preterm infants to maintain arterial pO_2 levels below 100 mm Hg and preferably between 50 and 70 mm Hg.

5. If capillary samples (arterialized, warmed-heel samples) are used, the pO_2 should be maintained between 35 and 50 mm Hg by adjusting the environmental oxygen concentration.

6. Inspired oxygen concentration should be lowered relatively slowly in a stepwise fashion. The usual maximum increment is 5%, but if PaO_2 is very high, faster reduction may be possible. It may also be possible to reduce the oxygen concentration more quickly when pO_2 is being recorded continuously (by transcutaneous oxygen tension [$tcpO_2$] or an intraarterial device).

7. Stabilization for 10 to 15 minutes after a change is made is sufficient time to allow equilibration (before obtaining blood gases), but continuous recording eliminates this requirement.

8. Frequent clinical observations combined with blood gas determinations determine how slowly or quickly concentrations can be lowered (or raised again).

9. Use of greatly elevated inspired oxygen concentrations should be kept to a minimum by the earlier application of methods to deliver continuous distending airway pressure (with or without the assistance of a ventilator).

Use of Headbox

Because great fluctuations in inspired oxygen concentration may occur in incubators when increased oxygen is required, a headbox (hood) should be used if oxygen concentrations over 30% are required. This rule applies only when the baby is breathing spontaneously in an incubator without any form of respiratory assistance. It becomes mandatory when a baby is in an open bed under the same conditions or when procedures (e.g., lumbar puncture) are being performed with the incubator sides down.

BAG-AND-MASK VENTILATION

Resuscitation can frequently be performed using this method without resorting to endotracheal intubation. Two main types of anesthetic bag are used for this purpose: self inflating and non–self inflating. The former requires a carefully controlled "pop-off" to prevent the use of pressures greater than 30 to 40 cm H_2O. It may also give a false sense of security because the bag refills whether or not an adequate seal of the mask is present. The latter can only be used successfully when an adequate seal at the face has been achieved and is usually effective with a mixture of approximately 5 L/min of air or oxygen flowing into the bag. Adequate ventilation is achieved if the upper part of the chest wall is seen to rise slightly and the baby's color improves.

ENDOTRACHEAL INTUBATION

Endotracheal intubation may be needed in either the delivery room (see Resuscitation in the Delivery Room section under Chapter 2) or the nursery. In an emergency, the principles are the same as those for the delivery room. When an elective procedure is performed, it is best if two people participate, one to intubate and the other to maintain oxygenation. Intermittent bag-and-mask ventilation may maintain oxygenation between attempts (if necessary). Oxygen should be held close to the baby's mouth during intubation. An even better method is to attach a small catheter to the underside of the laryngoscope blade so that oxygen can be attached to the catheter and can be provided at the tip of the laryngoscope blade. Suctioning of the oropharynx should be carried out, if necessary to obtain a clear view, before intubation is attempted. To prevent bradycardia, attempts should be limited to 20 to 30 seconds.

Only straight endotracheal tubes should be used (i.e., no Cole tubes), with an internal diameter of 2.5, 3.0, or 3.5 mm, depending on the size of the baby (roughly 1-, 2-, and 3-kg birthweight). Occasionally, a larger tube is required for a very large baby. The depth to which the endotracheal tube should be inserted may be calculated by measuring the baby's total length in centimeters and dividing by 5. This figure gives the nasotracheal length, and 0.5 cm should be subtracted for an orotracheal tube.

> Example: A baby weighing approximately 2 kg is 43 cm long
> (crown-to-heel measurement)
> Distance to insert nasotracheal tube = 43/5 = 8.5 cm
> Distance to insert orotracheal tube = 8.5 − 0.5 = 8.0 cm
> (An alternative method is described on p. 491).

The tip of the endotracheal tube should now be located halfway between the vocal cords and the carina. Air entry should be equal in both lungs, but the position should be verified by x-ray study. After removal of an endotracheal tube, one should consider the possibility of postextubation atelectasis, which may produce lobar opacification on chest x-ray study. This problem may be minimized by using nasal continuous positive airway pressure (CPAP). The possibility of subglottic stenosis should also be considered with upper airway difficulty after extubation.

NASAL PRONGS AND FACE MASK

It is frequently possible to avoid endotracheal intubation when respiratory failure is imminent. Two methods of ventilation are used to avoid using an endotracheal tube: nasal prongs (or soft nasal cannulae in bigger babies), and face mask (usually hand held). With both these methods, it is possible to apply CPAP and even to assist ventilation with the respirator, although pop-off down the esophagus occurs with nasal prongs when pressures above 20 cm H_2O are used. It is usually necessary to insert an orogastric tube to prevent gastric distension.

The clinician should be sure to insert nasal prongs the right way up. A simple method of stabilizing them is by placing a disposable face mask over the occiput and attaching the ties to the flanges of the prongs (Fig. 36–1). When the soft nasal cannulae are used, they should be inserted far enough that the openings are directed toward the larynx when they are placed in the naso-pharynx.

It has been suggested that nasal prong CPAP increases the work of breathing, but this is clearly not always the case. One study showed that babies

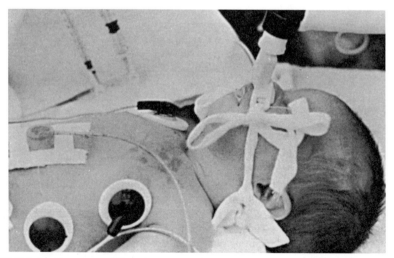

FIGURE 36–1. Continuous positive airway pressure being administered via nasal prongs. There is also a transcutaneous pO_2 electrode in place just above the umbilical artery catheter.

who do not tolerate nasal CPAP had increased levels of lactate within 10 to 15 minutes.

If either inadequate oxygenation (PaO_2 < 40 to 50 mm Hg in 80 to 100% oxygen) or inadequate ventilation (based on progressively increasing pCO_2 to > 60 mm Hg) is noted, endotracheal intubation should be initiated. Insertion of an endotracheal tube under these circumstances is not an emergency, but an elective, procedure.

NASAL CATHETER OR CANNULAE

We have found that a nasal catheter to supply oxygen is useful in the baby who is oxygen dependent. When the inspired oxygen requirement is approximately 30%, a flow of 0.75 to 1.0 L of oxygen per minute can maintain normal pO_2 values. Lower flow rates can be used when the oxygen requirement is lower. Oxygen requirement can be documented with $tcpO_2$ monitoring or pulse oximetry and may allow home management in selected cases. It may also facilitate nursing care and parent-infant interaction while an infant is still in the hospital. More recently, we have used small nasal cannulae, which protrude into the nares from tubing placed across the upper lip. This method eliminates irritation of the naris, which can occur if a catheter is inserted too deeply. Flow rates can be decreased to very low rates by use of special low-flow meters. Most nurseries use flow meters recording down to 0.1 L/min, and some have meters that can record values as low as 0.025 L/min.

ASSISTED VENTILATION

It is not possible to give details of ventilator management in a book of this size, but the reader is referred to Appendix 7 for useful guidelines. Suffice it to say that there are two main types of positive-pressure ventilators: (1) pressure-limited (e.g., BABYbird, Sechrist), and (2) volume-limited (e.g., Bourns). The latter has the advantage of delivering whatever volume is requested but may generate high pressures in doing so. The pressure-limited device is limited in the volume it can deliver.

If the baby is not breathing spontaneously, the machine controls the baby's ventilation. If the baby is breathing spontaneously but rather ineffectively, it may be desirable to have the machine perform a limited number of ventilations every minute, e.g., 10/min. This is referred to as intermittent mandatory ventilation. Frequently, rates as high as 60 to 100/min are used. When a resistance is applied to complete expiration this produces positive end-expiratory pressure. By convention, use of this term is reserved for when the ventilator is assisting the baby. If the baby is breathing entirely spontaneously against a resistance to complete expiration, the baby is said to be on CPAP. Independent devices (see Fig. 36–1) were used initially for this purpose, but modern ventilators allow rapid changes (if necessary) from CPAP to intermittent mandatory ventilation (with or without positive end-expiratory pressure).

In addition to positive-pressure devices, there are negative-pressure ventila-

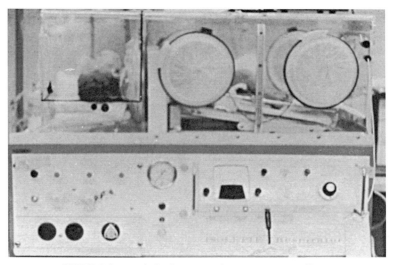

FIGURE 36–2. Larger baby in a negative-pressure ventilator.

tors (Fig. 36–2) that avoid endotracheal intubation, but they may be more difficult to use in the smaller baby (weighing < 1250 g). With newer modifications, some centers have had good success with intermittent negative-pressure (as well as continuous negative-pressure) even in the very small baby, but most centers have little or no experience with this technique.

Positive-pressure ventilators are now considered conventional ventilation, but more recently, several forms of high-frequency ventilation have moved from the research arena to routine clinical use. Initially, there seemed to be little advantage of high-frequency ventilation over conventional ventilation, but different devices and more experience suggest that some babies can be treated with high-frequency ventilation who could not be treated successfully with conventional ventilation. It may prevent the need for extracorporeal membrane oxygenation in some babies with persistent pulmonary hypertension and seems to have been particularly valuable in treating tiny babies with pulmonary interstitial emphysema.

There are several different types of high-frequency ventilation, and some may have advantages over others. The three main types are high-frequency oscillatory ventilation, high-frequency jet ventilation, and high-frequency flow interruption. Evaluation of these devices is ongoing.

EXTRACORPOREAL MEMBRANE OXYGENATION

Extracorporeal membrane oxygenation is available in many regional centers. Details of this technique are beyond the scope of this book, but the principle of extracorporeal membrane oxygenation is that blood is exteriorized from the body and passes through a device that allows the blood to be oxygenated (and carbon dioxide to be removed). Most cases have been performed using the common carotid artery and the internal jugular vein (i.e., arteriovenous access), but some cases have been performed with venovenous access. At most centers, eligibility criteria include a birthweight of 2 kg or more.

The future of extracorporeal membrane oxygenation remains somewhat cloudy at the time of this writing, in view of alternative strategies emerging for persistent pulmonary hypertension.

CHEST PHYSIOTHERAPY

Two techniques are used with appropriate positioning: (1) percussion, which may be performed with a small cup fashioned from the base of a feeding nipple, and (2) vibration, which is most easily accomplished with a battery-operated vibrator. When performed carefully, chest physiotherapy is effective in removing secretions, but one must be aware of the potential for producing severe hypoxemia.

PHOTOTHERAPY

Light with a blue spectrum is effective in breaking down unconjugated bilirubin into nontoxic byproducts as well as changing the structure of bilirubin into photoisomers (photobilirubin), which may be even more important (see also Chapter 10). Phototherapy may be used in the following situations:

1. In premature infants when the bilirubin level is greater than 10 mg/dl
2. In term infants when bilirubin level is greater than 15 mg/dl (or 18 mg/dl without hemolysis)
3. In infants who have undergone exchange transfusion
4. In infants with definite evidence of Rh incompatibility from birth

Immediate use of phototherapy should be considered for any small premature infant (1500 g or less) who has asphyxia, acidosis, hypoglycemia, or severe bruising.

A search for the cause of the hyperbilirubinemia is almost always indicated in the first two situations, but it is not certain what levels of bilirubin are toxic in the absence of hemolytic disease of the newborn. Phototherapy frequently is started in term babies at inappropriately low levels.

Bilirubin should be checked at least once every 24 hours while the infant is receiving phototherapy and within 12 to 24 hours of discontinuation of phototherapy (within 12 hours in cases of blood group incompatibility) because of rebound.

There are many ways of using phototherapy, but we generally use it continuously, except for feeding times. This usually means that phototherapy is given for 16 to 18 hours in the day in term infants (Fig. 36–3). Adequacy of phototherapy irradiance may be measured with a light meter. Damage to the retina is a potential problem, and the eyes should be covered. The eye blinders

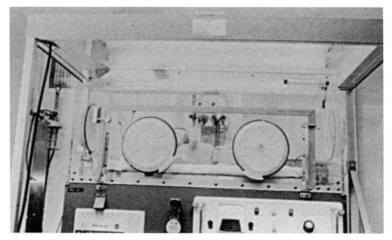

FIGURE 36–3. Phototherapy unit used with the baby in an incubator.

are removed during feeding times, or the eyes are inspected (for infection) at frequent intervals (with the light off) in premature infants on parenteral feeding. Abdominal distension has been seen in some babies receiving phototherapy and has been attributed to occlusion of the eyes.

An alternative method of providing phototherapy eliminates the need to cover the eyes: this is a fiberoptic device that can be wrapped around term babies. It may be necessary in preterm infants to use the device as a mattress because the device is not sufficiently pliable to wrap around smaller babies.

Phototherapy increases water loss from both the skin and the bowel; therefore, fluid intake should be increased by approximately 25 ml/kg/day. Temperature may also become elevated unless care is taken. The increased bowel water loss has been attributed to a temporary deficiency of intestinal lactase or irritation from bile acids in stool.

Phototherapy frequently produces a skin rash resembling erythema toxicum that rapidly subsides when the therapy is stopped. A peculiar skin color (bronze baby) may ensue when phototherapy is used in babies with elevated levels of conjugated bilirubin (see Chapter 25).

CIRCUMCISION

Circumcision was not discussed under routine procedures because it is not considered a routine procedure. Parents should understand that the major advantage is easier hygiene, which may have some relevance in warmer climates. Parents should be provided with enough information, before the baby is born, to make a decision based on facts rather than fancy. The Committee on Fetus and Newborn of the American Academy of Pediatrics has stated that

"... there are no valid medical indications for circumcision in the neonatal period." An Ad Hoc Task Force also considers that "... education leading to continuing good personal hygiene would offer all the advantages of routine circumcision without the attendant surgical risk." More recently, data suggest that urinary tract infections are more common in the first year in uncircumcised male infants, although the incidence (0.24%) is low. This information should be presented to parents to help them make an informed decision. When circumcision is performed, it is done with a Gomco clamp or the Plastibell.

PARACENTESIS

Insertion of a needle into a space may be either diagnostic or therapeutic. Thoracis (chest) is used for emergency treatment of pneumothorax (see Chapter 9). Abdominis (abdomen) may relieve pressure on the diaphragm in massive ascites, such as occurs in severe hemolytic disease of the newborn.

ANTIBIOTICS AND OTHER DRUGS

See Chapter 37.

FLUID ADMINISTRATION

See Chapter 11.

PREVENTING HEAT LOSS

See Chapter 5.

BIBLIOGRAPHY

Blood

Foley, W. J., and McGinn, T. J.: Jehovah's Witnesses and the question of blood transfusion. *Postgrad. Med.* 1973, 53:109.
Shigeoka, A., Hall, R. T., and Hill, H. R.: Blood transfusion in group B streptococcal sepsis. *Lancet* 1978, i:636.
Courtney, S. E., Hall, R. T., and Harris, D. J.: Effect of blood transfusion on mortality in early-onset group-B streptococcal septicemia. *Lancet* 1979, ii:462.
Scanlon, J. W., and Krakaur, R.: Hyperkalemia following exchange transfusion. *J. Pediatr.* 1980, 96:108–110.
Sagi, E., Eyal, F., Armon, Y., et al.: Exchange transfusion in newborns via a peripheral artery and vein. *Eur. J. Pediatr.* 1981, 137:283–284.
Yeager, A. S., Grumet, F. C., Hafleigh, E. B., et al.: Prevention of transfusion acquired cytomegalovirus infections in newborn infants. *J. Pediatr.* 1981, 98:281–287.

Black, V. D., and Lubchenco, L. O.: Neonatal polycythemia and hyperviscosity. *Pediatr. Clin. North Am.* 1982, 29:1137–1148.

Chudwin, D. S., Ammann, A. J., Wara, D. W., et al.: Posttransfusion syndrome. Rash, eosinophilia, and thrombocytopenia following intrauterine and exchange transfusions. *Am. J. Dis. Child.* 1982, 136:612–614.

Adler, S. P., Chandrika, T., Lawrence, L., and Baggett, J.: Cytomegalovirus infections in neonates acquired by blood transfusions. *Pediatr. Infect. Dis.* 1983, 2:114–118.

Blazer, S., Linn, S., Hocherman, I., et al.: Acute increase in serum toxicity following exchange transfusion: Increased risk for the very low birthweight infant during the first 48 hours of life. *Acta Paediatr. Scand.* 1990, 79:1182–1185.

Levy, G. J., Strauss, R. G., Hume, H., et al.: National survey of neonatal transfusion practices: I. Red blood cell therapy. *Pediatrics* 1993, 91:523–529.

Respiratory Support

Coldiron, J. S.: Estimation of nasotracheal tube length in neonates. *Pediatrics* 1968, 41:823.

Wung, J. T., Stark, R. I., Indyk, L., and Driscoll, J. M.: Oxygen supplement during endotracheal intubation of the infant. *Pediatrics* 1977, 59:1046.

Etches, P. C., and Scott, B.: Chest physiotherapy in the newborn: Effect on secretions removed. *Pediatrics* 1978, 62:713.

Finer, N. N., and Boyd, J.: Chest physiotherapy in the neonate: A controlled study. *Pediatrics* 1978, 61:282.

Fox, W. W., Schwartz, J. G., and Shaffer, T. H.: Pulmonary physiotherapy in neonates: Physiologic changes and respiratory management. *J. Pediatr.* 1978, 92:977.

Cats, B. P.: Nasal prongs and work of breathing (Letter). *Pediatrics* 1980, 65:1195–1196.

Johnson, B., Ahlstrom, H., Lindroth, M., and Svenningsen, N. W.: Continuous positive airway pressure: Modes of action in relation to clinical applications. *Pediatr. Clin. North Am.* 1980, 27:687–699.

Ciszek, T. A., Modanlou, H. D., Owings, D., and Nelson, P.: Mean airway pressure— Significance during mechanical ventilation in neonates. *J. Pediatr.* 1981, 99:121–126.

Engelke, S. C., Roloff, D. W., and Kuhns, L. R.: Postextubation nasal continuous positive airway pressure. A prospective controlled study. *Am. J. Dis. Child.* 1982, 136:359–361.

Ratner, I., and Whitfield, J.: Acquired subglottic stenosis in the very-low-birth-weight infant. *Am. J. Dis. Child.* 1983, 137:40–43.

Koops, B. L., Abman, S. H., and Accurso, F. J.: Outpatient management and follow-up of bronchopulmonary dysplasia. *Clin. Perinatol.* 1984, 11:101–122.

Boros, S. J., Bing, D. R., Mammel, M. C., et al.: Using conventional infant ventilators at unconventional rates. *Pediatrics* 1984, 74:487–492.

Preis, O.: A new fiberoptic guide for endotracheal intubation. *Am. J. Dis. Child.* 1984, 138:861–862.

Clark, R. H.: High-frequency ventilation. *J. Pediatr.* 1994, 124:661–670.

Kanto, W. P., Jr.: A decade of experience with neonatal extracorporeal membrane oxygenation. *J. Pediatr.* 1994, 124:335–347.

Walsh-Sukys, M., Stork, E. K., and Martin, R. J.: Neonatal ECMO: Iron lung of the 1990's? *J. Pediatr.* 1994, 124:427–430.

Phototherapy

Dobbs, R. H., and Cremer, R. J.: Phototherapy. *Arch. Dis. Child.* 1975, 50:833.

Bakken, A. F.: Temporary intestinal deficiency in light-treated jaundiced infants. *Acta Paediatr.* 1977, 66:91.

Preis, O., and Rudolph, N.: Abdominal distension in newborn infants on phototherapy— Role of eye occlusion. *J. Pediatr.* 1979, 94:816.

McDonagh, A. F.: Phototherapy: A new twist to bilirubin. *J. Pediatr.* 1981, 99:909–911.

Lewis, H. M., Campbell, R. H. A., and Hambleton, G.: Use or abuse of phototherapy for physiological jaundice of newborn infants. *Lancet* 1982, ii:408–410.

Berant, M., Diamond, E., Brik, R., and Yurman, S.: Phototherapy–associated diarrhea: The role of bile salts. *Acta Paediatr.* 1983, 72:853–855.

Watchko, J. F., and Oski, F. A.: Bilirubin 20 mg/dl = Vigintiphobia. *Pediatrics* 1983, 71:660–663.

Holtrop, P. C., Madison, K., and Maisels, M. J.: A clinical trial of fiberoptic phototherapy vs. conventional therapy. *Am. J. Dis. Child* 1992, 146:235–237.

Holtrop, P. C., Ruedisueli, K., and Maisels, M. J.: Double versus single phototherapy in low birth weight newborns. *Pediatrics* 1992, 90:674–677.

Kjartansson, S., Hammarlund, K., and Sedin, G.: Insensible water loss from the skin during phototherapy in term and preterm infants. *Acta Paediatr. Int. J. Paediatr.* 1992, 81:764–768.

Circumcision

Committee on Fetus and Newborn, American Academy of Pediatrics: Report of the Ad Hoc Task Force on Circumcision. *Pediatrics* 1975, 56:610.

Osborn, L. M., Metcalf, T. J., Mariani, E. M.: Hygienic care in uncircumcised infants. *Pediatrics* 1981, 67:365–367.

Boyce, W. J.: Care of the foreskin. *Pediatr. Rev.* 1983, 5:26–30.

Wiswell, T. E., and Geschke, D. W.: Risks from circumcision during the first month of life compared with those for uncircumcised boys. *Pediatrics* 1989, 83:1011–1015.

37
MINI-PHARMACOPEIA

In routine neonatal care, it is unusual to have to prescribe more than about a dozen drugs. It may be necessary to write specific orders about the use of oxygen and quantities of whole blood (15 to 20 ml/kg) or packed cells (10 ml/kg). Table 37–1 provides information on the most commonly used drugs in most nurseries, and Table 37–2 provides information on the drugs commonly used for neonatal intensive care.

In the first 5 to 7 days, it is usual to administer drugs (usually antibiotics) every 12 hours or twice daily. After 7 days until 2 or 3 weeks, dosage every 8 hours or three times per day is usual, and thereafter, four times per day. Variability in frequency of dosage primarily relates to delayed urinary excretion.

Pharmacokinetic studies are useful to document drug levels in situations where potential toxicity exists (e.g., gentamicin, theophylline).

TABLE 37-1. Drugs Commonly Used (or Available) in Newborn Nurseries

Drug	Route	Dosage		Comment
		First Week	*1–4 Weeks*	
ANTIBIOTICS				
Penicillin (aqueous)	IM/IV For meningitis	50,000 U/kg/day (b.i.d.) 100,000 U/kg/day (b.i.d.)	100,000 U/kg/day (t.i.d.) 150,000–250,000 U/kg/day (t.i.d. or q.i.d.)	May need higher dosage for GBS infection
Ampicillin	IM/IV (oral) For meningitis	50–100 mg/kg/day (b.i.d.) 100–200 mg/kg/day (b.i.d.)	100–150 mg/kg/day (t.i.d.) 200 mg/kg/day (t.i.d.)	Oral route may produce diarrhea; higher dosage for GBS
Cloxacillin/oxacillin	IM/IV (oral)	50 mg/kg/day (b.i.d.)	100–150 mg/kg/day (t.i.d.)	
Methicillin/nafcillin	IM/IV	50 mg/kg/day (b.i.d.)	100–150 mg/kg/day (t.i.d.)	
Carbenicillin	IM/IV	225–300 mg/kg/day (t.i.d. or q.i.d.)	400 mg/kg/day (q.i.d.)	Reserve for *Pseudomonas*
Kanamycin	IM (?IV) < 2000 g > 2000 g	15 mg/kg/day (b.i.d.) 20 mg/kg/day (b.i.d.)	15 mg/kg/day (b.i.d.) 30 mg/kg/day (t.i.d.)	May be given IV over 20 min
Gentamicin	IM (?IV)	5 mg/kg/day (b.i.d.)	7.5 mg/kg/day (t.i.d.)	May be given IV over 20 min; 29–34 w. gest.: 2.5 mg/kg every 18 h $\leq$ 28 w. gest.: 2.5 mg/kg every 24 h
Amikacin	IM/IV	15 mg/kg/day (b.i.d.)	15 mg/kg/day (t.i.d.)	
Chloramphenicol	IM/IV	25 mg/kg/day (daily)	50 mg/kg/day (b.i.d.)	Excessive dosage may result in gray baby syndrome (and possible death)
Neomycin	Oral	100 mg/kg/day (t.i.d. or q.i.d.)	100 mg/kg/day (t.i.d. or q.i.d.)	To sterilize the gut, e.g., in NEC
Cefotaxime	IV	50 mg/kg/day (b.i.d.)	75 mg/kg/day (t.i.d.)	Leukopenia or neutropenia (in adults)
Ceftriaxone	IM/IV	50–75 mg/kg/dose		Frequency varies with gestational age and postnatal age
Ticarcillin/piperacillin	IV	225–300 mg/kg/day (b.i.d. or t.i.d.)	400 mg/kg/day (q.i.d.)	
Vancomycin	IV	20 mg/kg/day (b.i.d.)	30 mg/kg/day (t.i.d.)	Give slowly (1 hour); decrease dose or frequency in infants <1000 g

Drug	Route	Dosage	Comment
FOR METABOLIC PROBLEMS			
Sodium bicarbonate	IV	2 mEq/kg (in emergency) or calculate from base deficit (mEq NaHCO$_3$ = wt (kg) × 0.3 × base deficit)	Give slowly (1 mEq/min): hyperosmolar; give ONLY if ventilation adequate
Calcium gluconate	Oral	1 mEq/kg/feeding	
	IV	100–200 mg/kg t.i.d./q.i.d. or by constant infusion at a dosage of 250 mg/kg/day (or higher, if necessary)	Give slowly: may produce bradycardia if given quickly
Glucose (dextrose)	IV	8 mg/kg/min of 10% solution (possibly to 12 mg/kg/min)	For hypoglycemia producing symptoms
Glucagon	SC/IM	100 μg/kg	For hypoglycemia
Prednisone	Oral	2 mg/kg/day	For refractory hypoglycemia
Pyridoxine (vitamin B$_6$)	Oral therapy	2–5 mg/day	Used in conjunction with electroencephalography
	IV (test for dependency)	50 mg	
Naloxone (Narcan)	IM/IV	0.1–0.2 mg/kg (0.25–0.5 ml/kg)	For narcotic depression; duration of action is short (< hr)
CARDIORESPIRATORY DRUGS			
Aminophylline (see Theophylline)			
Chlorothiazide (Diuril)	Oral	10–20 mg/kg/day (b.i.d.)	May cause electrolyte problems
Dexamethasone	IM/IV	0.5–1.0 mg/kg/day (b.i.d.)	For bronchopulmonary dysplasia; gradual reduction if used for more than 4 days
Digoxin	IM/IV	0.03–0.05 mg/kg ½ immediately ¼ 6–8 hr later ¼ further 6–8 hr later	May need further doses to digitalize completely; monitor serum concentrations (may get toxicity > 2 μg/ml, more likely > 4 μg/ml)
	Oral	Maintain with ¼–⅕ of digitalizing dose (b.i.d.) Alternative is to use 0.016 mg/kg/day as maintenance dosage from the start	Watch for falsely elevated levels (immunoreactivity)

Table continued on following page

399

TABLE 37-1. Drugs Commonly Used (or Available) in Newborn Nurseries (Continued)

Drug	Route	Dosage	Comment
Furosemide (Lasix)	IM/IV	1 mg/kg/dose	Action within 1 hr; duration 6 hr
Spironolactone (Aldactone)	Oral	0.5–1.0 mg/kg/day (t.i.d.)	May produce hyperkalemia (use with chlorothiazide)
Theophylline	IV	5 mg/kg/dose × 2,12 hr apart, then 2 mg/kg/day (b.i.d.)	Variable half-life; monitor serum levels (therapeutic range 8–15 µg/ml); for aminophylline dose, multiply by 1.25
ANTICONVULSANTS			
Phenobarbital	IM/IV (oral)	20 mg/kg (load); 3–5 mg/kg/day (maintenance)	Divide loading dose if baby not on assisted ventilation
Phenytoin (Dilantin)	IV	10–20 mg/kg (load)	Give slowly with saline flushes. Difficult to achieve adequate levels with oral administration
Diazepam (Valium)	IM/IV	0.3–0.5 mg/kg	May also be used rectally; adequate serum levels achieved within 5 min with 0.5–1.0 mg/kg. For IV use, dilute and give slowly. May produce respiratory depression, and benzoate competes with bilirubin for albumin binding.
Paraldehyde	Rectal	0.3 ml/kg 10% solution; 1 part to 9 parts mineral oil q 1h, up to 6 doses	For refractory seizures. Use glass syringe and rubber rectal tube
Dexamethasone (Decadron)	IM/IV	0.5–1.0 mg/kg t.i.d. or q.i.d.	May be helpful in cases of cerebral edema
Paregoric	Oral	1–3 drops/kg q.i.d.	For narcotic withdrawal

SEDATIVES/ANALGESICS

Chloral hydrate	Oral-rectal	50–100 mg/kg	For sedation; extreme caution needed for repeat doses
Morphine sulfate	IV	0.1 mg/kg q 4–6h	For pain

TOPICAL APPLICATIONS

Nystatin	Oral	100,000 U q.i.d.	For thrush
	Cream	2% q.i.d.	For monilial diaper rash
Bacitracin	Ointment	t.i.d.	
Silver nitrate	Ophthalmic solution	1–2 drops of 1%	Delay up to 1 hr after birth
Erythromycin	Ophthalmic ointment	0.5%	Delay up to 1 hr after birth
Cyclopentolate			
0.5% Neosynephrine	Ophthalmic solutions	1–2 drops, 1%	For retinal examination
0.5% Mydriacil		1 drop of each	For retinal examination

SUPPLEMENTS

Iron (Fer-in-Sol)	Oral	2–4 mg/kg elemental iron/day	In premature infants after 4–6 weeks
Vitamins	Oral	0.3 ml/day of solution containing vita-mins A, C, D, and E	For premature infants *before* iron therapy, probably within 1 week of birth
Folic acid	Oral	25 µg (0.3 ml)/day	For premature infants

b.i.d. = twice a day; GBS = group B streptococcal; IM = intramusculary; IV = intravenously; NaHCO₃ = sodium bicarbonate; NEC = necrotizing enterocolitis; q.i.d. = four times a day; t.i.d. = three times a day; SC = subcutaneous.

TABLE 37-2. Some Drugs Used in Neonatal Intensive Care

Drug	Dosage	Indication
Acyclovir	10 mg/kg/dose t.i.d by I.V. infusion over 1h	Herpes simplex infection
Adenosine	50 µg/kg rapid I.V. push Flush with saline	Paroxysmal SVT
Atropine	0.01–0.03 mg/kg/dose	Bradycardia; AV block
Dopamine	2–5 µg/kg/min to start; frequently need 10 µg/kg/min or more	Shock; hypotension
Epinephrine (1:10,000 solution)	0.25 ml for < 1500 g 0.50 ml for 1500–2500 g 1.0 ml for > 2500 g	During cardiopulmonary resuscitation (via ET tube)
Fentanyl	1 to 4 µg/kg IV	For sedation/analgesia
Hyaluronidase	1 ml SC/intradermal as 5 separate 0.2 ml around periphery	Extravasation of IV infusion *except* pressor agents
Hydralazine	0.15 mg/kg q 4h IM/IV	Hypertension
Indomethacin	0.2 mg/kg oral/IV, repeat 12 and 24 hr later	For closure of PDA (caution required)
Insulin	0.01–0.1 U/kg/hr	Hyperglycemia, despite decrease in glucose load
Pancuronium bromide (Pavulon)	0.1 mg/kg IV push	For paralysis on assisted ventilation
Phentolamine (Regitine)	1 ml SC around affected area	Extravasation of pressor agents (eg. dopamine)
Propranolol (Inderal)	0.5–2.0 mg/kg/day divided t.i.d. or q.i.d.	Hypertension (not with congestive heart failure)
Prostanglandin E₁ (Prostin)	Initial dose, 0.05 µg/kg/min down to 0.01 µg/kg/min IV infusion	For ductus-dependent cyanotic congenital heart disease
Tolazoline (Priscoline)	1 mg/kg IV bolus 1 mg/kg/hr IV infusion	Persistent pulmonary hypertension
Defibrillation	2 Wsec/kg up to 10 Wsec/kg	Ventricular fibrillation

AV = atrioventricular; ET = endotracheal; IM = intramuscularly; IV = intravenously; PDA = patent ductus arteriosus; SC = subcutaneous.

BIBLIOGRAPHY

Aranda, J. V., Cohen, S., and Neims, A. H.: Drug utilization in a newborn intensive care unit. *J. Pediatr.* 1976, 89:315.

Langslet, A., Meberg, A., Bredesen, J. E., and Lunde, P. K. M.: Plasma concentrations of diazepam and N-desmethyldiazepam in newborn infants after intravenous, intramuscular, rectal and oral administration. *Acta Paediatr. Scand.* 1978, 67:699.

Painter, M. J., Pippenger, C., MacDonald, H., and Pitlick, W.: Phenobarbital and diphenylhydantoin levels in neonates with seizures. *J. Pediatr.* 1978, 92:315.

Mulhall, A., DeLouvois, J., and Hurley, R.: Chloramphenicol toxicity in neonates: Its incidence and prevention. *B.M.J.* 1983, 287:1424–1427.

Pudek, M. R., Seccombe, D. W., and Whitfield, M. F.: Digoxin-like immunoreactivity in premature and full-term infants not receiving digoxin therapy. *N. Engl. J. Med.* 1983, 308:904–905.

Editorial: Neonatal paralysis. *Lancet* 1984, i:831–832.

Lindemann, R.: Resuscitation of the newborn: Endotracheal administration of epinephrine. *Acta Paediatr. Scand.* 1984, 73:210–212.

Hallidie-Smith, K. A.: Prostaglandin E_1 in suspected ductus dependent cardiac malformation. *Arch. Dis. Child.* 1984, 59:1020–1026.

Alpert, G., Campos, J. M., Harris, M. C., et al.: Vancomycin dosage in pediatrics reconsidered. *Am. J. Dis. Child.* 1984, 138:20–22.

Kasik, J. W., Jenkins, S., Leuschen, M. P., and Nelson, R. M., Jr.: Post-conceptional age and gentamicin elimination half-life. *J. Pediatr.* 1985, 106:502–505.

Padbury, J. F., Agata, Y., Baylen, B. G., et al.: Pharmacokinetics of dopamine in critically ill newborn infants. *J. Pediatr.* 1990, 117:472–476.

Bhatt, D. R., Reber, D. J., Wirtschafter, D. D., et al.: *Neonatal Drug Formulary,* 3rd ed. Neonatal Drug Formulary, Los Angeles, 1993.

Young, T. E., and Mangum, O. B.: *Neofax '93: A Manual of Drugs Used in Neonatal Care,* 6th ed. Ross Laboratories, Columbus, Ohio, 1993.

Quizzes

38

PICTORIAL QUIZ

The following cases are examples of relatively uncommon disorders, most of which fit into the "once seen, never forgotten" category. They should be considered as an integral part of this book rather than an interesting afterthought. For other, more extensive case discussions, please see Philip, A. G. S.: *Neonatology Case Studies: A Compilation of 75 Clinical Studies.* Medical Examination Publishing Co., Inc., Garden City, NY, 1982.

CASE 1

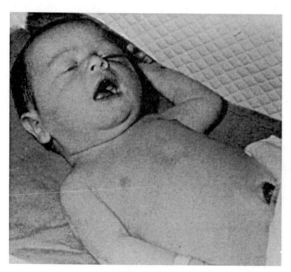

FIGURE 38–1

1. What abnormality is being shown here?
2. What is the differential diagnosis?

CASE 2

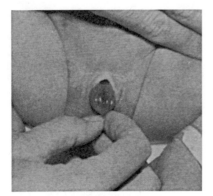

FIGURE 38–2

1. What is being demonstrated? (Look *very* carefully!)
2. How is this presumed to arise?

CASE 3

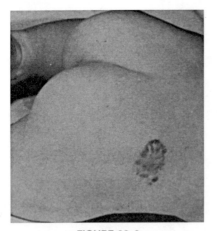

FIGURE 38–3

1. What is this lesion?
2. What is the natural history?

CASE 4: This baby is 7 days old.

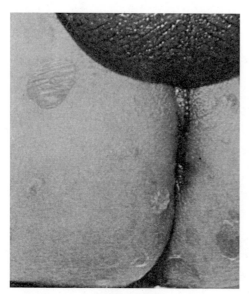

FIGURE 38–4

1. What is being demonstrated?
2. What is the etiology?
3. How would you treat this?

CASE 5: At birth, this baby showed the findings demonstrated.

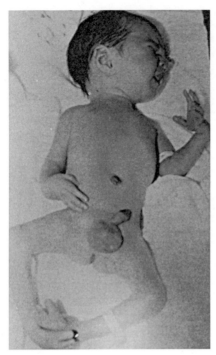

FIGURE 38–5

1. What is the diagnosis?
2. Another diagnosis is sometimes linked closely to it. What is it?
3. What is the presumed etiology of this diagnosis?
4. What comment may be elicited from the mother about her pregnancy?

CASE 6

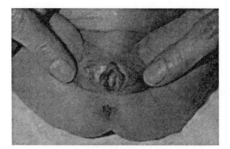

FIGURE 38–6

1. What is being demonstrated?
2. What should be done about it?
3. If unrecognized in the neonatal period, how may this present later?

CASE 7

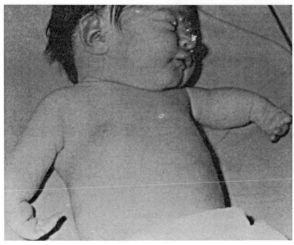

FIGURE 38–7

1. How is this abnormality categorized (designated)?
2. What is the possible etiology, and when did it occur?
3. What other abnormalities might be associated?

CASE 8

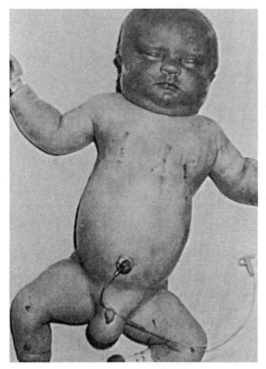

FIGURE 38–8

1. What happened here? Diagnosis, please.
2. Trace a probable course of events that would culminate in this diagnosis.

CASE 9

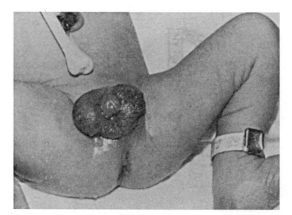

FIGURE 38–9

1. Describe the abnormality in this small for gestational age baby.
2. What should be considered in the differential diagnosis?
3. How would you arrive at a definitive diagnosis?

CASE 10

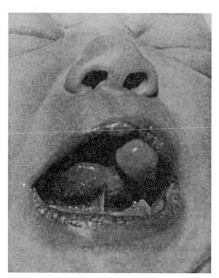

FIGURE 38–10

1. What is this?
2. With what might it be confused?
3. How would you manage it?

CASE 11

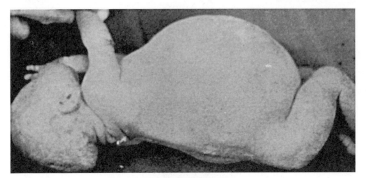

FIGURE 38–11

1. What abnormalities are present?
2. What are the major differential diagnoses?

CASE 12: This baby is female.

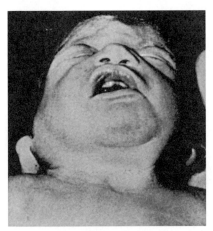

FIGURE 38–12

1. What is being demonstrated?
2. What is your diagnosis (plus any alternative)?
3. How would you confirm this?

CASE 13

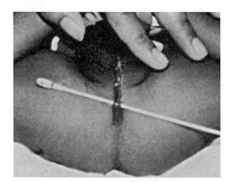

FIGURE 38–13

1. What is being demonstrated?
2. What other abnormalities might be associated?

CASE 14: This baby was 3 days old when this picture was taken.

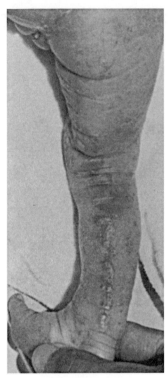

FIGURE 38–14

1. Describe the lesion.
2. What is the most likely diagnosis?
3. Suggest any other possible diagnosis.

CASE 15: Same baby, day 1 *(A)* and day 5 *(B)*.

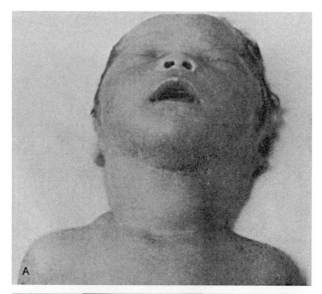

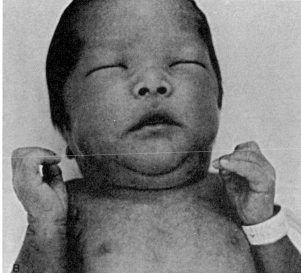

FIGURE 38–15

1. What condition is being demonstrated?
2. What problems may arise?
3. What is the most likely precipitating factor?

CASE 16

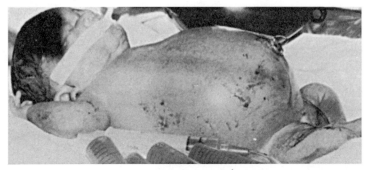

FIGURE 38–16

1. What is being demonstrated?
2. What is the most likely diagnosis?
3. What other possible diagnoses are there?

CASE 17

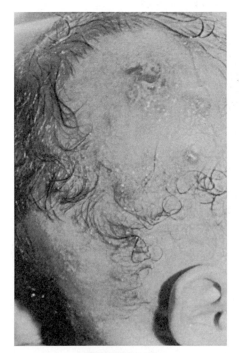

FIGURE 38–17

1. What are these lesions?
2. What is the probable etiology?
3. How might this have been prevented?

CASE 18

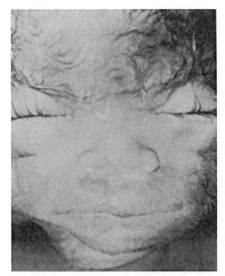

FIGURE 38–18

1. What is your diagnosis?
2. What is the alternative name for this condition and what is known of its etiology?

CASE 19

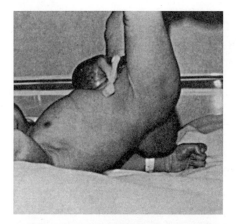

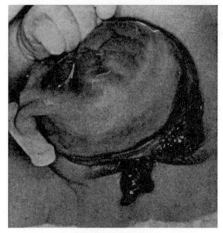

FIGURE 38–19

1. What abnormalities are demonstrated?
2. What does this add up to (total picture)?

CASE 20

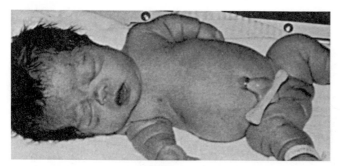

FIGURE 38–20

1. What is your diagnosis?
2. What is the mode of inheritance?
3. How is the diagnosis established (supported) clinically?

CASE 21

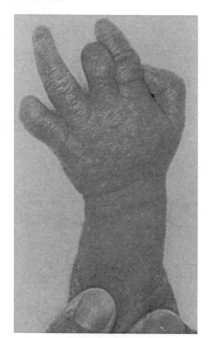

FIGURE 38–21

1. What abnormality is represented?
2. How does this arise?
3. What other name has been applied?

CASE 22

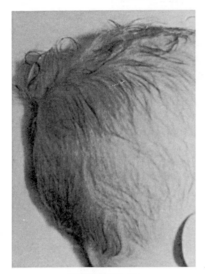

FIGURE 38–22

1. What is this?
2. What broad category does this fit into?
3. What alternative diagnoses are there?

CASE 23

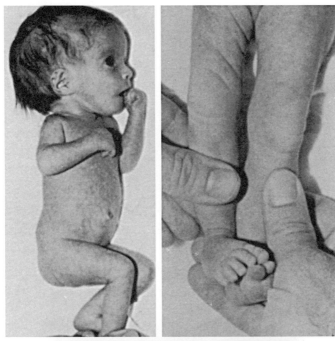

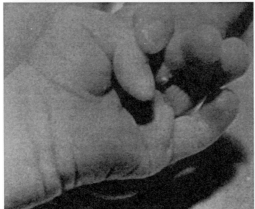

FIGURE 38–23

1. What abnormalities may be noted?
2. What syndrome does this add up to?

CASE 24

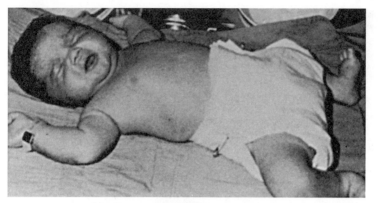

FIGURE 38–24

1. How might this baby be classified?
2. What problems could be anticipated?

CASE 25

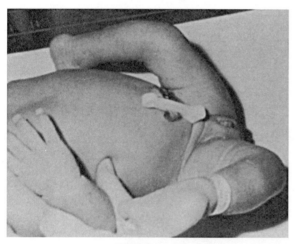

FIGURE 38–25

1. What descriptive term has been applied to this abnormality?
2. What might produce it?
3. How may it be treated?

CASE 26

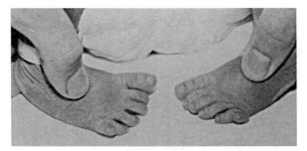

FIGURE 38–26

1. What abnormality is demonstrated?
2. In what group is it more common?
3. With what may this be associated?

CASE 27

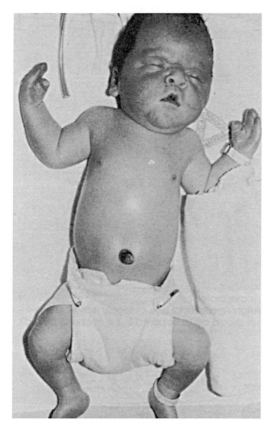

FIGURE 38–27

1. What features are apparent?
2. What name is attached?

CASE 28

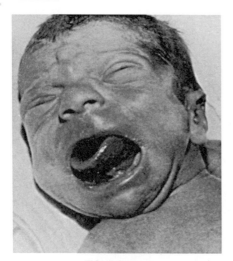

FIGURE 38–28

1. What abnormal feature is shown?
2. What name is associated?
3. What birth weight–gestational age category is most likely?
4. What problem should be anticipated in the neonatal period?

CASE 29

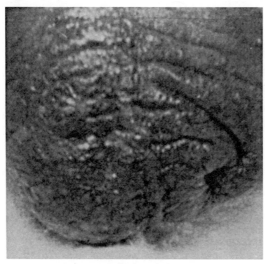

FIGURE 38–29

1. What may be wrong here?
2. What should be done about it?

CASE 30

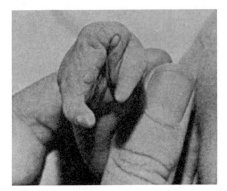

FIGURE 38–30

1. Describe the appearance of this baby's hand.
2. What is the descriptive diagnosis?
3. What is the probable etiology?

CASE 31

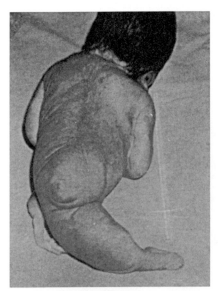

FIGURE 38–31

1. What is this abnormality?
2. What other name might be used?
3. How might it have arisen?

CASE 32

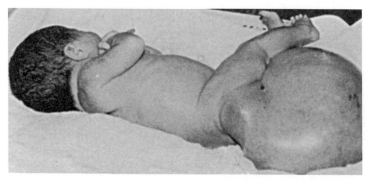

FIGURE 38–32

1. What is this rare disorder?
2. What should be done about it?

CASE 33

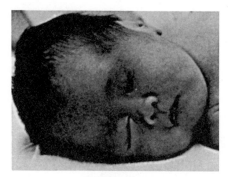

FIGURE 38–33

1. What abnormality is demonstrated?
2. What factors may play a role in its etiology?

CASE 34

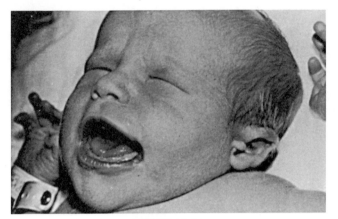

FIGURE 38–34

1. What abnormalities are visible?
2. What problem should one anticipate in the first month of life?
3. Who should be consulted?

CASE 35: This baby had laxness of the abdominal musculature in addition to the limb defect.

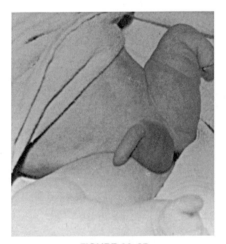

FIGURE 38–35

1. Describe the abnormality.
2. What might the etiology be?

CASE 36

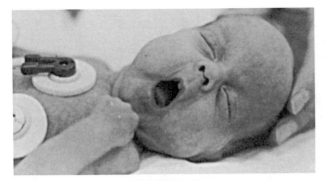

FIGURE 38–36

1. What is wrong here?
2. How do you think this might have arisen?

CASE 37

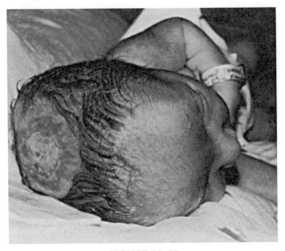

FIGURE 38–37

1. What is this abnormality?
2. With what chromosomal anomaly is it associated?

CASE 38: The spots found on this baby had a bluish-purple appearance and were slightly raised.

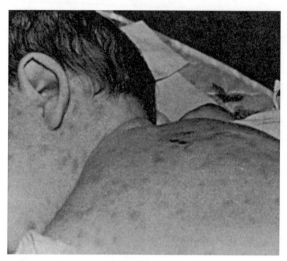

FIGURE 38–38

1. What do you think the dark spots over the upper back are?
2. What is the probable diagnosis?
3. How might this be confirmed?
4. What possible treatment is available?

CASE 39

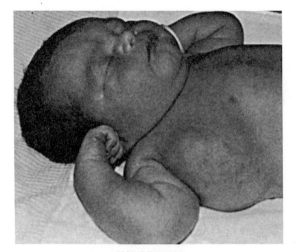

FIGURE 38–39

1. What is this?
2. Is it usually found in this location?
3. With what might it be confused?
4. How might one simply differentiate the two?

CASE 40

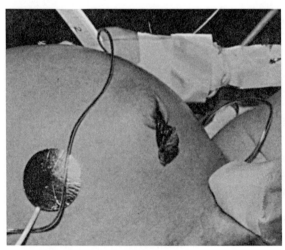

FIGURE 38–40

1. What is being demonstrated?
2. What are the most likely diagnoses?
3. What tests could be helpful in differentiating these diagnoses?

CASE 41: This baby is being treated for respiratory difficulty under a radiant warmer.

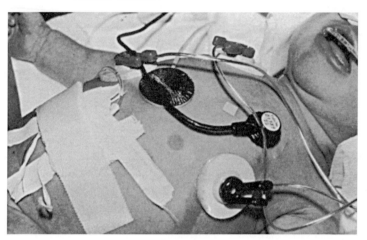

FIGURE 38–41

1. What is the spot close to the xiphoid?
2. Will more of these spots appear?
3. How long do you estimate it will be until the spot fades?

CASE 42

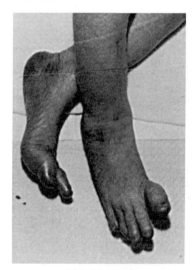

FIGURE 38–42

1. What is being demonstrated?
2. What is the most likely associated diagnosis?
3. What is the prevalence of this diagnosis and its sex ratio?

CASE 43

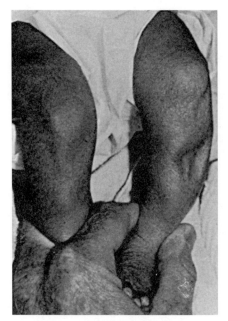

FIGURE 38–43

1. What is being demonstrated?
2. In the absence of heart disease, what are the most likely diagnoses?

CASE 44

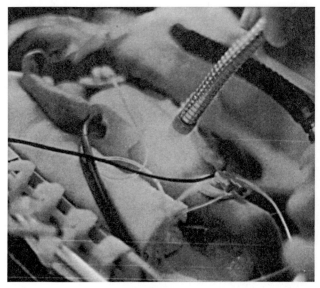

FIGURE 38–44

1. What is being demonstrated?
2. How might this arise *in this baby?*
3. What should be done about it?

CASE 45: The skin was very erythematous in the affected areas in this 1-day-old baby.

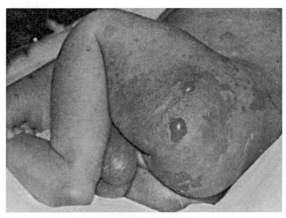

FIGURE 38–45

1. What is your diagnosis?
2. What alternative diagnosis might be considered?
3. What other information might clarify the diagnosis?

CASE 46: This x-ray was taken at 12 hours of age.

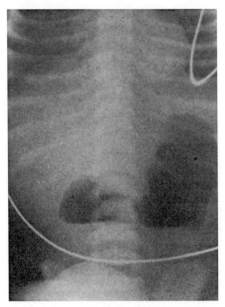

FIGURE 38–46

1. What is being shown?
2. What diagnosis is indicated?
3. With what other condition may this be associated?

CASE 47

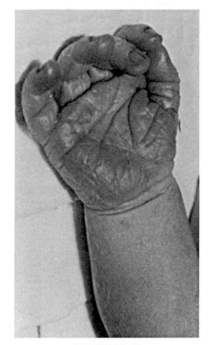

FIGURE 38–47

1. Describe what you see.
2. What can be inferred from these findings?

CASE 48: This term baby was approximately 10 days old at the time this photograph was taken.

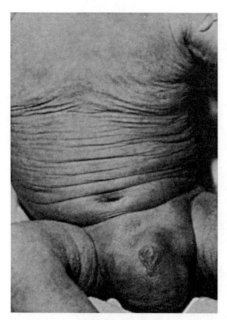

FIGURE 38–48

1. What abnormalities are visible?
2. If a skin biopsy were performed, what would it be likely to show?
3. Can you suggest any associated abnormalities?

CASE 49: Obviously these photographs (*top, bottom*) were obtained post mortem.

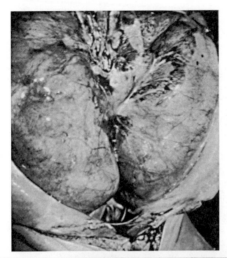

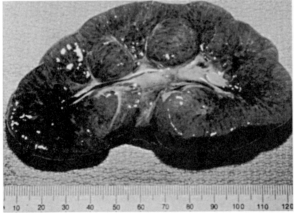

FIGURE 38–49

1. Why do you think the baby died?
2. What is the abnormality demonstrated?
3. What is the mode of inheritance?

CASE 50: This finding was noted immediately after birth.

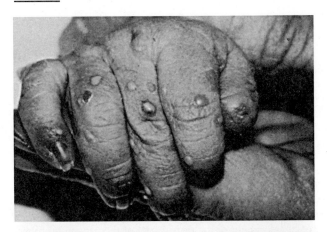

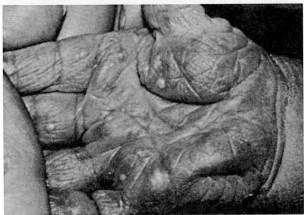

FIGURE 38–50

1. What is this disorder?
2. What other possibilities should come to mind if this had been noted first at 5 days after birth?
3. What is the treatment?

ANSWERS

Case 1

1. In a term baby who is lying quietly, the right arm is lying in extension while the left arm is obviously flexed.
2. The most likely diagnoses are:
   a. Right Erb's palsy (right brachial nerve palsy)
   b. Right fractured clavicle
   Both may result from traumatic delivery.

Case 2

1. This is a male infant with complete epispadias (the identity band says "boy" on it).
2. This rare abnormality reveals the urethral orifice or groove on top of the penis. It is probably the result of failure of infraumbilical mesoderm, with resultant deficiency of development of the dorsal part of the urogenital tubercle.

Case 3

1. This is a strawberry hemangioma (raised capillary nevus).
2. It usually resolves spontaneously over several months. Intervention is only rarely necessary, usually for rapid growth that compromises surrounding structures.

Case 4

1. These are scattered lesions of bullous impetigo.
2. They are staphylococcal in origin and are related to certain phage types, e.g., type 71.
3. Treatment is usually with systemic antibiotic, e.g., methicillin, cloxacillin, depending on culture and sensitivities.

Case 5

1. Arthrogryposis multiplex congenita (amyoplasia congenita)
2. Werdnig-Hoffmann disease (progressive spinal muscular atrophy)
3. A variety of adverse prenatal situations, usually involving neuromuscular disorders or imbalance
4. Mother may have noticed lack of fetal movement.

Case 6

1. Imperforate hymen, leading to hydrocolpos (hydrometrocolpos)
2. Surgical consultation (urologic or gynecologic) should be obtained and the obstruction to outflow relieved.
3. Most commonly this will present as primary amenorrhea, with a suprapubic mass and abdominal pain at puberty. Rarely, a cystic swelling may produce urologic symptoms due to obstruction of the ureters, producing hydroureter and hydronephrosis.

Case 7

1. Confusion reigns, but this is usually designated as bilateral hemimelia (NOT phocomelia). The use of the term *distal phocomelia* may be acceptable.
2. This is NOT the classic thalidomide embryopathy (phocomelia IS: hands originating close to the shoulder). Maternal riboflavin deficiency has also been implicated. The effect is determined before 45 days of gestation.
3. a. Thrombocytopenia
   b. Anomalies of the VATER association (vertebral, anal, tracheoesophageal fistula, renal)

Case 8

1. Subcutaneous emphysema, which was probably secondary to a traumatic intubation and communication of subcutaneous space with trachea
2. More likely to have meconium aspiration syndrome, with pneumothorax with or without pneumomediastinum and eventual decompression into the neck, etc.

Case 9

1. There appears to be an incomplete phallus separating two scrotal masses, which appear to contain gonads (i.e., ambiguous genitalia).
2. a. This may be (and was) a male with hypospadias and small phallus.
   b. Could be virilized female, with either edema of labia or scrotal ovaries (adrenogenital syndrome or secondary to progestogens).
   c. True hermaphroditism
3. a. Careful physical examination (testes in scrotum)
   b. Buccal smear (early interpretation is questionable)
   c. Chromosomal analysis
   d. Serum electrolytes
   e. Urine for excretion of 17-ketosteroids and pregnanetriol
   f. Biopsy of gonad, etc.

Case 10

1. Congenital epulis
2. Epignathus or hemangioma
3. Surgical excision

Case 11

1. Abdominal distention; microcephaly; purpura with or without petechiae
2. a. Cytomegalovirus infection (which this was)
   b. Toxoplasmosis
   c. Other viral infection
   d. Hydrops fetalis (for any reason)
   e. Ascites secondary to urinary tract abnormality, with teratogen affecting brain growth, etc.
   f. Meconium peritonitis, with microcephaly, etc.

Case 12

1. Webbing of the neck (and there was edema of the feet)
2. Turner's syndrome seems most likely but it was NOT. Baby had congestive cardiac failure, secondary to truncus arteriosus, and had webbing of the neck INCIDENTALLY.
3. Turner's is confirmed by XO constitution on chromosomal analysis (buccal smear *may* help). Cardiac problem confirmed via cardiac catheterization.

Case 13

1. Imperforate anus, with congenital band extending to the scrotum
2. May be part of the VATER association, includes vertebral, radial, and renal anomalies as well as tracheoesophageal fistula.

Case 14

1. There is a jagged linear lesion over the extensor surface of the right leg, which is pigmented and slightly vesicular.
2. Mastocytosis (urticaria pigmentosa/incontinentia pigmenti)
3. Somewhat similar lesions have been described in a few cases of varicella-zoster infection in the newborn.

Case 15

1. Neonatal (congenital) goiter
2. May be associated with upper airway obstruction (requiring endotracheal tube for relief); may have associated hypothyroidism or hyperthyroidism, but usually euthyroid.
3. Maternal ingestion of antithyroid medication or iodides (in cough/asthma preparations)

Case 16

1. Ascites (and ascitic fluid in syringes), plus edema of face, etc., with endotracheal tube in place
2. Hydrops fetalis—secondary to Rh incompatibility
3. Hydrops may also be due to:
   a. α-Thalassemia
   b. Kell incompatibility
   c. Congenital syphilis
   d. Obstructive uropathy, etc.

Case 17

1. Vesicobullous lesions of the scalp
2. This is due to herpes simplex (herpesvirus hominis)
3. Delivery by cesarean section *may* prevent infection of the neonate.

Case 18

1. Cornelia de Lange syndrome
2. Typus degenerativus amstelodamensis. The etiology is uncertain—it is probably gene mutation, but subtle chromosomal abnormality is possible.

Case 19

1. a. Omphalocele (exomphalos)
   b. Exstrophy of bladder
   c. Imperforate anus
   d. Hydromyelia (lumbosacral spina bifida)
2. Exstrophy of the cloaca

Case 20

1. Achondroplasia
2. Autosomal-dominant, about 90% fresh mutations
3. Apart from the facial features and short upper segment of the limbs, the upper:lower body segment ratio is usually >2:1.

Case 21

1. Congenital amputation
2. This seems to be the result of congenital constriction (amniotic) bands.
3. Streeter's dysplasia

Case 22

1. Occipital encephalocele
2. Neural tube defects
3. Hemangioma, lipoma, hematoma; but these are unlikely in this location

Case 23

1. Hemihypertrophy (or hemiatrophy) in an infant who appears to have intra-uterine growth retardation, with a large head and small body, with incurved little finger
2. Russell-Silver dwarf (syndrome)

Case 24

1. Large for gestational age, or infant of diabetic mother
2. Hypoglycemia, hypocalcemia, hyperbilirubinemia, and possibly respiratory distress syndrome

Case 25

1. Genu recurvatum
2. A cramped intrauterine environment, resulting in "dislocation" at the knee
3. Correction of position and simple splint (in slight flexion)

Case 26

1. Polydactyly
2. Greatly increased frequency in the black population
3. Several syndromes (Ellis-van Creveld, Carpenter's, trisomy 13, etc.)

Case 27

1. Syndactyly and unusually shaped head (acrocephaly)
2. Apert's syndrome

Case 28

1. Macroglossia
2. Beckwith's syndrome
3. Large for gestational age
4. Hypoglycemia

Case 29

1. There is puckering of the scrotum, suggesting pathology.
2. Surgery is required and, in this baby, revealed bilateral testicular torsion (Fig. 38–51).

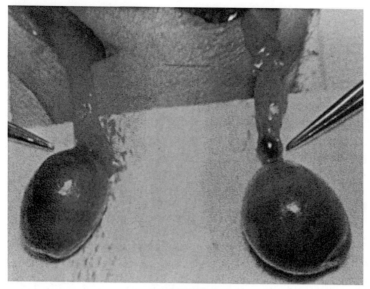

FIGURE 38–51

Case 30

1. There are apparently only two digits (one of which looks like a thumb) and a rudimentary digit between.
2. Lobster-claw hand
3. This is most likely familial and therefore genetic in origin. It may be associated with ectodermal dysplasia.

Case 31

1. Sirenomelia (severe caudal axis deficit)
2. Mermaid syndrome
3. Presumably the consequence of a wedge-shaped early deficit of the posterior axis mesoderm during the third week. No specific cause is known.

Case 32

1. Sacrococcygeal teratoma (cystic)
2. It should be surgically removed, and if all tissue can be excised the long-term outlook is good.

Case 33

1. Microphthalmia (left eye)
2. Radiation has been most frequently incriminated, but genetic and viral factors should be considered.

Case 34

1. Macrostomia; abnormally shaped ear with preauricular appendage (there was also a thoracic deformity).
2. Deafness
3. A plastic surgeon

Case 35

1. The lower part of the left leg is absent. The stump attached to the femur has an apparent constriction ring but has a small appendage.
2. The appendage suggests that this is not the result of an amniotic band. A drug etiology is possible—oral contraceptives have been implicated (and antiemetics suggested).

Case 36

1. There is a furrow of the nasal septum.
2. This baby was extremely premature and had relatively prolonged therapy with CPAP by nasal prongs, which produced a pressure necrosis (the long-term result was good).

Case 37

1. This is a huge scalp defect.
2. Trisomy 13 (as in this baby)

Case 38

1. These were produced by skin biopsy of two nodules.
2. Congenital leukemia (myelogenous)—the presence of nodules of this color in a pale baby is almost pathognomonic.
3. CBC, skin biopsy, and bone marrow
4. Vincristine and prednisone, but therapy is not usually very successful.

Case 39

1. This is a cystic hygroma.
2. The majority are found involving the face and neck, but approximately 10 to 20% are in this location.
3. It could be confused with a large (cavernous) hemangioma (see Fig. 30–6) or possibly a hamartoma.
4. This cystic mass transilluminated widely.

Case 40

1. Marked abdominal distention
2. One can estimate that this is a term infant, so Hirschsprung's disease, meconium plug syndrome, meconium ileus/peritonitis, or volvulus is perhaps most likely (see also pp. 312 to 313).
3. Abdominal x-ray, barium (Gastrografin) enema, anorectal manometry

Case 41

1. The circular erythematous spot is the result of heating the skin under the transcutaneous pO_2 electrode (over the upper chest).
2. Undoubtedly—the electrode is moved every 3 to 4 hours.
3. 24 hours (approximately)

Case 42

1. Bilateral short hallux
2. Trisomy 18
3. 1:3000 with a 3:1 preponderance of females to males

Case 43

1. Marked pitting edema
2. Milroy's disease (congenital lymphedema); Turner's syndrome; blockage of venous (or lymphatic) return; possibly fluid overload

Case 44

1. Pneumoperitoneum is being demonstrated by transillumination.
2. This was associated with a right-sided pneumothorax (notice the chest tubes) and was not due to a perforated viscus.
3. Conservative management (i.e., surgery is not indicated)

Case 45

1. Epidermolysis bullosa (probably nonscarring)
2. Toxic epidermal necrolysis or staphylococcal scalded skin syndrome (S_4); bullous congenital ichthyosiform erythroderma
3. Family history (mother had similar problem as a baby, with easy peeling later); day of onset makes staphylococcal etiology unlikely; culture; skin biopsy

Case 46

1. A double-bubble sign, with a gastric and duodenal bubble
2. Duodenal atresia
3. Down's syndrome

Case 47

1. This baby's right hand is shown. There is thickening and peeling of the skin.
2. The baby is most likely past term (more than 42 weeks of gestation).

Case 48

1. Bilateral inguinal hernias are very evident, and there are many redundant folds of skin, which suggest the diagnosis of cutis laxa (or cutis inelastica). Incidentally, the skin appears somewhat mottled, and the nipples may be somewhat widely spaced.
2. As implied above, the problem is one of *absence* (or marked decrease) of elastic tissue in the skin. The skin biopsy performed in this infant showed no evidence of elastic fibers.
3. If you guessed incorrectly that this is Ehlers-Danlos syndrome (cutis elastica), you might wonder about a bleeding tendency. The associated abnormalities in this baby were intrauterine growth retardation, laxity of joints, and congenital dislocation of the hips. This constellation is rare in males. Gastrointestinal diverticulae and pulmonary emphysema have also been reported.

Case 49

1. The most likely explanation is ventilatory failure, as a result of either limitation of lung expansion or true hypoplasia (structural defect) of the lung.
2. Polycystic disease of the kidney (Potter's type I). It has also been called infantile sponge kidney. Although not very clear in this black and white reproduction (see Fig. 38–49, *bottom*), the cut surface shows numerous minute cysts of variable size and is sometimes referred to as a honeycomb appearance.
3. This is an autosomal-recessive disease, in contrast to cystic dysplasia of the kidney (Potter's type II), which is not hereditary.

Case 50

1. Pustular melanosis (in a white infant)—you can also put "transient neonatal" before pustular if you wish; some prefer "pustulosis."
2. Although not a typical site, i.e., palmar involvement, the possibility of staphylococcal pyoderma should be considered, and cutaneous candidiasis has been reported to look quite similar.
3. "Masterly inactivity" (i.e., nothing)

REFERENCES

Case 1. Greenwald et al: *J. Pediatr. Orthop.* 1984, 4:689–692.
Case 2. Duckett. *Urol. Clin. North Am.* 1978, 5:107–126.
Case 3. Illingworth: *Arch. Dis. Child.* 1976, 51:138–140.
Case 4. Melish & Glasgow: *J. Pediatr.* 1971, 78:958–967.
Case 5. Beckerman & Buchino: *Pediatrics* 1978, 61:417–422

Case 6. McCusick et al.: *JAMA* 1964, 189:813.
Case 7. Warkany: *Congenital Malformations*. Year Book Medical Publishers, Chicago, 1971, pp. 939–941.
Case 8. Mandansky et al.: *Am. Rev. Respir. Dis.* 1979, 120:729–737.
Case 9. Kottmeier & Velcek: *Clin. Perinatol.* 1978, 5:163–176.
Case 10. Rainey & Smith: *J. Pediatr. Surg.* 1984, 19:305–306.
Case 11. Pass et al.: *Pediatrics* 1980, 66:758–762.
Case 12. Uchida & Soltan: *Pediatr. Clin. North Am.* 1963, 10:409.
Case 13. Boles: *Clin. Perinatol.* 1978, 5:149–161.
Case 14. Solomon & Esterly: *Neonatal Dermatology*. W. B. Saunders Co., Philadelphia, 1973, pp 147–148.
Case 15. Streeto: *Lancet* 1970, 2:212.
Case 16. Griscom et al.: *Am. J. Roentgenol* 1977, 128:961–969.
Case 17. Whitley & Hutto: *Pediatr. Rev.* 1985, 7:119–126.
Case 18. Gellis (ed.): *Year Book of Pediatrics*. Year Book Medical Publishers, Chicago, 1963–1966 Series, pp. 472–474.
Case 19. Hayden et al.: *Am. J. Dis. Child.* 1973, 125:879–883.
Case 20. Mukherji & Moss: *Postgrad. Med. J.* 1977, 53:204–211.
Case 21. Stock & Stock: *Obstet Gynecol.* 1979, 53:592–598.
Case 22. Fisher & Smith: *Pediatrics* 1981, 68:480–483.
Case 23. Cassidy et al.: *Am. J. Dis. Child.* 1986, 140:155–159.
Case 24. Vohr et al.: *J. Pediatr.* 1980, 97:196–199.
Case 25. Clarren & Smith: *Pediatr. Clin. North Am.* 1977, 24:665–677.
Case 26. Warkany: *Congenital Malformations*. Year Book Medical Publishers, Chicago, 1971, pp. 978–980.
Case 27. Warkany: *Ibid.*, pp. 899–901.
Case 28. Greenwood et al.: *Am. J. Dis. Child.* 1977, 131:293–294.
Case 29. Sieber et al.: *Clin. Perinatol.* 1978, 5:135–147.
Case 30. Smith & Lipke: *N. Engl. J. Med.* 1979, 300:344–349.
Case 31. Duhamel: *Arch. Dis. Child.* 1961, 36:152
Case 32. Havranek et al.: *J. Pediatr Surg.* 1992, 27:1447–1450.
Case 33. Murphy: *Am. J. Obstet. Gynecol.* 1979, 18:179.
Case 34. Setzer et al.: *J. Pediatr.* 1981, 98:88–90.
Case 35. Janerich et al.: *N. Engl. J. Med.* 1974, 291:697–700.
Case 36. Risemberg et al.: *Johns Hopkins Med. J.* 1974, 135:171–177.
Case 37. Kosnik & Sayers: *J. Neurosurg.* 1975, 42:32–36.
Case 38. Wolk et al.: *Am. J. Dis. Child.* 1974, 128:866.
Case 39. Chervenak et al.: *N. Engl J. Med.* 1983, 309:822–825.
Case 40. Klein et al.: *J. Pediatr. Surg.* 1984, 19:370–374.
Case 41. Boyle & Oh: *Pediatrics* 1980, 65:333–334.
Case 42. Nyhan: *Cytogenetic Disease*. Ciba Clinical Symposia 1983, 35:1–32.
Case 43. Barnes et al.: *Molec. Aspects Med.* 1977, 1:187–282.
Case 44. Wyman & Kuhns: *Am. J. Dis. Child.* 1976, 130:1237–1238.
Case 45. Adashi et al.: *J. Pediatr.* 1980, 96:443–446.
Case 46. Gee & Abdulla: *Br. Med. J.* 1978, 2:1265.
Case 47. Clifford: *J. Pediatr.* 1954, 44:1.
Case 48. Philip: *J. Pediatr.* 1978, 93:150–151.
Case 49. Osathanondh & Potter: *Arch Pathol.* 1964, 77:459–509.
Case 50. Merlob et al.: *Am. J. Dis. Child.* 1982, 136:521–522.

39

WRITTEN QUIZ

MULTIPLE-CHOICE QUESTIONS

DIRECTIONS: Each of the questions or incomplete statements below is followed by five (occasionally six) suggested answers or completions. Select the *answer(s)* that is/are best in each case.

1. With which of the following are elevated levels of maternal serum alpha-fetoprotein associated?
   A. Open meningomyelocele
   B. Isolated hydrocephalus
   C. Omphalocele
   D. Twins
   E. All of the above

2. With which of the following are decreased levels of maternal serum alpha-fetoprotein associated?
   A. Open meningomyelocele
   B. Down's syndrome (trisomy 21)
   C. Omphalocele
   D. Trisomy 13
   E. All of the above

3. Prenatal ultrasonography has been valuable in which of the following circumstances?
   A. To identify many forms of congenital heart disease
   B. To detect ventral wall defects of the fetus
   C. To define gestational age in the third trimester
   D. To detect fetal hydrocephalus
   E. All of the above

4. Cordocentesis (percutaneous umbilical blood sampling) has been used to assess which of the following?
   A. Anemia associated with Rhesus incompatibility
   B. Fetuses with intrauterine growth retardation
   C. Intrauterine infection with toxoplasmosis
   D. Fetal thrombocytopenia
   E. All of the above

5. Maternal toxemia has been associated with which of the following problems in the neonate?
   A. Hyperkalemia
   B. Hypermagnesemia
   C. Neutropenia
   D. Anemia
   E. All of the above

6. In making the transition from fetal to neonatal existence, which of the following statements is/are TRUE?
   A. 60 ml of placental blood may pass to the baby in 60 seconds.
   B. The ductus arteriosus closes within 1 hour of delivery.
   C. Pulmonary artery pressures remain the same as systemic artery pressures.
   D. Under normal circumstances, the systemic arterial oxygen tension increases from 25 to 30 mm Hg to 80 to 100 mm Hg.
   E. None of the above

7. During neonatal resuscitation, which of the following statements is/are TRUE?
   A. A baby who gasps cannot be in secondary apnea.
   B. Naloxone (Narcan) can counteract narcotic depression.
   C. Spontaneous breathing within 40 minutes of delivery has a uniformly good prognosis.
   D. Most very preterm infants have decreased Apgar scores because of poor muscle tone.
   E. None of the above

8. Polyhydramnios may accompany which of the following?
   A. Bilateral renal agenesis
   B. Esophageal atresia
   C. Defective swallowing by the fetus
   D. Severe intrauterine growth retardation
   E. All of the above

9. Which of the following has a swelling on the head as the presenting feature?
   A. Subgaleal hemorrhage
   B. Cephalhematoma
   C. Subarachnoid hemorrhage
   D. Subdural hemorrhage
   E. None of the above

10. Which of the following statements is/are TRUE for the term newborn?
    A. Fractures of the clavicle require careful orthopedic evaluation.
    B. A posterior cleft palate is inconsequential.
    C. Erb's palsy involves the lower extremity.
    D. Bilateral simian creases always indicate a chromosomal anomaly.
    E. None of the above

11. Which of the following statements about nursery practices is/are TRUE?
    A. Overgowns are as important as handwashing in the prevention of infection.
    B. The prone position prevents sudden infant death syndrome.
    C. Silver nitrate eye drops are effective in preventing gonococcal ophthalmitis but cause chemical conjunctivitis.
    D. Good response to diphtheria-tetanus-pertussis vaccine has been seen in preterm infants 2 months after delivery.
    E. Vitamin K prophylaxis is no longer considered appropriate.

12. Fever in the newborn may be caused by which of the following?
    A. An incubator temperature over 35°C in a term infant
    B. A rebound response after cooling in the delivery room
    C. Epidural anesthesia of the mother
    D. Overhydration with intravenous fluids
    E. None of the above

13. Which of the following statements about thermoregulation in the newborn is/are TRUE?
    A. Summit metabolism is the highest metabolic rate achieved when a baby is warmed above normal temperature.
    B. Premature (preterm) infants are at a disadvantage with respect to conserving body temperature.
    C. Evaporative heat loss is important in the delivery room.
    D. The neutral thermal environment is the same for all babies.
    E. Infant servocontrol devices cannot be used in preterm babies.

14. Gestational age assessment after birth provides which of the following?
    A. A more accurate assessment than an early (at 14 weeks) prenatal ultrasound evaluation
    B. Confirmation of gestational age by last menstrual period when it is within 2 weeks of that estimate
    C. Help in predicting neonatal problems
    D. An accurate assessment (within 1 week), no matter what the gestational age
    E. None of the above

15. With regard to transport of the fetus/neonate to a regional center, which of the following statements is/are FALSE?
    A. Prenatal ultrasound has not had an impact on the care provided.
    B. When cyanotic congenital heart disease is suspected, prostaglandin E should be used.
    C. Maternal-fetal transfer is preferred to infant transfer.
    D. With extremely low-birth-weight (< 1000 g) infants, immediate transfer is more important than stabilization.
    E. Many infant transfers can be conducted without a physician in attendance.

16. Which of the following statements about Down's syndrome is/are TRUE?
   A. Bilateral simian creases are always present.
   B. Severe hypotonia is almost invariably seen.
   C. Duodenal atresia is not infrequently seen.
   D. Congenital heart disease is uncommon.
   E. None of the above

17. Which of the following are associated with trisomy 13?
   A. Scalp defects (cutis aplasia)
   B. Cleft lip/palate
   C. Large for gestational age
   D. Heterochromia of the iris (irises of different color)
   E. All of the above

18. With which of the following has tracheoesophageal fistula been frequently associated?
   A. Scalp defects (cutis aplasia)
   B. Clubfeet
   C. Vertebral abnormalities
   D. Imperforate anus
   E. All of the above

19. Which of the following statements about neural tube defects (NTDs) is/are FALSE?
   A. There is no correlation with maternal serum alpha-fetoprotein levels.
   B. Periconceptional folic acid supplementation markedly reduces the risk of NTDs.
   C. Hydrocephalus is frequently associated with meningomyelocele.
   D. Most NTDs are detectable with prenatal ultrasound.
   E. None of the above

20. Which of the following have been associated with uniparental disomy?
   A. Down's syndrome
   B. Turner's syndrome
   C. Angelman's syndrome
   D. Prader-Willi syndrome
   E. None of the above

21. Which of the following statements about respiratory distress syndrome is/are TRUE?
   A. It is predominantly encountered in infants < 33 weeks' gestation.
   B. Dyspnea starts at or soon after birth.
   C. The primary problem is inhalation of amniotic fluid.
   D. Exogenous surfactant can be used for "rescue" therapy.
   E. Radiographic findings cannot be distinguished from those seen with meconium aspiration syndrome.

22. Which of the following treatments seems to be beneficial in cases of persistent pulmonary hypertension?
    A. Digoxin
    B. Corticosteroids
    C. Theophylline
    D. Hyperventilation to produce alkalemia
    E. All of the above

23. Which of the following treatments may be beneficial in cases of bronchopulmonary dysplasia?
    A. Adenosine
    B. Corticosteroids
    C. Naloxone
    D. Hyperventilation to produce alkalemia
    E. None of the above

24. With which of the following has choanal atresia been associated?
    A. Imperforate anus
    B. Coloboma
    C. Duodenal atresia
    D. Heart defects
    E. All of the above

25. Glucuronyl transferase activity may be affected by which of the following?
    A. Phenobarbital administration
    B. Increasing levels of bilirubin
    C. Phenytoin administration
    D. Increased levels of creatinine
    E. None of the above

26. Persistent jaundice beyond 1 week of age may be caused by which of the following?
    A. Tracheoesophageal fistula
    B. Maple syrup urine disease
    C. Congenital hypothyroidism
    D. Congenital biliary atresia
    E. All of the above

27. Which of the following statements about retained fetal lung fluid syndrome is/are TRUE?
    A. It is more common after cesarean section than after vaginal delivery.
    B. It is indistinguishable from respiratory distress syndrome.
    C. It never persists beyond 24 hours after delivery.
    D. It is seen predominantly in post-term infants.
    E. None of the above

28. Which of the following statements about the use of phenobarbital in the treatment of hyperbilirubinemia is/are TRUE?
    A. It has no effect on glucuronyl transferase activity.
    B. Prenatal use may be beneficial to minimize the effects of glucose-6-phosphate dehydrogenase deficiency.
    C. It may be helpful in encouraging excretion of bile.
    D. Some babies with Crigler-Najjar syndrome respond to it.
    E. It is extremely beneficial in congenital biliary atresia.

29. Which of the following statements about breast-feeding and jaundice is/are FALSE?
    A. Breast-fed babies are less likely than formula-fed babies to develop jaundice.
    B. Some cases of "breast-milk jaundice" are associated with increased amounts of β-glucuronidase in the milk.
    C. Some cases of "breast-milk jaundice" have shown increased levels of substances in the milk that inhibit glucuronyl transferase.
    D. Breast-feeding *must* be stopped in the presence of clinically apparent jaundice.
    E. All of the above

30. With regard to breast-feeding, which of the following statements is/are TRUE?
    A. The majority of milk is ingested in the first 5 to 10 minutes.
    B. Colostrum looks more yellow than milk produced at 2 weeks.
    C. The baby should be encouraged to feed for as long as possible.
    D. Unless breast-feeding is initiated within 24 hours of delivery, it will not be successful.
    E. None of the above

31. When using parenteral nutrition, which of the following is important in calculating the fluid requirements?
    A. Medications administered to the baby
    B. Insensible loss
    C. Use of phototherapy
    D. Use of continuous positive airway pressure
    E. All of the above

32. In order to increase caloric intake with parenteral nutrition, which of the following should help?
    A. Adding amino acids, while decreasing glucose concentration
    B. Decreasing amino acids, while increasing glucose concentration
    C. Adding lipid, keeping amino acids and glucose constant
    D. Decreasing lipid, increasing amino acids, keeping glucose constant
    E. None of the above

33. To which of the following does "minimal enteral feeding" refer?
    A. The lowest volume of bolus gavage feeding tolerated by a baby
    B. The smallest amount of gavage feeding that results in no residual gastric aspirate
    C. The lowest volume of gavage feeding that results in weight gain
    D. Small amounts of continuous gavage feeding that stimulate gut enzymes
    E. None of the above

34. Which of the following errors of metabolism relate to protein metabolism?
    A. Galactosemia
    B. Hypothyroidism
    C. Phenylketonuria
    D. Maple syrup urine disease
    E. Zellweger syndrome

35. Which of the following problems are seen more frequently in very preterm (premature) infants?
    A. Meconium aspiration syndrome
    B. Inguinal hernia
    C. Diaphragmatic hernia
    D. Retinopathy (retrolental fibroplasia)
    E. All of the above

36. With regard to follow-up of very-low-birth-weight infants, which of the following statements is/are TRUE?
    A. Over 90% of infants will have severe neurologic deficits.
    B. The incidence of cerebral palsy has decreased universally.
    C. Eye problems are more common than in term infants.
    D. Hearing loss need not be evaluated.
    E. None of the above

37. Which of the following problems are commonly encountered in extremely low-birth-weight infants?
    A. Retinopathy of prematurity
    B. Anemia of prematurity
    C. Hyperkalemia
    D. Respiratory distress syndrome
    E. All of the above

38. Which of the following has been associated with twins?
    A. An increased incidence of group B streptococcal infection
    B. The parabiotic syndrome
    C. Biotinidase deficiency
    D. An increased incidence of gastroschisis
    E. An increased incidence of single umbilical artery

39. Which of the following is/are TRUE concerning parent-infant interaction?
    A. Early contact of mother and baby is to be discouraged.
    B. Contributing breast milk for a very preterm baby can relieve a feeling of helplessness.
    C. Many preterm babies need a "personal prescription" of intervention.
    D. How parents react determines the baby's behavior.
    E. None of the above

40. The grief response has been associated with which of the following?
    A. Birth of a baby with congenital malformations
    B. Birth of a baby with suspected sepsis
    C. Birth of a stillborn baby
    D. Birth of an extremely preterm baby
    E. All of the above

41. Which of the following organisms is/are frequently associated with neonatal sepsis at the present time?
    A. *Proteus mirabilis*
    B. *Streptococcus agalactiae*
    C. *Staphylococcus epidermidis*
    D. *Haemophilus influenzae* type B
    E. *Streptococcus viridans*

42. Group B streptococcus may cause which of the following in the neonate?
    A. Sepsis
    B. Pneumonia
    C. Meningitis
    D. Osteomyelitis
    E. All of the above

43. Which of the following is/are associated with increased susceptibility to neonatal infection?
    A. Phenylketonuria
    B. Gaucher's disease
    C. Galactosemia
    D. Maple syrup urine disease
    E. None of the above

44. Which of the following are considered late manifestations of neonatal sepsis/meningitis?
    A. Abdominal distention
    B. Temperature instability
    C. Seizures
    D. Sclerema
    E. Apneic episodes

45. Which of the following tests have proved useful in the diagnosis of neonatal sepsis?
    A. Fibrinogen
    B. Nitroblue tetrazolium
    C. C-reactive protein
    D. Immature/total neutrophil ratio
    E. All of the above

46. Which of the following tests have shown promise for early diagnosis of neonatal infection?
    A. Neutrophil elastase
    B. Interleukin-1α
    C. Interleukin-6
    D. Tumor necrosis factor-α
    E. All of the above

47. With which of the following has congenital toxoplasmosis been associated?
    A. Dogs
    B. Cats
    C. Chorioretinitis
    D. Scalp vesicles
    E. All of the above

48. Which of the following is/are TRUE of perinatally acquired hepatitis B?
    A. The risk is negligible with mothers who are surface antigen positive.
    B. There is no protection from administration of hepatitis B immune globulin.
    C. Hepatitis B vaccine is recommended to be given to all babies.
    D. Risk of transmission is high in Asia.
    E. None of the above

49. With which of the following neonatal disorders has cytomegalovirus been associated?
    A. Endocardial fibroelastosis
    B. Retrolental fibroplasia
    C. Intracranial calcification
    D. Chronic lung disease
    E. Microcephaly

50. Which of the following is/are seen more frequently in infants of diabetic mothers than in infants of nondiabetic mothers?
    A. Hypocalcemia
    B. Congenital heart disease
    C. Hypoglycemia
    D. Hyperbilirubinemia
    E. All of the above

51. Which of the following statements are TRUE concerning infants with intrauterine growth retardation?
   A. Many infants have a low ponderal index.
   B. High hematocrits are very uncommon.
   C. The incidence is higher in infants born at high altitude.
   D. Chromosomal problems do not need to be considered in the etiology.
   E. None of the above

52. Which of the following have been used in an attempt to prevent intraventricular hemorrhage?
   A. Vitamin D
   B. Ethamsylate
   C. Indomethacin
   D. Ethacrynic acid
   E. None of the above

53. With which of the following presentations has herpes simplex infection in the newborn been associated?
   A. Vesicles on the scalp
   B. Encephalitis
   C. Multiple organ system involvement
   D. Sepsis-like picture with asymptomatic mother
   E. All of the above

54. Which of the following laboratory findings are seen frequently in very-low-birth-weight infants with intrauterine growth retardation?
   A. Marked increase in neutrophil counts
   B. Marked increase in eosinophil counts
   C. Low blood glucose levels
   D. Increased nucleated red blood cell counts
   E. All of the above

55. Which of the following have been associated with hydrops fetalis?
   A. Congenital biliary atresia
   B. Rhesus incompatibility
   C. α-Thalassemia (Bart's hemoglobin)
   D. Parvovirus B 19 infection
   E. None of the above
   F. All of the above

56. How many milligrams of bilirubin result from the degradation of 1 gram of hemoglobin?
   A. 35
   B. 350
   C. 200
   D. 125
   E. 75

57. Which of the following may be seen with hypoglycemia?
    A. Jitteriness
    B. Hypotonia
    C. Abdominal distention
    D. Bulging fontanel
    E. All of the above

58. Which of the following statements about hypocalcemia is TRUE?
    A. Convulsions invariably result in brain damage.
    B. Hypoglycemia is often associated.
    C. Clinical manifestations are clearly distinguishable from those of hypoglycemia.
    D. It produces a prolonged Q_oT_c.
    E. All of the above

59. Which of the following are considered inborn errors of metabolism?
    A. Phenylketonuria
    B. Galactosemia
    C. Maple syrup urine disease
    D. Kernicterus
    E. All of the above

60. Metabolic acidosis may be associated with:
    A. Asphyxia
    B. Hypoglycemia
    C. Excessive protein intake
    D. Sepsis
    E. Elevated pCO_2

61. Which of the following problems is NOT usually associated with prematurity?
    A. Respiratory distress syndrome
    B. Wilson-Mikity syndrome
    C. "Late" edema
    D. Intraventricular hemorrhage
    E. Meconium aspiration syndrome

62. Prolonged administration of magnesium sulfate to the mother may produce which of these problems in the neonate?
    A. Meconium plug syndrome
    B. Intraventricular hemorrhage
    C. Hemolytic anemia
    D. Respiratory depression
    E. Hypothermia

63. Which of the following statements about breast-feeding is/are TRUE?
    A. The gums should grasp the nipple, not the areola.
    B. Delivery before 35 weeks' gestation is a contraindication to breast-feeding.
    C. Breast milk provides protection against infection.
    D. Ten bowel movements a day may be normal.
    E. Milk may spurt from the nipple before feeding when the mother hears the infant cry.

64. The usual artificial feeding (simulated human milk) has a caloric content of:
    A. 35 cal/100 ml
    B. 44 cal/100 ml
    C. 67 cal/100 ml
    D. 85 cal/100 ml
    E. 100 cal/100 ml

65. Gavage feeding should be carried out in which of the following situations?
    A. Infants with gestational age less than 32 weeks
    B. Infants with abdominal distention and blood in the stool
    C. Infants who are vomiting
    D. Infants with a defective swallowing mechanism
    E. All of the above

66. Which of the following have been used to *augment* caloric input with intravenous feeding?
    A. Ringer's lactate
    B. Amino acids and dextrose solutions
    C. Fructose solutions
    D. Soybean emulsion
    E. Cod liver oil

67. Which of the following is/are TRUE of parent-infant interaction?
    A. Immediate "skin-to-skin" contact may have a long-lasting effect.
    B. When babies are very sick the parents should be excluded from the nursery.
    C. It is unwise to show a mother a baby with serious congenital abnormalities.
    D. Transfer of a sick infant to a regional center may induce a "grief response."
    E. None of the above

68. Which of the following may show increased levels with neonatal bacterial infections?
    A. C-reactive protein
    B. Haptoglobin
    C. Erythrocyte sedimentation rate
    D. α_1-Acid glycoprotein (orosomucoid)
    E. All of the above
    F. None of the above

69. Which of the following problems are considered frequent in infants of diabetic mothers?
    A. Hypothermia
    B. Hypoglycemia
    C. Hyperbilirubinemia
    D. Hypernatremia
    E. All of the above

70. Infants of diabetic mothers are more likely to have respiratory distress syndrome because of:
    A. Insulin action on the liver
    B. Infant too big for surfactant production
    C. Insulin suppression of cortisol stimulation
    D. Cortisol suppression of insulin stimulation
    E. None of the above

71. In a preterm infant who is small for gestational age, which of the following complications could be anticipated?
    A. Pulmonary hemorrhage
    B. Subdural effusion
    C. Renal vein thrombosis
    D. Pneumothorax
    E. Hypoglycemia

72. Which of the following problems are common to both infants of diabetic mothers and those who are intrauterine growth retarded?
    A. Hypertonicity
    B. Hypoglycemia
    C. Respiratory distress syndrome
    D. Hypocalcemia
    E. All of the above

73. Which of the following is associated with intrauterine growth retardation?
    A. Rubella
    B. Toxoplasmosis
    C. Chronic alcohol ingestion
    D. Group B streptococcal infection
    E. "Placental insufficiency"

74. Both hypoglycemia and hypocalcemia may be anticipated in which of these infants?
    A. Asphyxiated small for date infants
    B. Infants with Down's syndrome
    C. Infants with central nervous system damage
    D. Infants with Beckwith's syndrome
    E. Infants of diabetic mothers

75. The common link in neonatal hypocalcemia seems to be:
    A. A renal tubular defect
    B. Vitamin D deficiency
    C. A and B above
    D. Transient hypoparathyroidism
    E. None of the above

76. Which of the following have been implicated in the etiology of necrotizing enterocolitis?
    A. Intestinal ischemia
    B. Breast-milk feeding
    C. Bacterial infection
    D. High hematocrit (hyperviscosity)
    E. Hypomagnesemia

77. Under which of the following circumstances is surgery indicated in necrotizing enterocolitis?
    A. Blood in the stool
    B. Excess reducing substance in the stool
    C. Pneumatosis intestinalis
    D. Disseminated intravascular coagulation (consumptive coagulopathy)
    E. Pneumoperitoneum

78. Which of the following drugs have been shown to compete for albumin-binding sites?
    A. Phenobarbital
    B. Diazepam benzoate
    C. Penicillin
    D. Long-acting sulfonamides
    E. Salicylates

79. Maternal ingestion of which of the following has been associated with a specific pattern of congenital abnormalities?
    A. Alcohol
    B. Ampicillin
    C. Chlorothiazide
    D. Chloramphenicol
    E. Warfarin (Coumadin)

80. Which of the following drugs ingested by a mother has been associ-
ated with a hemorrhagic tendency in her newborn?
A. Tetracyclines
B. Phenothiazines
C. Diazepam benzoate
D. Long-acting sulfonamides
E. None of the above

81. With what type of abnormality was thalidomide associated?
A. Neural tube defect
B. Cleft palate
C. Renal agenesis
D. Phocomelia
E. Clubfoot (talipes equinovarus)

82. Which of the following factors have shown demonstrable effect on
low-birth-weight rates?
A. Previous stillbirth
B. Low prepregnancy weight (< 50 kg)
C. Living at high altitude
D. First-trimester bleeding
E. None of the above

83. All of the following are characteristic of premature infants, EXCEPT:
A. Head appears larger than trunk
B. Thin extremities
C. Breast engorgement
D. Minimal subcutaneous fat
E. Limbs not well flexed

84. Decreased breath sounds are found on one side of the thorax during
a newborn examination. The most likely cause is:
A. Bronchopneumonia
B. Retained lung fluid syndrome
C. Respiratory distress syndrome
D. Pneumothorax
E. Hyaline membrane disease

85. Which of the following are appropriate measures in caring for infants
with a diaphragmatic hernia?
A. Endotracheal intubation
B. Position on affected side, with chest elevated with respect to pelvis
C. Gastric decompression
D. A and C above
E. All of the above

86. Choanal atresia is a congenital anomaly characterized by:
    A. Episodic respiratory distress
    B. Drooling
    C. Gasping in delivery room
    D. Vomiting
    E. All of the above

87. Which of the following relate to phenylketonuria (PKU)?
    A. Inherited inborn error of metabolism
    B. No clinical signs demonstrated in newborn
    C. Inherited disorder of central nervous system
    D. Associated with marked mental retardation
    E. B, C, and D above
    F. A, B, and D above

88. Staphylococcal colonization usually starts at which of the following sites?
    A. Respiratory tract
    B. Circumcision
    C. Gastrointestinal tract
    D. Umbilical cord
    E. None of the above

89. The normal range for a newborn heart rate is:
    A. 60–80
    B. 80–100
    C. 110–150
    D. 140–200

90. Which of the following are NOT important predisposing causes of neonatal sepsis?
    A. Prolonged rupture of membranes
    B. Eclampsia
    C. Premature onset of labor
    D. Prenatal or perinatal maternal infection
    E. Cesarean section

91. A lethargic newborn may have:
    A. Hypoxia
    B. Severe infection
    C. Congenital cerebral defect
    D. Sedation from maternal analgesia
    E. All of the above

92. Which of the following statements is/are TRUE?
    A. Isolation of an infant suspected of being infected can be effectively accomplished by placing the infant in a closed incubator and employing strict handwashing techniques.
    B. One should always be on the lookout for infection in infants born prematurely.
    C. Infected infants often present with any combination of the following: poor temperature control, irritability, jaundice, abdominal distention.
    D. Women with evidence of herpes infection of the cervix or vulva at term should never be delivered by cesarean section.
    E. All of the above

93. All of the following are commonly observed in the postmature infant, EXCEPT:
    A. Abundance of lanugo
    B. Dry, peeling skin
    C. Long nails
    D. Abundance of scalp hair
    E. None of the above

94. In the first week after birth, group B streptococcal infection frequently presents as:
    A. Pneumonia
    B. Meningitis
    C. Mastoiditis
    D. Sepsis
    E. Any of the above

95. Yellowish-green color of the skin in an infant at birth is probably due to:
    A. Infectious hepatitis
    B. Carotenemia
    C. Meconium staining
    D. Syphilis
    E. Hyperbilirubinemia

96. Which of the following are complications of cold stress (hypothermia)?
    A. Depletion of energy stores
    B. Increased oxygen consumption
    C. Metabolic acidosis
    D. A and C above
    E. All of the above

97. Which of the following are evidences of respiratory distress syndrome in a newborn?
   A. Dilated nares
   B. Expiratory grunt
   C. Intercostal retractions
   D. Xiphoid retractions
   E. A, B, and C above only
   F. All of the above

98. Which of the following are secondary complications that can result from meconium aspiration?
   A. Pneumothorax
   B. Pneumonitis
   C. Pneumomediastinum
   D. Pulmonary hemorrhage
   E. All of the above

99. First feedings should:
   A. Be given between 4 and 6 hours
   B. Consist of sterile water/breast milk
   C. Consist of 10% glucose and water
   D. A and B above
   E. None of the above

100. Which of the following is/are FALSE when a tracheoesophageal fistula is present?
   A. The stomach is markedly distended.
   B. Pneumonia is quite common.
   C. X-rays are helpful in diagnosis.
   D. Stridor or "crowing" respirations are present.
   E. Most can be corrected surgically.

DIRECTIONS: Each group of questions below consists of a list of lettered headings followed by a list of numbered words, phrases, or statements. For each numbered word, phrase, or statement, select the lettered heading(s) most closely associated with it. Each lettered heading may be selected once, more than once, or not at all.

Questions 101–105

A. VATER association
B. Polyhydramnios
C. Trisomy 13 and 18
D. Double-bubble on x-ray
E. "Dextrocardia"

101. Single umbilical artery

102. Tracheoesophageal fistula

103. Duodenal atresia

104. Diaphragmatic hernia

105. Imperforate anus

Questions 106–110

A. Small for gestational age
B. Large for gestational age
C. Post-term (postmature)
D. Preterm (premature)

106. Beckwith's syndrome

107. Trisomy 18

108. Meconium aspiration syndrome

109. Pulmonary hemorrhage

110. Antepartum hemorrhage

Questions 111–114

A. Poor peripheral pulses
B. Bounding peripheral pulses
C. Pulsatile liver
D. Cyanosis
E. Above average birth weight

111. Patent ductus arteriosus

112. Tricuspid atresia

113. Hypoplastic left heart syndrome

114. Transposition of great vessels

Questions 115–119

A. Pierre Robin syndrome
B. Abduction splint
C. Edema of the extremities
D. Copious amounts of mucus
E. "Dextrocardia"

115. Tension pneumothorax on left

116. Tracheoesophageal fistula

117. Cleft palate

118. Congenital dislocation of hip

119. Turner's syndrome

Questions 120–123

A. Prolonged Q_oT_c interval
B. Coma
C. Lethargy
D. Jitteriness
E. Meconium plug syndrome

120. Hypoglycemia

121. Hypocalcemia

122. Hypermagnesemia

123. Hyperammonemia

Questions 124–127

A. Right-sided diaphragmatic hernia
B. Late-onset meningitis
C. Brain abscess
D. Pustules in the groin

124. *Citrobacter diversus*

125. Group B streptococci

126. *Staphylococcus aureus*

127. *Listeria monocytogenes*

Questions 128–132

A. Syndrome of inappropriate ADH
B. Beckwith's syndrome
C. Ornithine transcarbamoylase (OTC) deficiency
D. Meconium plug syndrome
E. Jitteriness

128. Hypoglycemia

129. Hyponatremia

130. Hypermagnesemia

131. Hypocalcemia

132. Hyperammonemia

Questions 133–137

A. Confined by suture lines
B. Crosses suture lines
C. Face mask application in tiny baby
D. Asphyxia in preterm infant
E. Difficult forceps delivery

133. Subdural hemorrhage

134. Subarachnoid hemorrhage

135. Cerebellar hemorrhage

136. Subgaleal hemorrhage

137. Cephalhematoma

Questions 138–142

A. Seizures
B. Bile-stained vomitus
C. Pallor
D. Gasping respiration
E. Gaseous abdominal distention

138. Subcapsular hemorrhage of liver

139. Subarachnoid hemorrhage

140. Volvulus

141. Neonatal sepsis

142. Choanal atresia

Questions 143–146

A. Drainage from the umbilicus
B. Sometimes associated with chromosomal disorders
C. Emerges to the right of umbilicus
D. May be associated renal anomalies
E. None of the above

143. Omphalocele

144. Gastroschisis

145. Prune-belly syndrome

146. Persistent urachus

Questions 147–151

A. Defect of skull bones
B. Associated deafness
C. Maternal ingestion of iodides
D. Potter's facies
E. Trisomy 13

147. Bilateral renal agenesis

148. Congenital goiter

149. Craniotabes

150. Coloboma of iris

151. Cutis aplasia

Questions 152–159

A. Increased level of C-reactive protein
B. Test dose of naloxone
C. Test dose of neostigmine
D. May need higher dosage of ampicillin
E. Hypotonia
F. Test dose of pyridoxine
G. Treat with theophylline
H. Test dose of pancuronium

152. Group B streptococcal sepsis

153. Refractory seizures

154. Respiratory depression at birth

155. *Escherichia coli* meningitis

156. Myasthenia gravis

157. Werdnig-Hoffmann disease

158. Asynchronous breathing on respirator

159. Apnea of prematurity

Questions 160–164

A. Chorioretinitis
B. Myocarditis
C. Scalp vesicles
D. Cataract
E. Hemorrhagic tendency
F. Deafness
G. Congenital heart disease

160. Rubella

161. Toxoplasmosis

162. Cytomegalovirus

163. Herpes simplex

164. Coxsackie B

Questions 165–168

A. Thrombocytopenia
B. Edema
C. Vitamin E deficiency
D. Vitamin K deficiency
E. Rhesus incompatibility
F. Decreased fibrinogen

165. Hemolytic disease of the new-born

166. Hemorrhagic disease of the newborn

167. Hemolytic anemia of prematurity

168. Disseminated intravascular coagulation

Questions 169–175

A. 37–42 weeks' gestation
B. Thin gelatinous skin
C. Hypoglycemia, trisomy 18
D. Diabetic mother
E. Lack of recoil
F. Bacterial infection
G. <2500 grams
H. Plantar creases over two-thirds of sole
I. 3500-gram term infant

169. AGA

170. SGA

171. LGA

172. Preterm

173. Term gestation

174. Post-term

175. Low birth weight

ANSWERS

1. A, C, D	18. C, D	35. B, D
2. B, D	19. A	36. C
3. A, B, D	20. C, D	37. E
4. E	21. A, B, D	38. A, B, E
5. B, C	22. D	39. B, C
6. A, D	23. B	40. A, C, D
7. B, D	24. B, D	41. B, C
8. B, C	25. A, B	42. E
9. A, B	26. C, D	43. C
10. E	27. A	44. C, D
11. C, D	28. B, C, D	45. C, D
12. A, C	29. A, D	46. A, C
13. B, C	30. A, B	47. B, C
14. B, C	31. B, C	48. C, D
15. A, D	32. C	49. C, D, E
16. B, C	33. D	50. E
17. A, B	34. C, D	51. A, C

52. B, C	94. A, D	135. C
53. E	95. C	136. B
54. C, D	96. E	137. A, E
55. B, C, D	97. F	138. C
56. A	98. A, B, C	139. A
57. A, B	99. D	140. B, E
58. B, D	100. A, D	141. C, E
59. A, B, C	101. C	142. D
60. A, C, D	102. A, B	143. B
61. E	103. B, D	144. C
62. A, D	104. E	145. D
63. C, D, E	105. A	146. A
64. C	106. B	147. D
65. A, D	107. A	148. C
66. B, D	108. C	149. A
67. A, D	109. A	150. B
68. E	110. D	151. E
69. B, C	111. B	152. A, D
70. C	112. C, D	153. F
71. A, E	113. A, D	154. B
72. B, D	114. D, E	155. A, D
73. A, B, C, E	115. E	156. C, E
74. A, C, E	116. D	157. E
75. D	117. A	158. H
76. A, C, D	118. B	159. G
77. D, E	119. C	160. D, F, G
78. B, D, E	120. C, D	161. A
79. A, E	121. A, C, D	162. A, F
80. E	122. C, E	163. C, E
81. D	123. B	164. B
82. B, C	124. B, C	165. B, E
83. A, C	125. A, B	166. D
84. D	126. D	167. B, C
85. E	127. B	168. A, F
86. A, C	128. B, E	169. I
87. F	129. A	170. C
88. B, D	130. D	171. D
89. C	131. E	172. B, E, F
90. B, E	132. C	173. A
91. E	133. E	174. H
92. A, B, C	134. D	175. C, G
93. A		

Appendices

Appendix 1

TECHNIQUE FOR PLACEMENT, SAMPLING, AND REMOVAL OF UMBILICAL ARTERY CATHETER

PLACEMENT

1. Full aseptic precautions should be taken. This is most easily accomplished with the baby under the infant warmer and a headbox (hood) or ventilator to maintain appropriate oxygen concentration.

2. A special umbilical artery tray is usually available and should always be used.

3. The cord and abdomen should be "prepped" with povidone-iodine (Betadine) before covering with drapes.

4. Heparinized saline should be prepared and flushed through the umbilical artery catheter to be used. Use a 3.5-F catheter in infants under 1500 g and a 5-F catheter when weight is over 1500 g.

5. A pursestring suture (4-0 silk) is next inserted around the cord as superficially as possible and as close to the abdomen as possible. Care should be taken not to perforate any vessels, and the skin should be avoided.

6. The suture is tied loosely so that it can be pulled tight if bleeding occurs.

7. With the suture protected, the cord is cut across horizontally with a scalpel blade. A clean cut does not usually bleed, but the arteries go into spasm.

8. The lumen of one artery should be dilated by dropping the tips of iris forceps (nontoothed) into it and letting them spring open (Fig. A1–1). After several attempts the lumen will remain dilated.

9. The iris forceps are then used to stabilize the artery by placing one blade in the lumen and grasping the edge of the cord with the other blade (Fig. A1–2).

10. The catheter is then inserted into the artery twice the distance between the symphysis pubis and the middle of the umbilicus plus any umbilical stump (Fig. A1–3). (Example: distance from symphysis to midumbilicus is 3.5 cm and umbilical stump is 1.5 cm; length of catheter is (3.5 × 2) + 1.5 = 8.5 cm) (Fig. A1–4).

11. The tip of the catheter should now lie opposite L3–4 vertebrae, i.e.,

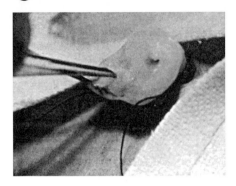

FIGURE A1–1. Iris forceps dilating the lumen of an umbilical artery.

FIGURE A1–2. After the artery is well dilated, one limb of the forceps is inserted into the lumen and stability is obtained by grasping the umbilical cord wall with the other limb.

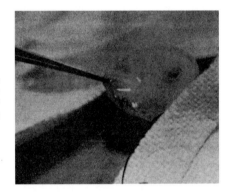

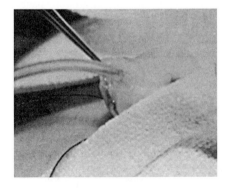

FIGURE A1–3. Catheter being inserted into the umbilical artery after the procedure described in Figure A1–2.

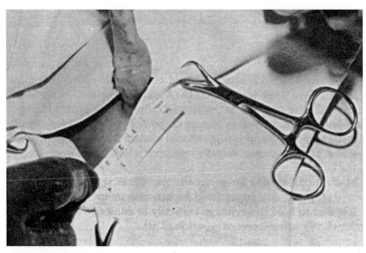

FIGURE A1–4. Calculation of distance to insert umbilical artery catheter. The distance from the middle of the umbilicus to the symphysis pubis is measured and doubled.

below the main branches of the aorta but above the bifurcation. (For high placement [T6–10], measure the distance between the umbilicus and the shoulder.) Catheter position should always be confirmed with x-ray of the abdomen (or with ultrasound) and repositioned if necessary.

12. There should be free flow of blood in the catheter, and arterial pulsation is usually noted. If there is no arterial pulsation, the catheter should be removed.

13. If difficulties are encountered, further efforts with that artery should be discontinued and an attempt made with the other artery.

14. Fixation of the catheter is achieved with taping. Two T pieces are applied to the abdomen parallel to each other on either side of the catheter. Two strips of tape are used to enclose the catheter and the vertical stems of the T pieces. A "flag" is placed on the catheter (Fig. A1–5). In small babies with friable skin, an alternative method is to place an adhesive band on the catheter, just above the umbilicus, and suture it to the umbilical cord.

SAMPLING

A "double-stopcock setup" should be used for withdrawing blood (Fig. A1–6). Two three-way stopcocks (A and B) are placed in the infusion line, immediately attached to the arterial catheter. The proximal stopcock A and syringe (i.e., the ones closest to the baby) are used for sampling. The distal stopcock B and syringe should contain a small amount of saline into which blood is drawn initially and from which blood is injected back into the baby.

Medications should be given via the distal stopcock to leave the proximal stopcock uncontaminated for accurate sampling.

It is best to hold the syringes vertically to minimize the admixture of blood and saline and prevent injection of air.

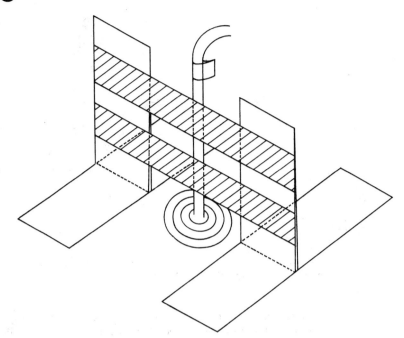

FIGURE A1–5. Method of taping the umbilical artery catheter in place.

Although speed is not essential, it is advisable to carry out sampling reasonably quickly to prevent clotting in the system.

When sampling for blood gases and pH, the sampling syringe should be heparinized (just enough to fill the connecting space). If air is inadvertently drawn into the syringe, it should be removed at the time of sampling (after the syringe is removed from the stopcock) by inverting the syringe, placing a needle on the end, and ejecting the air.

REMOVAL

The equipment needed consists primarily of a small curved hemostat, some suture material, and some gauze wipes (swabs).

Hemorrhage is the major complication. This may be avoided by removing the catheter SLOWLY—particularly for the last 3 to 4 cm—to allow the artery to go into spasm. Continuing pulsation indicates that communication with the major vessels persists.

After removing the tape from the abdomen, the catheter is slowly withdrawn (with one hand) with the hemostat (in the other hand) astride the vessel. Assistance in restraining the baby's limbs is usually required. The last 3 cm should be removed at the rate of 1 cm/min. In the event that spasm does not occur, the hemostat can be clamped on the artery at the moment of complete removal and suture material knotted below the hemostat.

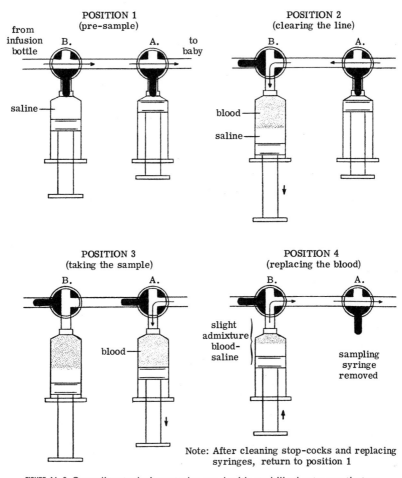

FIGURE A1–6. Sampling technique to be used with umbilical artery catheters.

Appendix 2
EXCHANGE TRANSFUSION TECHNIQUE

The procedure should be carried out as for insertion of an umbilical artery catheter, but the catheter is inserted into the umbilical vein. If flow of blood is not free, the position of the catheter tip should be checked with AP and lateral x-rays. In critically ill babies, placement of an arterial catheter may be valuable to monitor the status of the baby. A special exchange transfusion pack is used, and the following points should be noted:

1. A 2-volume exchange is usually carried out (2 × 80 ml/kg), which achieves 80 to 85% turnover (exchange) of blood.

2. The blood should be warmed before injection into the baby (preferably with a special warmer or a waterbath).

3. Calculation of the distance to insert the catheter is most easily estimated by measuring the distance from the umbilicus to the xiphoid process. The *free flow* of blood must be ensured before starting the exchange because of the possibility of entering the portal system.

4. Venous pressure should be checked before beginning and after every 100 ml. A gradually increasing deficit may be desirable if the initial venous pressure is greatly elevated. (Normal venous pressure is approximately 6 to 7 cm of blood.)

5. When using citrated blood, calcium gluconate is often given, approximately every 100 ml (1 ml of 10% solution). This should be given slowly and the heart rate carefully monitored.

6. Pre- and postexchange samples are sent for hemoglobin, hematocrit, and bilirubin determinations (and possibly total protein).

If the need arises, exchange transfusion can be performed through an umbilical artery catheter. Some use a continuous exchange method (with a two-sided constant infusion pump) to simultaneously remove blood from the artery and administer blood through vein.

Appendix 3
WEIGHT CONVERSION

TABLE A3–1. Gram Equivalents for Pounds and Ounces

Weight Conversion

Pounds	\	Ounces														
	0	1	2	3	4	5	6	7	8	9	10	11	12	13	14	15
0		28	57	85	113	142	170	198	227	255	283	312	340	369	397	425
1	454	482	510	539	567	595	624	652	680	709	737	765	794	822	850	879
2	907	936	964	992	1021	1049	1077	1106	1134	1162	1191	1219	1247	1276	1304	1332
3	1361	1389	1417	1446	1474	1503	1531	1559	1588	1616	1644	1673	1701	1729	1758	1786
4	1814	1843	1871	1899	1928	1956	1984	2013	2041	2070	2098	2126	2155	2183	2211	2240
5	2268	2296	2325	2353	2381	2410	2438	2466	2495	2523	2551	2580	2608	2637	2665	2693
6	2722	2750	2778	2807	2835	2863	2892	2920	2948	2977	3005	3033	3062	3090	3118	3147
7	3175	3203	3232	3260	3289	3317	3345	3374	3402	3430	3459	3487	3515	3544	3572	3600
8	3629	3657	3685	3714	3742	3770	3799	3827	3856	3884	3912	3941	3969	3997	4026	4054
9	4082	4111	4139	4167	4196	4224	4252	4281	4309	4337	4366	4394	4423	4451	4479	4508
10	4536	4564	4593	4621	4649	4678	4706	4734	4763	4791	4819	4848	4876	4904	4933	4961
11	4990	5018	5046	5075	5103	5131	5160	5188	5216	5245	5273	5301	5330	5358	5386	5415
12	5443	5471	5500	5528	5557	5585	5613	5642	5670	5698	5727	5755	5783	5812	5840	5868
13	5897	5925	5953	5982	6010	6038	6067	6095	6123	6152	6180	6209	6237	6265	6294	6322
14	6350	6379	6407	6435	6464	6492	6520	6549	6577	6605	6634	6662	6690	6719	6747	6776
15	6804	6832	6860	6889	6917	6945	6973	7002	7030	7059	7087	7115	7144	7172	7201	7228
16	7257	7286	7313	7342	7371	7399	7427	7456	7484	7512	7541	7569	7597	7626	7654	7682
17	7711	7739	7768	7796	7824	7853	7881	7909	7938	7966	7994	8023	8051	8079	8108	8136
18	8165	8192	8221	8249	8278	8306	8335	8363	8391	8420	8448	8476	8504	8533	8561	8590
19	8618	8646	8675	8703	8731	8760	8788	8816	8845	8873	8902	8930	8958	8987	9015	9043
20	9072	9100	9128	9157	9185	9213	9242	9270	9298	9327	9355	9383	9412	9440	9469	9497
21	9525	9554	9582	9610	9639	9667	9695	9724	9752	9780	9809	9837	9865	9894	9922	9950
22	9979	10007	10036	10064	10092	10120	10149	10177	10206	10234	10262	10291	10319	10347	10376	10404

Appendix 4
ACID-BASE NOMOGRAM

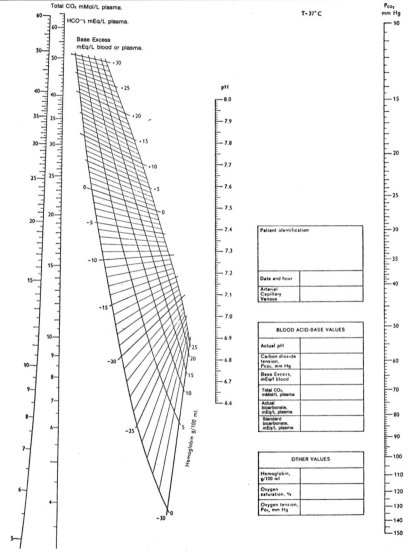

FIGURE A4–1. Acid-base nomogram. (Reproduced from the Siggaard-Andersen Acid-Base Nomogram, by Radiometer A/S. EMDRUPVEJ. DK-2400, Copenhagen NU, Denmark, 1962, with permission of the publisher.)

GROWTH RECORD FOR INFANTS

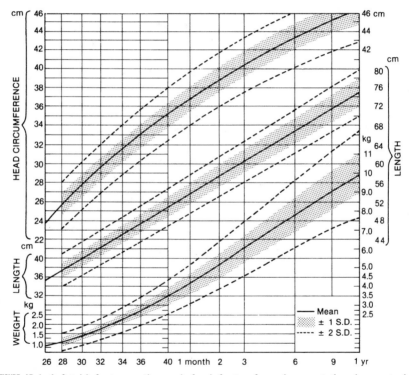

FIGURE A5–1. A fetal-infant growth graph for infants of varying gestational ages to be used for plotting growth from birth until 1 year of age after "term" has been reached. (Reproduced from Babson, S. G., and Benda, G. I.: Growth graphs for the clinical assessment of infants of varying gestational age. *J. Pediatr.* 1976, 89:814–820, with permission of the publisher.)

Appendix 6
BLOOD PRESSURE IN THE NEWBORN

TABLE A6–1. Systolic and Diastolic Blood Pressures in Term Infants*

	Systolic		Diastolic	
	Doppler	*Direct Arterial*	*Doppler*	*Direct Arterial*
Arm	60 ± 10.3	55 ± 9.0	38 ± 9.4	35 ± 9.0
Leg	54 ± 9.6	56 ± 9.4	38 ± 8.6	34 ± 9.7

*Based on Dweck, H. S., Reynolds, D. W., and Cassidy, G.: *Am. J. Dis. Child.* 1974, 127:492.

TABLE A6–2. Change in Systolic Blood Pressure* In Term Infants During First 6 Weeks†

Age	Mean Systolic Blood Pressure (n = 99)
2 days	70 mm Hg
14 days	84 mm Hg
6 weeks	93 mm Hg

*Doppler.
†See Earley, A., et al.: *Arch. Dis. Child.* 1980, 55:755–758.

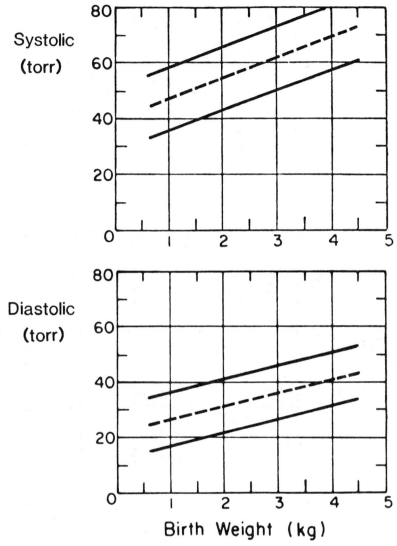

FIGURE A6–1. Mean values and 95% confidence limits for systolic, diastolic, mean, and pulse blood pressures during the first 12 hours of life. (Reproduced from Versmold, H. T., et al.: Aortic blood pressure during the first 12 hours of life in infants with birth weight 610 to 4220 grams. *Pediatrics* 1981, 67:607–613, with permission of the publisher.)

Illustration continued on following page

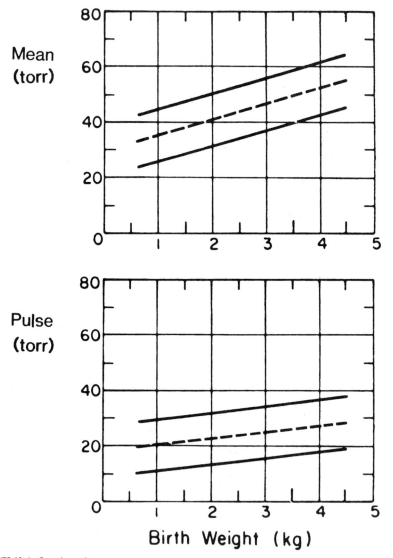

FIGURE A6–1. *Continued*

"FOOL'S GUIDE" TO VENTILATOR MANAGEMENT OF THE NEONATE

Although this subject is frequently complex, the following oversimplification may be helpful for initiating care or making changes.

1. To produce an increase in pO_2 either:
   a. Increase inspired O_2 concentration
   b. Increase end-expiratory pressure
   c. Increase I/E ratio (prolong inspiration)
   d. Increase minute volume (see below)
   e. Increase mean airway pressure

2. To produce a decrease in pCO_2 either:
   a. Increase minute volume (see below)
   b. Decrease I/E ratio (prolong expiration)
   c. Increase end-expiratory pressure in worsening lung disease
   d. Decrease end-expiratory pressure in recovery phase

3. To lower pO_2 decrease 1a, b, c, d, or e

4. To increase pCO_2 decrease minute volume.

> Minute volume = tidal volume (volume per breath) × rate per minute.
> With volume-limited ventilators: volume can be calculated (use tidal volume = 6 ml/kg)
> With pressure-limited ventilators: increasing peak inspiratory pressure results in increased volume.
> A reasonable starting point with a pressure-limited ventilator would be:
> Respiration rate = 40/min
> Peak inspiratory pressure = 25 cm H_2O (18–20 cm H_2O if lungs normal)
> I/E ratio = 1:2
> PEEP = 4–5 cm H_2O
> Inspired oxygen concentration = 40–50%
> Changes can be made according to changes in transcutaneous or blood gas measurements. Oxygen saturation monitoring can guide inspired oxygen concentration.
> A simple guide to depth of insertion of an endotracheal tube is to use the "tip-to-lip" distance of 7, 8, or 9 cm for babies weighing 1, 2, or 3 kg (Tochen, M. L.: *J. Pediatr.* 1979, 95:1050).

Appendix 8
NORMAL VALUES

TABLE A8-1.

	Normal Values			
Determination	Blood/Serum/Plasma	Urine	Cerebrospinal Fluid	SI Conversion
Ammonia	90–150 µg/ml*			$\times$ 0.587 = µmol/L
Bilirubin	<12 mg/dl			$\times$ 17.1 = µmol/L
Blood cells				
white	5000–30,000/mm³	Few	0–30/mm³	$\times 10^6 = 10^9$/L
red	4.5–6 million/mm³	Few	Up to 675/mm³	$\times 10^6 = 10^{12}$/L
Calcium	Cord: 9.3–12.2 mg/dl First week 9.2–11.2 mg/dl (breast) 8.0–10.6 mg/dl (bottle)	First day 0.1–0.3 mg/24 hr Seventh day 0.1–0.3 mg/4 hr		$\times$ 0.25 = mmol/L
Chloride	90–114 mEq/L	17–85 mEq/L	109–123 mEq/L	$\times$ 1.0 = mmol/L
Creatinine	Cord 0.6–1.7 mg/dl Later 0.6–1.2 mg/dl	10–20 mg/kg/24 hr†		mg $\times$ 8.84 = µmol/L
Fibrinogen	1–2 days 120–290 mg/dl 3–7 days 200–400 mg/dl			$\times$ 0.01 = g/L
Fibrin split products	2.3–19.5 µg/ml			$\times$ 1 = mg/L
Glucose	40–80 mg/dl		30–75 mg/dl	$\times$ 0.056 = mmol/L
Hematocrit	Cord 40–60% Fifth day 40–65%			
Hemoglobin	Cord 14–20 g/dl Fifth day 13–21 g/dl			$\times$ 0.155 = mmol/L

Table continued on following page

TABLE A8-1. *Continued*

Determination	Blood/Serum/Plasma	Normal Values Urine	Cerebrospinal Fluid	SI Conversion
Magnesium	1.50–2.10 mg/dl	First day 0–0.4 mg/24 hr Seventh day 0–1 mg/24 hr	2.2–3.2 mg/dl	× 0.41 = mmol/L
Osmolality	280–300 mOsm/kg	Birth 79–118 mOsm/kg Later 150–250 mOsm/kg	Same as serum	× 1.0 = mmol/kg
pCO_2	35–45 mm Hg		38–63 mm Hg	× 0.133 = kPa
pH	7.35–7.45	5.1–6.8†	7.32–7.37	
pO_2	80–100 mm Hg			
Phosphorus	First week 5.8–9.0 mg/dl Second week 4.9–8.9 mg/dl	First day 0.06–0.18 mg/kg/24 hr Seventh day 0.07–0.7 mg/kg/24 hr	0.7–3.1 mg/dl	× 0.133 = kPa × 0.323 = mmol/L
Platelets	150,000–300,000/mm³			
Potassium	Early 4.3–7.6 mEq/L 1 mo 3.5–5.6 mEq/L	First day 0.08–0.64 mg/kg/24 hr Seventh day 0–2.25 mEq/kg/24 hr	2.1–3.9 mEq/L	× 1.0 = mmol/L
Protein (total)	4.6–7.7 g/dl*	8–12 mg/24 hr	30–200 mg/dl†	

At Birth	At 1 Month (Serum)	
IgG 650–1300 mg/dl*	270–850 mg/dl	× 0.01 = g/L
IgA 0–15 mg/dl	4–36 mg/dl	
IgM 0–30 mg/dl	25–56 mg/dl	
Prothrombin time	12–21 sec	
Partial thromboplastin time	50–90 sec†	
Reticulocytes	1–2 days 3–7%	
	3–7 days 0–4%	
Sedimentation rate (mini-ESR)	1–2 days <2 mm/1st hr	
	3–7 days <10 mm/1st hr	
Sodium	136–148 mEq/L	First day 0.11–0.39 mEq/kg/24 hr	× 1.0 = mmol
		Seventh day up to 4.4 mEq/kg/24 hr
Urea nitrogen	5–25 mg/dl†	First day 25 ml (0–100)	× 0.357 = mmol/L
Volume	Blood 70–100 ml/kg	Seventh day 150 ml (50–300)	40–60 ml
	RBC 25–50 ml/kg	2 weeks 225 ml (200–250)
	Plasma 30–50 ml/kg	

*May be lower in premature (immature) infants.

†May be higher in premature (immature) infants.

This information was gleaned from several sources, principally Belton, N. R.: In *Textbook of Paediatrics*, Forfar, J. O., and Arneil, G. C. (eds.). Churchill Livingston, Edinburgh, 1979, Chapter 40. See also Meites, S., et al.: *Pediatric Clinical Chemistry*. American Association for Clinical Chemistry, Inc., Washington, D.C., 1977.

Appendix 9
NEONATAL MORTALITY

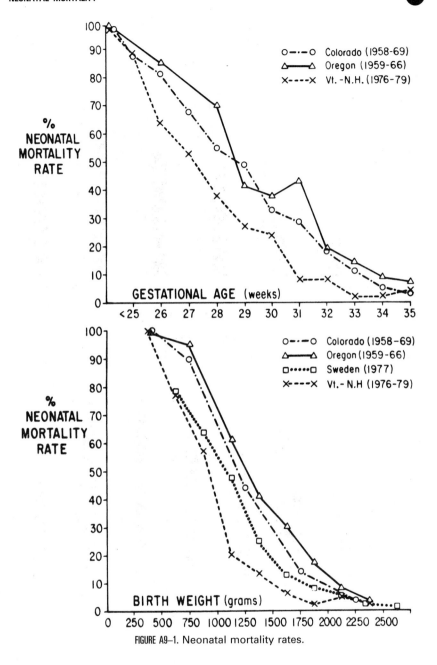

FIGURE A9–1. Neonatal mortality rates.

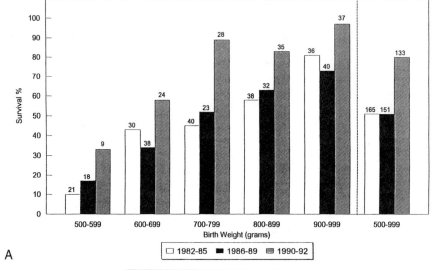

A

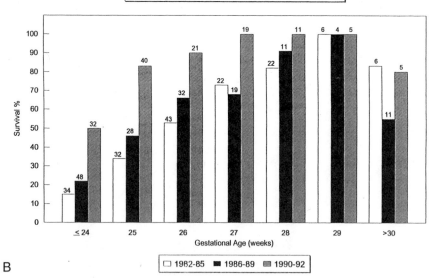

B

FIGURE A9–2. The survival of extremely low-birth-weight (< 1000 g) infants in the Maine Medical Center NICU is compared over time, by gestational age *(A)* and by birth weight *(B),* showing a marked improvement in 1990 to 1992. The numbers above each column indicate the denominator from which the percentages were derived in each category.

TABLE A9-1. NEONATAL MORTALITY*

Birth Weight (grams)	Gestational Age (weeks)											
	≤25	26	27	28	29	30	31	32	33	34	35	≤35
2250–2499								†	8	2	0	2 (111)
2000–2249						†	†	7	3	0	8	5 (151)
1750–1999							0	5	0	1	3	2 (210)
1500–1749			†	†		0	9	8	5	3	0	6 (205)
1250–1499			†	25	33	26	5	11	0	0	†	13 (168)
1000–1249	60	†	30	26	19	16	12	11	0	17		20 (168)
750–999	90	67	58	64	25	56	†	17		†	†	57 (95)
500–749	96	67	†	†	†	†		†		†		77 (48)
≤2499	89 (38)	64 (28)	53 (36)	38 (69)	27 (48)	24 (93)	8 (107)	8 (199)	2 (161)	2 (220)	4 (158)	

*Neonatal mortality (%) for admissions to intensive care nurseries in Vermont/New Hampshire (1976–79) by birth weight/gestational age groups.
†Fewer than five admissions in a group.
Note: Figures in parentheses indicate the number of admissions in each group.

Appendix 10
GLUCOSE RATE CALCULATOR

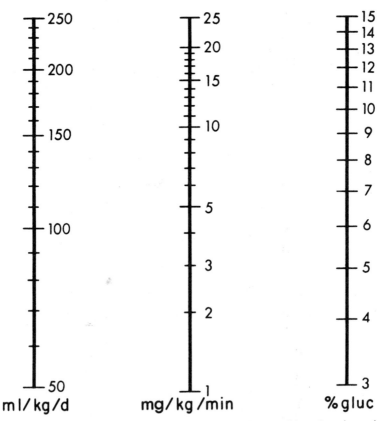

FIGURE A10–1. Glucose rate calculator. Use a straightedge to determine the volume required per 24 hours. (Reproduced from Klaus, M., and Fanaroff, A. A.: *Care of the High Risk Neonate,* 3rd ed. Philadelphia, W. B. Saunders Company, 1979, with permission.)

SUGGESTED READING

Many subjects are not covered in detail in this book, and the following are suggested as references for more detailed information.

GENERAL NEONATOLOGY

Avery, G. B.: *Neonatology: Pathophysiology and Management of the Newborn,* 3rd ed. J. B. Lippincott, Philadelphia, 1987.

Fanaroff, A. A., and Martin, R. J.: *Neonatal-Perinatal Medicine: Diseases of the Fetus and Infant,* 5th ed. Mosby Year Book, St. Louis, 1992.

Taeusch, H. W., Ballard, R. A., and Avery, M. E.: *Schaffer and Avery's Diseases of the Newborn,* 6th ed. W. B. Saunders, Philadelphia, 1991.

FETAL AND NEONATAL PHYSIOLOGY

Dawes, G. S.: *Foetal and Neonatology Physiology: A Comparative Study of the Changes at Birth.* Year Book Medical Publishers, Chicago, 1968.

Smith, C. A., and Nelson, N. M.: *The Physiology of the Newborn Infant,* 4th ed. Charles C Thomas Publishers, Springfield, Ill., 1976.

Polin, R. A., and Fox, W. W.: *Fetal and Neonatal Physiology.* W. B. Saunders, Philadelphia, 1992.

CONGENITAL MALFORMATIONS

Bergsma, D. (ed.): *Birth Defects: Atlas & Compendium,* 2nd ed. Williams & Wilkins, Baltimore, 1979.

Jones, K. L.: *Smith's Recognizable Patterns of Human Malformation,* 4th ed. W. B. Saunders, Philadelphia, 1988.

Goodman, R. M., and Gorlin, R. J.: *The Malformed Infant and Child.* Oxford University Press, New York, 1983.

Feingold, M., and Pashayan, H.: *Genetics and Birth Defects in Clinical Practice.* Little, Brown & Company, Boston, 1983.

SURGERY

Welch, K. J., Randolph, J. G., Ravitch, M. M., et al.: *Pediatric Surgery,* 4th ed. Year Book Medical Publishers, Chicago, 1986.

Holder, T. M., and Ashcraft, K. W.: *Pediatric Surgery.* W. B. Saunders, Philadelphia, 1980.

PATHOLOGY

Potter, E. L., and Craig, J. M.: *Pathology of the Fetus and the Infant,* 3rd ed. Year Book Medical Publishers, Chicago, 1975.

Larroche, J. C.: *Developmental Pathology of the Neonate.* Elsevier-North Holland Biomedical Press, Amsterdam, 1977.

Wigglesworth, J. S.: *Perinatal Pathology.* W. B. Saunders, Philadelphia, 1984.

Reed, G. B., Claireaux, A. E., and Bain, A. D.: *Diseases of the Fetus and Newborn: Pathology, Radiology and Genetics.* C. V. Mosby, St. Louis, 1989.

INDEX

Note: Page numbers in *italics* refer to illustrations;
page numbers followed by (t) refer to tables.

Abdomen, distention of, 288, 312–313
  emergency and, 288
  gasless, 361–362
  scaphoid, 313
  wall of, blueness of, 289
    defects of, 88, *314*, 315, *315, 316*
Abdominal sign(s), 309–317
  blood in stool and, 311–312
  constipation and, 312
  delayed passage of meconium and, 312
  diarrhea and, 311
  single umbilical artery and, 309
  umbilical drainage and, 317
  vomiting and, 309–310
    blood and, 310
ABO incompatibility, 143–144, 143(t), 386
Abortion law(s), 259
Achondroplasia, 353, 354
Acid-base nomogram, 486
Acidosis, bilirubin and, 139
  metabolic, 284, 218–220
  respiratory, 358
Acquired immunodeficiency syndrome
  (AIDS), 196–197
Acrocephaly, 324
Acrocyanosis, 295
Acyanotic congenital heart disease, 97–98,
  98(t)
Addiction and drug withdrawal, 252–253
Adenomatoid malformations, 129
Adrenal hemorrhage, 313
Adrenal hyperplasia, congenital, 348–350,
  349, 350
Adrenaline. See *Epinephrine.*
AGA. See *Appropriate-for-gestational-age
  baby.*
Aganglionosis of colon, 93–94
Age, gestational. See *Gestational age.*
AIDS, acquired immunodeficiency
  syndrome, 196–197
Airway obstruction, 290
Albumin-bilirubin binding, 135–136
Aldactone. See *Spironolactone.*
Alkalosis, metabolic, 220
Amikacin, 398(t)
Aminoglycoside(s), 188

Aminophylline. See *Theophylline.*
Ammonia, 224, 386, 493(t)
Amniocentesis, 4
Amniotic fluid, culture and, 100
  examination of, 4, 5–6
  meconium staining of, 16–17
Ammonia, 493(t)
Ampicillin, 398(t)
  intrauterine pneumonia and, 113
  meningitis and, 188
  sepsis and, 186
Analgesia, labor and, 249
Analgesics, 401(t)
Anemia(s), pallor and, 284
  prematurity and, 238–240
  screening for, 40(t)
Anencephaly, 82, 84, *84*
Anesthesia, effects of, 249(t)
  labor and, 249–250
Antepartum hemorrhage, 17
Antibiotic(s), 117, 398(t)
Anticonvulsant(s), 400(t)
Anti-D globulin, 140
Antihistamine(s), 248
Antithyroid drug(s), 248
α_1-Antitrypsin, 149
Anus, imperforate, *30*, 88–89, *89*
Aorta, coarctation of, 99(t)
  stenosis of, 99(t)
Apert's syndrome, 324
Apgar scoring system, 14, 14(t)
Apnea, 298–299
  monitoring of, 365, *366*
  respirograph and, 376
Appropriate-for-gestational-age baby
  (AGA), 58, 96–97
Apt test, 380
Arm, normal, 25
Arrest, cardiopulmonary, 285–286
Arrhythmia, 286–287, 305–306
Arterial oxygen tension, cyanosis and, 295
  oxygen therapy and, 387
  persistent pulmonary hypertension and,
    123
Arterialized blood gas(es), 358. See also
  Blood gas(es).

Artificial feeding, 155
Ascites, 289
ASD. See *Atrial septal defect (ASD)*.
Asphyxia, bilirubin and, 139
    emergency and, 281–283, *282*
    intrauterine growth retardation and, 210
    meconium aspiration syndrome and, 117
Aspirate, pharyngeal, 378
Aspiration, 115–117
Aspirin, 248, 249(t)
Assisted ventilation, *389*, 390–391, *391*, 491
Asymmetry, of facial movements, 327, *328*
Atelectasis, 306
Atresia, biliary, 148–149
    choanal, 128–129, 281–282
    duodenal, 71
    esophageal, 90, 290, 361–362
    tricuspid, 97, 98(t)
Atrial flutter, 286
Atrial septal defect (ASD), 70–71, 99(t)
Atropine, 402(t)
Autosomal disorder(s), 71–74, 101
Axillary temperature, 34–35

BABYbird respirator, 390
Bacitracin, 401(t)
Back, normal, 29–30, *30*
Bacterial infection(s), 182–192
    conjunctivitis and, 190, *190*
    enteritis and, 191
    meningitis and, 187–189
    omphalitis and, 189
    osteomyelitis and, 191
    otitis media and, 192
    peritonitis and, 191
    sepsis and, 182–187
    tetanus and, 192
    tuberculosis and, 192
    urinary tract and, 190–191
Bag-and-mask ventilation, 388
Bag-to-tube ventilation, 15
Ballard modification, of Dubowitz score,
    54, *55*, *56*
Barbiturate(s), 249(t), 250
Barium enema, 94
Barlow's maneuver, 95
Bathing, 37
Bathing trunk nevus, *338*, 338–339
Beckwith's syndrome, 353, *353*
Benzyl alcohol, 252
Betamethasone, 250
Beta-sympathomimetic agent(s), 8
Beta-thalassemia, 39(t)
Bicarbonate, acidosis and, 220
Bile-stained vomitus, 289
Biliary atresia, 148–149

Bilirubin, breast feeding and, 138
    conjugated, 148–149
    encephalopathy and, 145–146, *146*
    exchange transfusion and, 386
    kernicterus and, 145–146, *146*
    prematurity and, 139
    metabolism of, 134–149
        albumin-bilirubin binding in, 135–136
        Crigler-Najjar syndrome and, 147
        encephalopathy and, 145–146, *146*
        erythroblastosis fetalis and, 139–143
        hyperbilirubinemia and, 137, 138(t)
        kernicterus and, 145–146, *146*
        prematurity and, 139
    normal laboratory values for, 493(t)
    phototherapy and, 392
    tests for, 359
    toxicity and, 145–146, *146*. See also
        Kernicterus.
    unconjugated, 134–135, *135*, 147–148
Bilirubinometry, transcutaneous, 380–381
Binding, albumin-bilirubin, 135–136
Biopsy, chorionic villi, 4
Biotinidase deficiency, 39(t)
Biparietal diameter, 3
Birth weight, intrauterine growth
    retardation and, 258
    low, 258
    mortality risk and, 54–58, *57*
Birthmark, 338–339, *338*, *339*
Bladder, exstrophy of, 291
Bleeding. See *Hemorrhage*.
Bleeding time, 360
Blister(s), 340
Blood, 238–244
    anemia and, pallor and, 284
        prematurity and, 238–240
        screening for, 40(t)
    cells and, 493(t)
    coagulation disorder of, 244
    culture and, 368
        transport to regional center and, 64
    fetomaternal hemorrhage and, 244
    glucose and, intrauterine growth retarda-
        tion and, 211
    metabolic disorder and, 215
    mother-to-fetus gradient and, 204
    screening and, 36
    hemorrhagic disease of newborn and,
        240–241, 241(t)
    hyperviscosity syndrome and, 242–243
    normal laboratory values of, 493(t)
    phlebotomy and, 386–387
    stool and, 311–312
    transfusion of. See *Transfusion(s)*.
    urine and, 354
    vomitus and, 310
Blood gas(es), 358–359
    acidosis and, 219

Blood gas(es) (Continued)
  measurement of, 374–375
  prior to transport, 66
Blood group incompatibility, ABO,
  143–144, 143(t)
  Rh, 140–143, 142, 143(t)
Blood pressure, congenital heart disease
  and, 98–99
  elevated. See Hypertension.
  in newborn, 488t–490t
  low, 307–308
  monitoring of, 366–367, 367
Blood volume, 495(t)
Blue color disorder(s), 295
Blueberry muffin baby, 342
Blueness of abdominal wall, neonatal
  emergency and, 289
Blue-purple color disorder(s), 295
Body temperature, 47. See also
  Temperature; Thermoregulation.
Bone(s), osteomyelitis and, 191
Bone marrow, 380
Bottle feeding, 155
Bourns respirator, 390
Bowel. See Intestine.
Bowel movement, breast-feeding and, 154.
  See also Stool.
BPD. See Bronchopulmonary dysplasia (BPD).
Bradycardia, 286, 298, 305–306
Brazelton evaluation, 30, 178–179
Breast, Dubowitz score and, 53(t)
  hypertrophy of, 24, 25
Breast-feeding, 152–155
  drugs and, 251, 251(t)
  jaundice and, 138
  necrotizing enterocolitis and, 229
Breathing. See also Respiratory entries.
  apnea and, 298–299
  difficulty in, 299–301
  fetal, 6
Breech delivery, 16
  perinatal mortality and, 260
Broken apnea, 298
Bronchopulmonary dysplasia (BPD),
  125–128, 126(t), 127
Bronze color disorder, 296
Brown fat, 45
Bruising, 342–343
Brushfield's spots, 68, 70
Burnout, 64

Calcium, 493(t)
Calcium gluconate, 399t
Candida albicans, 199, 200
Cannula(e), 390
Capillary blood gas(es), 358. See also Blood
  gas(es).

Capillary hemangioma(s), 338
Capillary nevus, 338
Car seat(s), 41
Carbenicillin, 398(t)
Carbon dioxide tension (pCO$_2$), normal
  laboratory values and, 494(t)
  oxygen therapy and, 491
Carbon dioxide transcutaneous tension,
  376
Cardiac. See also Heart entries.
Cardiac sign(s), 305–308
Cardiomyopathy, hypertrophic, 206
Cardiopulmonary arrest, 285–286
Cardiorespiratory drug(s), 399t–400t
Cataract(s), 332, 333
Catheter(s), nasal, 390
  umbilical artery, blood gases and, 374,
  375
    placement technique for, 477–480, 478
    479, 480
    position of, 479, 480
Cavernous hemangioma(s), 338
Cefotaxime, 398(t)
Ceftriaxone, 398(t)
Cell culture, amniocentesis and, 100
Central nervous system (CNS), dyspnea
  and, 300
  hyperviscosity syndrome and, 242
Cephalhematoma(s), 21, 22, 325, 326
  jaundice and, 144–145
Cephalic ultrasound, 372, 372, 373
Cerebrospinal fluid (CSF), circulation of,
  blockage in, 85–86, 86, 87
  culture and, 368–369
  meningitis and, 188
Cesarean section, 16
CHARGE Association, 129, 282
Chemoprophylaxis, 187
Chemstrip bG, 36
Chest, normal, 24, 25
  physiotherapy of, 392
  transillumination of, 376–378, 377
  x-ray of, 307, 360–361
Chloral hydrate, 401(t)
Chloramphenicol, 398(t)
  effects of, 249(t)
  meningitis and, 188
Chloride, normal laboratory values for,
  493(t)
Chloroquine, 249(t)
Chlorothiazide, 399(t)
Chlorpropamide, 248
Choanal atresia, 128–129
  emergency treatment of, 281–282
Choledochal cyst(s), 148
Chorionic villi biopsy, 4
  genetic counseling and, 101
Chromosome(s), analysis of, 4
  disorder of, 74–76, 101

Chromosome(s) *(Continued)*
  sex, 74–76
Chronic pulmonary insufficiency of
  prematurity (CPIP), 165
Cigarette smoking. See *Smoking.*
Circulation, persistent fetal, 122–124
Circumcision, 393–394
Cleansing agent(s), 252
Cleft lip, 76–78, *76, 77, 78*
Cleft palate, 23, *23,* 76–78, *76, 77, 78*
Clotting factor deficiency(ies), 287
Cloudy cornea, 332, *333*
Cloxacillin, 398(t)
Clubfoot, 28–29, 79–80, *79, 80*
CMV (cytomegalovirus), 192, *194*
CNS. See *Central nervous system (CNS).*
Coagulation, defects of, 244, 287
  disseminated intravascular, 244, 287
  study of, 360
Coarctation of aorta, 99(t)
Cold, injury from, emergency and, 284–285
  stress of, 45, 47
Colitis, necrotizing, 228–231
Collapse of lung. See *Pneumothorax.*
Colon, aganglionosis of, 93–94
Color disorder(s), 293–296
  blue or blue-purple, 295
  bronze, 296
  cyanosis in, 295
  gray, 295–296
  green, 296
  jaundice in, 293–294
  pallor in, 294
  plethora in, 294–295
  red or red-purple, 294–295
  tanning in, 296
  white, 294
  yellow-orange, 293–294
Community hospital(s), 64
Complete heart block, 305–306
Computed tomography scan (CT scan),
  370, 371, 371–372
  hydrocephalus and, 85
Congenital condition(s), 68–103
  adrenal hyperplasia as, 348–350, *349, 350*
  biliary atresia as, 148–149
  central nervous system and, 242
  choanal atresia as, 128–129
  cystic adenomatoid malformation as, 129
  emergency and, 290–291
  examination and investigation of, 89–100
  heart block as, 305–306
  heart disease as, 96–100, 98(t), 99(t)
    screening for, 40(t)
  hip dislocation as, 26, 95–96
  hip dysplasia as, 40(t)
  lobar emphysema as, 129
  malaria as, 199
  megacolon as, 93–94

Congenital condition(s) *(Continued)*
  neonatal death and, 257
  observation and, 68–89
  perinatal mortality and, 259
  pneumonia as, 112–114, *114*
  recurrence risk and, 102–103, 103(t)
  tuberculosis as, 192
Conjugated bilirubin, 148–149
Conjunctiva(e), hemorrhage in, 333–334
  infection and, 190, *190*
  gonorrheal, 36–37
Constipation, 312
Continuous positive airway pressure
  (CPAP), 389–390
  in respiratory distress syndrome, 110
  meconium aspiration syndrome and, 117
Contraceptive(s), oral, 249(t)
Convulsion(s), 319–320, 320(t)
  neonatal emergency and, 289–290
Cooling, 44–47, *45,* 47(t). See also
  Thermoregulation.
Cord. See *Umbilical cord.*
Cordocentesis, 6
Cornea, cloudy, 332, *333*
Corticosteroid(s), in respiratory distress
  syndrome, 112
Coughing, 303
Coumadin, 249(t)
Counseling, genetic, 100–103
Coxsackie B virus, 198
CPAP. See *Continuous positive airway
  pressure (CPAP).*
CPIP (chronic pulmonary insufficiency of
  prematurity), 165
Crash or crump, neonatal emergency and,
  283
C-reactive protein, 185, 186
Creatinine, 493(t)
Cri-du-chat syndrome, 74
Crigler-Najjar syndrome, 147, 223
Cry disorder(s), 322
Cryptochordism, 76, 350–351
CSF. See *Cerebrospinal fluid (CSF).*
CT scan. See *Computed tomography scan (CT
  scan).*
Culture(s), amniotic fluid and, 100
  blood, 368
  cerebrospinal fluid, 368–369
  urine, 368
Cutis aplasia, 340, *341.* See also *Skin.*
Cutis marmorata, 343
Cyanosis, 295
  congenital heart disease and, 97–98, 98(t)
  hyperviscosity syndrome and, 242
  neonatal emergency and, 285
  persistent pulmonary hypertension and,
    123
Cyclopentolate, 401(t)
Cyst(s), choledochal, 148

Cyst(s) *(Continued)*
  vaginal, 26, *27*
Cystic adenomatoid malformation, 129
Cystic fibrosis, 223
Cystic hygroma, 329, *329*
Cytomegalovirus (CMV), 192, *194*

Death. See *Mortality.*
Decadron. See *Dexamethasone.*
Deceleration of fetal heart, 5
Delivery, breech, 16, 260
  midforceps, 17
  premature rupture of membrane and,
    260
  traumatic, 260
  vacuum-extractor and, 17
Delivery room, 13–17
Demand feeding schedule, 153
Deterioration, neonatal, sudden, 283
Dexamethasone, 399(t), 400(t)
  beneficial effects of, 250
  convulsions and, 189
Dextrocardia, 306
  diaphragmatic hernia and, 91
Dextrose, 399(t)
Dextrostix, 36
Diabetes, fetal growth and, 7
  growth and, 204–207, *206*
  large-for-gestational-age infant and, 353
Diagnostic technique(s), 365–381
  Apt test and, 380
  bone marrow and, 380
  cephalic ultrasound and, 372, *372, 373*
  chest wall transillumination and, 376–
    378, *377*
  computed tomography and, *370, 371,*
    371–372
  hyperoxia test and, 376
  infection and, 368–369
  Kleihauer technique and, 380
  magnetic resonance imaging and, 372
  monitoring and, 365–367
  neurologic, 369–374
  pharyngeal aspirate evaluation and, 378
  pulse oximetry and, 375
  radiology and, 371–372, *370, 371, 372,*
    373
  respiratory evaluation and, 374–378
  respirography and, 76
  stool and, 379
  transcutaneous bilirubinometry and,
    380–381
  transcutaneous tension and, carbon diox-
    ide, 376
    oxygen, 375–376
  urine and, 378–379
  x-ray and, 381

Diameter, biparietal, 3
Diaphragm, eventration and, 93
  hernia and, 91–93, *92, 93*, 290–291, 348(t)
  paralysis and, 93
Diarrhea, 311
Diastolic blood pressure, 488(t)
Diazepam, 400(t)
  convulsions and, 290
  effects of, 249(t), 250
DIC (disseminated intravascular
    coagulation), 244, 287
Diethylstilbestrol, 248
DiGeorge's syndrome, 102
Digoxin, 100, 399(t)
Dilantin. See *Phenytoin.*
Discharge, from eyes, 333
  from hospital, 167–168
  from vagina, 26
Dislocation(s), of hip, 26, 95–96
Disseminated intravascular coagulation
    (DIC),244, 287
Distention, abdominal, 312–313
  neonatal emergency and, 288
Distress syndrome, respiratory. See
    Respiratory distress syndrome (RDS).
Diuril. See *Chlorothiazide.*
Dopamine, 402(t)
Doppler technique, for blood pressure, 367
Down's syndrome, 6, 39(t), 68–71, *69, 70*
Drainage, from umbilicus, 317
Drug(s). See also named drug or drug
    group.
  addictive, 252–253
  fetal effects of, adverse, 248, 249(t)
    in labor, 249–250
    nonproven, 248–249
    teratogenic, 246–248
  nursery procedures and, 398(t)–401(t)
  overdose of, exchange transfusion and,
    386
  withdrawal from, 252–253
Dubowitz score, Ballard modification of,
    54, *55, 56*
  criteria for, external, 53(t)–54(t)
    neurologic, *50, 51,* 52(t)
  defined, 49
Duodenal atresia, 71
Dwarfism, presenting signs and, 353–354
Dysgenesis, gonadal, 74–76
Dysostosis, mandibulofacial, 77, *78*
Dysplasia, bronchopulmonary, 125–128,
    126(t), *127*
  congenital hip, 40(t)
Dysrhythmia, 286–287

Ear(s), abnormal position of, 19
  Dubowitz score and, 54(t)

Ear(s) (Continued)
  trisomies and, 71–74
Echocardiography, congenital heart
    disease and, 99
Ectopia vesicae, 291
Edema, Dubowitz score and, 53(t)
  of head, 325, 326
  of neck, 329, 329, 330
  of scrotum, 290
  presenting signs and, 346, 347
Electrode(s), fetal scalp, 17
Electrolyte(s), 359
Ellis–van Creveld syndrome, 353–354
Emergency(ies), acute abdominal
    distention as, 288
  arrhythmia as, 286–287
  ascites as, 289
  bile-stained vomitus as, 289
  birth asphyxia as, 281–283, 282
  cardiopulmonary arrest as, 285–286
  congenital abnormalities as, 290–291
  convulsions as, 289–290
  cyanosis as, 285
  dysrhythmia as, 286–287
  scrotal swelling as, 290
  shock as, 283–285
  sudden deterioration as, 283
Emphysema, congenital lobar, 129
  pulmonary interstitial, 122
Encephalocele, 329, 329, 330
Encephalopathy, bilirubin, 145–146, 146
Enclosed hemorrhage, jaundice and,
    144–145
Endotracheal intubation, 388–389
Enema, barium, 94
Enteritis, 191
Enteroviruses, 198, 198
Environment(s), temperature of, 45–46, 46t
Epidermolysis bullosa, 341
Epinephrine, 252, 402(t)
Erb's palsy, 25
Erythema toxicum, 336, 337
Erythroblastosis fetalis, 39(t), 139–143, 142
  perinatal mortality and, 260
Erythromycin, 401(t)
Esophageal atresia, 90, 290, 361–362
Eventration, diaphragmatic, 93
Exchange transfusion(s), 386
  technique of, 481
Exstrophy, of bladder, 291
  of cloaca, 440
Extracorporeal membrane oxygenation,
    391–392
Eye(s), cloudy cornea of, 332, 333
  conjunctival hemorrhage in, 333–334
  discharge from, 333
  iris of, 334
  lens opacity of, 332, 333
  normal, 22

Eye(s) (Continued)
  optic disc of, 334
  pupil of, light reflex in, 334
    membranous lesion behind, 332
  retina of, 335
  wide apart, 77, 77, 332

Face, asymmetrical movements of, 327, 328
  masks for, 389–390, 389
Fallot, tetralogy of, 97
Family planning, 261
Fat, brown, 45
Feces. See Stool.
Feeding, bottle, 155
  breast, 152–155
  gavage, 156–157, 157(t), 158
  parenteral, 158–160
  prematurity and, 164
Feet, 28–29
Fentanyl, 402(t)
Fer-in-Sol (ferrous sulfate), 401t
Fetal alcohol syndrome, 247, 247(t)
Fetomaternal hemorrhage, 244, 283
α-Fetoprotein, 6, 83–84, 100
Fetoscopy, 101
Fetus, assessment of, 3–6
  breathing movement of, 6
  death rate of, 257
  distress of, 210
  drug effects on. See Drug(s), fetal effects
    of.
  growth of, modification of, 7
    perinatal mortality and, 261–262
    retardation of. See Intrauterine growth
      retardation (IUGR).
  head/abdomen circumference ratio of, 3
  hemorrhage and, 244
  immaturity of, 259
  malnutrition of. See Intrauterine growth
      retardation (IUGR).
  management of, 7–9
  maternal screening and, 6
  monitoring of, heart rate and, 4–5
    scalp electrode and, 17
  persistent transitional circulation and,
      122–124
  scalp of, 5
    electrodes on, 17
  sex prediction and, 4
  surgery and, 9
  well-being of, test of, 5
Fever, 46. See also Thermoregulation.
Fibrin split products, 493(t)
Fibrinogen, 493(t)
Finger(s), extra, 80, 81
  flexing of, 72
  fusion of, 80, 81

Finger(s) *(Continued)*
  supernumerary, 80, *81*
Firm skin, 343
Fistula(s), rectovaginal, 88
  tracheoesophageal, 89–90
Flexing of fingers, 72
Floppy baby, 321–322, *322*
Fluid, retained, 117–118
Flush technique, for blood pressure, 367
Flutter, atrial, 286
Folate, deficiency of, 224
Folic acid, 401(t)
Fontanel, 326, *327*
Foot, 28–29
Formula feeding, 155
Fracture(s), 325
Fragilitas ossium, 328
Furosemide, 400(t)

Galactosemia, 222
  screening for, 39(t)
Ganglion cell(s), 94
Gas(es), blood, 358–359. See also *Blood
    gas(es)*.
Gasless abdomen, 361–362
Gastric feeding, 156–157
Gastrointestinal obstruction, 39(t)
Gastroschisis, 291, 315, *316*
Gavage feeding, 156–157, 157(t), *158*
Genetic counseling, 100–103
Genitalia, ambiguous, 291
    presenting signs of, 348–350, *349, 350*
  Dubowitz score and, 54(t)
  normal, 26–27, *27, 28*
Gentamicin, 113, 398(t)
Germinal matrix hemorrhage, 236
Gestational age, 49–62
  assessment of, 54–58, *57*
  estimation of, 49–62
  large for, 58
  mortality risk and, *57*
  small for, 58, *59, 60, 61*
Glossoptosis, 24, 129
Glucagon, 399t
  hypoglycemia and, 215
Glucose, 359, 399t
  blood. See also *Diabetes*.
    fetal growth and, 211
    hypoglycemia and, 211
    normal laboratory values for, 493(t)
    screening and, 3–6
  infusion feeding and, 159
  rate calculation for, *500*
  urine and, 378
Gonadal dysgenesis, 74–76
Gonorrheal conjunctivitis, 36–37
Gravity, specific, of urine, 379

Gray color disorder, 295–296
Green color disorder, 296
Grief response, 179–180
Growth, deviations of, 204–212
  diabetes and, 204–207, *206*
  intrauterine, deviations of, 204–212
    modifications of, 7
    retardation of. See *Intrauterine growth
      retardation* (IUGR).
  record of, *487*
Guthrie test, 39–40

Hair pattern, 325–326
Hand(s), normal, 25
  washing of, 33
Harlequin phenomenon, 336, *337*
Head, 324–330, *325–330*
  abnormal hair pattern on, 325–326
  anencephaly and, 82, 84, *84*
  asymmetrical movements of, 327, *328*
  bony defects of, 328
  cephalhematoma of, 21, *22*
    jaundice and, 144–145
  encephalocele and, 329, *329, 330*
  fontanel and, 326, *327*
  hydranencephaly and, 324
  hydrocephalus and, 85–86, *86, 87*
  intracranial hemorrhage and, 233–236,
    234(t)
  intracranial pressure monitoring and,
    374
  large, 324
  normal, 21–22, *22*
  odd-shaped, 324–325
  Potter's facies and, 326–327, *328*
  scalp and. See *Scalp*.
  small, 324, *325*
  swelling of, 325, *326*
  tilted or twisted, 329–330
  transillumination of, 370–371
Headbox, 387–388
Hearing, 40(t)
  loss of, prematurity and, 167–168
Heart. See also *Cardiac; Cardio-* entries.
  congenital disease of, 40(t), 96–100, 98(t),
    99(t)
  emergency and, 284
  large, 307
  murmur of, 305
  myopathy (hypertrophic) and, 206
  sounds of, 306–307
Heart block, 305–306
Heart rate, 305–306
  fetal, 4–5
    scalp electrode and, 17
Heel, warmed, blood gases and, 374–375
Hemangioma(s), capillary, 338

Hemangioma(s) *(Continued)*
  cavernous, 338
  of neck and chest, 329, *329*
  strawberry, 338
Hematocrit, 357
  congenital heart disease and, 99
  intrauterine growth retardation and, 210, 211
  hyperviscosity syndrome and, 242–243
  normal laboratory values for, 493(t)
Hematoma(s), cephalic, 21, *22*
  scrotal, 26–27, *28*
  sternomastoid muscle and, *24*
Hematuria, 354
Hemoglobin, 493(t)
Hemolytic disease of newborn, 139–143, *142*
  ABO incompatibility and, 143–144, 143(t)
  rhesus incompatibility and, 140–143, *142*, 143(t)
Hemorrhage, antepartum, 17
  conjunctival, 333–334
  enclosed, 144–145
  fetomaternal, 244, 283
  generalized, 287
  intracranial, 233–236, 234(t)
  intraventricular, 233
    neonatal death and, 259
  localized, 288
  periventricular, 233
  pulmonary, 210
  subgaleal, 325
  umbilical artery catheter and, 480
Hemorrhagic disease of newborn, 240–241, 241(t)
Hepatitis B immune globulin, 197
Hepatitis B vaccine, 38, 197
Hereditary disorder(s), 100–103
Hernia(s), diaphragmatic, 91–93, *92, 93*, 290–291
  inguinal, 165
  umbilical, 165
Heroin, 250
Herpes simplex, 196
  TORCH syndrome and, 195
Herpesvirus hominis, 339–340
High hematocrit syndrome, exchange transfusion and, 386
Hip(s), dislocation of, 26, 95–96
  dysplasia of, 40(t)
  normal, 26
  subluxable, 95–96
Hirschsprung's disease, 93–94
Hyaline membrane disease, 259. See also *Respiratory distress syndrome (RDS).*
Hyaluronidase, 402(t)
Hydantoin, 247
Hydralazine, 402(t)
Hydranencephaly, 324

Hydrocele(s), 350
Hydrocephalus, 85–86, *86, 87*
Hydrocolpos, 26–27, *27*
Hydrometrocolpos, 26
Hydrops fetalis, 141, *142*
  presenting signs and, 347–348, 348(t)
Hygroma(s), cystic, 329, *329*
Hymen, cyst and, 26
  imperforate, 26–27, *27*
Hyperammonemia, 224, 386
Hyperbilirubinemia, 137, 138(t). See also *Bilirubin.*
  conjugated, 148–149
  Crigler-Najjar syndrome and, 147
  drugs in, 147
  exchange transfusion and, 386
  phototherapy and, 392
  unconjugated, 147–148
Hypercalcemia, 218
Hyperglycemia, 216
Hyperkalemia, 221
Hypermagnesemia, 220–221
Hypernatremia, 221
Hyperoxia test, 376
  persistent pulmonary hypertension and, 123
Hyperplasia, adrenal, 348–350, *349, 350*
Hypertelorism, 77, *77*, 332
Hypertension, 307. See also *Blood pressure.*
  pregnancy-induced, 7
  pulmonary, meconium aspiration syndrome and, 116
  persistent, 122–124, 260–261
Hyperthyroidism, 223
Hypertrophic cardiomyopathy, 206
Hypertrophy, of breast, 24, *25*
Hyperviscosity syndrome, 242–243
  intrauterine growth retardation and, 210
Hypocalcemia, 216–218
  intrauterine growth retardation and, 210
Hypochondroplasia, 353, *353*
Hypoglycemia, 214–216
  intrauterine growth retardation and, 210
Hypokalemia, 222
Hypomagnesemia, 221
Hyponatremia, 221
Hypoplasia, pulmonary, 124–125
Hypospadias, 26, *27*
  incomplete phallus and, 351
  urethra and, 26–27, *27*
Hypotension, 307–308
Hypothermia, 47. See also *Thermoregulation.*
  emergency and, 284–285
Hypothyroidism, 223
  screening for, 38–39, 39(t)
Hypotonia, 321–322, *322*
Hypoxia, 233, 295
Hypovolemia, 283, 385

Ichthyosis, 341, *341*
Identification of neonate, 34
IDM. See *Infant of diabetic mother (IDM)*.
IgA, 495(t)
IgC, 495(t)
IgM, 495(t)
Illegitimacy, 258–259
Imaging. See specific modality.
Immaturity. See also *Prematurity*.
  of lung, 163. See also *Respiratory distress
    syndrome (RDS)*.
  of organ systems, 163
  neonatal death and, 259
  organ system, 163
Immune globulin hepatitis B, 197
Immune-mediated thrombocytopenia, 287
Immunization, 38, 169, 170
Immunoglobulin(s), 495(t)
Impedance monitoring, 365, *366*
Imperforate anus, *30*, 88–89, *89*
  omphalocele and, 291
Imperforate hymen, 26–27, *27*
Incompatibility, of blood, ABO, 143–144,
    143(t)
  Rh, 140–143, *142*, 143(t)
Incomplete phallus, 351
Incubator(s), temperature and, 45–46, 46t
  transport and, 64–66, *65*
Inderal, 402(t)
Indomethacin, 402(t)
Indurated skin, 343
Infant of diabetic mother (IDM), 204–207,
  206. See also *Diabetes*.
Infant mortality rate(s), 257–258, *497, 498*,
  499(t)
Infant-parent interaction(s), 175–179, *176,
  177, 178*
Infection(s), 182–203
  bacterial, 182–192
  central nervous system, 242
  death and, 259
  detection of, 368–369
  gonorrheal, 36–37
  herpes simplex, 196
  intrauterine, 112–114, *114*
  necrotizing enterocolitis and, 228–231,
    230
  nonbacterial, 192–200
  peritonitis and, 191
  pneumonia and, 112–115, *114*
  prematurity and, 164
  presenting signs and, 346–355
  staphylococcal, 183
  viral, 197–199
Infusion(s), feeding, 158–160
Inguinal hernia(s), 165
Injury, delivery and, 260
  due to cold, 284–285
Insulin, 402(t)

Insulin dependence, 207. See also *Diabetes*.
Intensive care nursery, 64
  parental visiting in, 175, *176, 177, 178*
Interstitial emphysema, 122
Intestine, aganglionosis and, 93–94
  dilated loops of, 362
  necrotizing enterocolitis of, 228–231, *230*
    abdominal distention and, 288, 312–
      313
  frothy appearance of, 362
  hyperviscosity syndrome and, 242
  intrauterine growth retardation and,
    210
Intracranial hemorrhage, 233–236, 234(t)
Intracranial pressure monitoring, 374
Intranatal history, 20
Intrapartum period, 16–17
Intrauterine growth retardation (IUGR),
    208–212, 209(t)
  birth weight and, 258
  diabetes and, 205
  multiple pregnancy and, 170–173, *171,
    172*, 172(t)
  presenting signs of, 352–353
  thermoregulation and, 44–45
Intrauterine infection(s), pneumonia and,
    112–114, *114*
Intravascular coagulation, disseminated,
    244, 287
Intraventricular hemorrhage, 233
  neonatal death and, 259
Intubation, endotracheal, 388–389
  asphyxia and, 281
  cardiopulmonary arrest and, 285–286
  diaphragmatic hernia and, 290–291
  prior to transport, 65
Iodide(s), 249(t)
Iris, 334
Iron, anemia and, 239
  supplement of, 401t
Isolation technique, 34
IUGR. See *Intrauterine growth retardation
    (IUGR)*.

Jaundice, 134–149, 293–294. See also
    Bilirubin, metabolism of.
  breast-milk, 138
  enclosed hemorrhage and, 144–145
  hyperviscosity syndrome and, 242
  physiologic, 136–137
Jaw, micrognathia and, 129
Jitteriness, 319, 320(t)

Kanamycin, 398(t)
Kernicterus, bilirubin metabolism and,
    145–146, *146*

Kernicterus *(Continued)*
  prematurity and, 139
Kidney(s), hematuria and, 354
  oliguria and, 354–355
Kleihauer technique, 380
Klinefelter's syndrome, 76, 351
Klippel-Feil syndrome, 24
Klumpke's paralysis, 25

Labor, arresting of, 8
  drugs in, 249–250
  premature, perinatal mortality and, 260
Laboratory test(s), 357–362
  bilirubin in, 359
  blood gases in, 358–359
  coagulation study in, 360
  electrolytes in, 359
  glucose in, 359
  hematocrit in, 357
  liver enzymes in, 360
  normal values for, 493(t)-495(t)
  nucleated RBC in, 357
  pH in, 358–359
  platelets in, 358
  total protein in, 359
  WBC in, 357–358
Lacrimal duct, 333
Lanugo, 53(t)
Large-for-gestational-age infant, 58
  presenting signs and, 353, *353*
Lasix. See *Furosemide.*
Leg(s), 27–28, *29*
Lens opacity, 332, *333*
Lethargy, 320–321
Leukocyte count, 357–358
Leukopenia, 184–185
LGA. See *Large-for-gestational-age infant.*
Light-for-date infant. See *Intrauterine
  growth retardation (IUGR).*
Limb pain, 355
Lip, cleft, 76–78, *76, 77, 78*
Liver, biliary atresia and, 148–149
  enzymes of, 360
Lobar emphysema, congenital, 129
Low-birth-weight infant. See also
  Intrauterine growth retardation (IUGR).
  discharge criteria and, 167–168
  perinatal mortality and, 258
  prematurity and, 165–167
Lumbar puncture, 369–370
  hydrocephalus and, 85–86
Lumbosacral meningomyelocele, 81–85, *82,
  83, 84*
Lung(s), chronic disease of, 125–128, 126(t),
  127. See also *Respiratory disorder(s).*
  collapse of, 119–121, *120, 121.* See also
  Pneumothorax.

Lung(s) *(Continued)*
  congenital lobar emphysema and, 129
  hemorrhage and, 210
  hypoplasia of, 124–125
  interstitial emphysema and, 122
  maturation of, 7–8
  pneumothorax and. See *Pneumothorax.*
  pulmonary hypertension and, meconium
    aspiration and, 115–117
    persistent, 122–124
  respiratory distress syndrome and. See
    Respiratory distress syndrome (RDS).
  retained fluid in, 117–118
  tuberculosis and, 192
Lyon hypothesis, 102

Macrocephaly, 324
Magnesium, 221, 250, 494(t)
Magnesium sulfate, 249(t)
Magnetic resonance imaging, 372
Malformation(s). See specific
  malformation.
Malmo splint, 95–96
Malnutrition, fetal. See *Intrauterine growth
  retardation (IUGR).*
Mandibulofacial dysostosis, 77, *78*
Maternal age, 258
Maternal medical problem(s), 259
Maternal screening, 6
Maturation, 7–8. See also *Immaturity.*
Measles virus, 199
Meconium, amniotic fluid and, 16–17
  aspiration of, 115–117
  delayed passage of, 312
  perinatal mortality and, 260
Mediastinal shift, 360
Mediastinum. See *Pneumomediastinum.*
Megacolon, 93–94
Melanosis, pustular, 339
Membrane disease, hyaline. See *Hyaline
  membrane disease.*
Membranous lesion, behind pupil, 332
Meningitis, 187–189
Meningomyelocele, lumbosacral, 81–85, *82,
  83, 84*
Mental retardation, 71
Mesomelic dwarfism, 353–354
Metabolic disorder(s), 214–227
  acidosis and, 218–220
  alkalosis and, 220
  bilirubin and. See *Bilirubin.*
  Crigler-Najjar syndrome and, 223
  cystic fibrosis and, 223
  drugs for, 399t
  galactosemia and, 222
  hyperammonemia and, 224
  hypercalcemia and, 218

Metabolic disorder(s) (Continued)
  hyperglycemia and, 216
  hyperkalemia and, 221
  hypermagnesemia and, 220–221
  hypernatremia and, 221
  hyperthyroidism and, 223
  hypocalcemia and, 216–218
  hypoglycemia and, 214–216
  hypokalemia and, 222
  hypomagnesemia and, 221
  hyponatremia and, 221
  hypothyroidism and, 223
  inborn, 222–223
  phenylketonuria and, 222
  vitamin deficiency and, 224–225
Methemoglobinemia, 295
Methicillin, 398(t)
Microcephaly, 324, 325
Micrognathia, 129
Midforceps delivery, 17
Milk, aspiration of, 115
  breast, 152–155
    drugs in, 251, 251(t)
    jaundice and, 138
    necrotizing enterocolitis and, 231
  witch's, 24, 25
Mini-pharmacopeia, 397–402. See also
    Pharmacopeia.
Mini-sedimentation rate, 369
Modified-demand feeding schedule, 153
Mongolian blue spot, 338–339
Mongolism, 6, 39(t), 68–71, 69, 70
Monilia, 199, 200
Monitoring, 365–367
  apnea and, 365, 366
  blood pressure and, 366–367, 367
  heart rate, 4–5, 365
  intracranial pressure and, 374
  perinatal mortality and, 260
  respiration and, 365, 366
  temperature and, 365–366, 367
Monosomy, 74
Morphine sulfate, 401(t)
Mortality, causes of, 259
  decline in, 259–261
  definitions of, 257–258
  family planning and, 261
  fetal growth and, 261–262
  grief response and, 179–180
  influences of, 258–259
  low birth weight and, 258
  nutrition and, 261
  rate of, 257–258, 497, 498, 499t
  regionalization and, 259–260
  smoking and, 262
Mother, age of, 258
  fetomaternal hemorrhage and, 244
  Rh-negative, 140
  screening of, for fetal disorder, 6

Mother-to-fetus blood glucose gradient,
    204
Mottling of skin, 343
Mouth, 23–24, 24
Mucoviscidosis, 223
Mucus, tracheoesophageal fistula and, 90
Muffled heart sounds, 306–307
Multiple pregnancy, 170–173, 171, 172,
    172(t)
Mumps virus, 199
Murmur, heart, 305
Mydriacil, 401(t)

Nafcillin, 398(t)
Nail(s), malformed, 29, 346, 347
Naloxone, 399t
  birth asphyxia and, 281
  resuscitation and, 16
  Narcan. See Naloxone.
Narcotic(s), birth asphyxia and, 231
  effects of, 249(t)
  withdrawal and, 252–253
Nasal catheter(s), 390
Nasal prongs, 389–390, 389
Natal teeth, 23–24, 24
NEC. See Necrotizing enterocolitis (NEC).
Neck, normal, 24, 24
  swelling in, 329, 329, 330
  tilted-twisted head and, 329–330
Necrosis, subcutaneous fat, 325
Necrotizing enterocolitis (NEC), 228–231,
    230
  abdominal distention and,
  frothy appearance of bowel and, 362
  hyperviscosity and, 242
  intrauterine growth retardation and, 210
Negative-pressure respirator, 390
Neomycin, 398(t)
Neosynephrine, 401(t)
Neural tube defect(s), 81–85, 82, 83, 84, 291
  screening for, 39(t)
Neurologic evaluation, 324–330
  cephalic ultrasound in, 372, 372, 373
  intracranial pressure monitoring in, 374
  lumbar puncture in, 309–310
  normal, 30
  spinal tap in, 369–370
  transillumination of skull in, 370–371
Neurologic sign(s), 319–322
  convulsion as, 319–320, 320(t)
  cry disorders as, 322
  floppy baby as, 321–322, 322
  hypotonia as, 321–322, 322
  jitteriness as, 319, 320(t)
  lethargy as, 320–321
  narcotic withdrawal and, 252–253
Nevus(i), 338–339, 338, 339

Nevus(i) *(Continued)*
  bathing trunk, *338,* 338–339
  capillary, 338
  sebaceous, 339, *339*
  strawberry, 338
New Ballard score, 54, *55, 56*
Nipple(s), Dubowitz score and, 53(t)
  stimulation test and, 5
Nomogram, acid-base, 486
Nonbacterial infection(s), 192–200
  candidiasis as, 199, *200*
  congenital malaria as, 199
  hepatitis B and, 197
  TORCH syndrome and, 192–196, *193,*
    194, 195(t)
  virus(es) in, Coxsackie B as, 198
    enterovirus as, 198, *198*
    herpes simplex as, 196
    influenza as, 199
    measles as, 199
    mumps as, 199
    parvovirus B19 as, 198
    respiratory syncytial as, 198–199
    varicella zoster as, 197
Nonshivering thermogenesis, 45
Nonstress test, 5
Nose. See also *Nasal* entries.
  catheter and, 390
  choanal atresia and, 128–129, 281–282
  normal, 22
  stuffy and runny, 302
Nucleated red blood cells, 210, 357
Nursery procedure(s), 33–41
  bathing as, 37
  blood glucose screening as, 36
  car seat information and, 41
  Chemstrip bG and, 36
  Dextrostix and, 36
  drugs and, 398(t)–401(t)
  identification and, 34
  immunization and, 38
  isolation technique in, 34
  nursery technique in, 33
  positioning for, 35–36
  prophylaxis and, 36–37
  respiratory distress syndrome and, 110–
    111
  screening techniques in, 38–40, 39t–40t
  umbilical cord care and, 37–38
  vital signs and, 34–35
  weighing as, 35
Nutrition, 258, 261. See also *Feeding.*
Nystatin, 401(t)

Obstetric history, 258
Obstruction(s), airway, 290
Obstruction(s) *(Continued)*
  apnea and, 298
  gastrointestinal, 39(t)
  urinary tract, 39(t)
Occipital encephalocele, 329, *329*
Occipitofrontal circumference, 21
Oliguria, 354–355
Omphalitis, 189
Omphalocele, 291, *314,* 315, *315*
One-way transport, 64
Opacity of lens, 332, *333*
Opisthotonos, 145, *146*
Optic disc(s), 334
Oral contraceptives, 249(t)
Orogastric tube(s), 92
Ortolani's procedure, 95
Oscillometry, 367
Osmolality, 494(t)
Osteogenesis imperfecta, 328
Osteomyelitis, 191
  limb pain and, 355
Osteopenia, 360
Otitis media, 192
Overdose, drug, exchange transfusion and,
  386
Oxacillin, 398(t)
Oxygen, 387
  prematurity and, 164
  resuscitation and, 16
  tachycardia and, 306
  transport incubator and, 64–66, *65*
Oxygen tension (pO_2), arterial, cyanosis
  and, 123
    persistent pulmonary hypertension
    and, 123
  hyperoxia test and, 376
  normal laboratory values for, 494(t)
  transcutaneous, 375–376
Oxygenation, extracorporeal membrane,
  391–392

Pain, with limb movement, 355
Palate, cleft, 76–78, *76, 77, 78*
  posterior defect of, *23,* 78
  trisomy 13 and, 71
Pallor, 284–285, 294
Palsy, Erb's, 25
Pancuronium bromide, 402(t)
Parabiotic syndrome, 171, *172*
Paracentesis, 394
Paraldehyde, 400(t)
Paralysis, diaphragmatic, 93
Paregoric, 400(t)
Parenteral feeding(s), 158–160
Parent-infant interaction(s), 175–180, *176,*
  177, 178

Parenting disorder(s), 40(t)
Partial thromboplastin time, 495(t)
Parvovirus B19, 198
Pavulon. See *Pancuronium bromide.*
pCO₂. See *Carbon dioxide tension (pCO₂).*
Peeling skin, 340–342, *341*
PEEP (positive end-expiratory pressure), 110
Penicillin, 398(t)
  in intrauterine pneumonia, 113
  meningitis and, 188
  sepsis and, 186
  syphilis and, 348(t)
Penis, hypospadias and, 26, *27*
  incomplete, 351
Perinatal mortality, 257–262. See also *Mortality.*
Peritonitis, 191
Periventricular hemorrhage, 233
Persistent pulmonary hypertension, 122–124, 260–261
Personnel, burnout among, 64
Petechia(e), 342
pH, 494(t)
  fetal, 5
  of blood gases, 358–359
  of urine, 379
  normal laboratory values for, 494(t)
Pharmacopeia, 397–402
  analgesics in, 401(t)
  antibiotics in, 398(t)
  anticonvulsants in, 400(t)
  cardiorespiratory drugs in, 399t–400t
  metabolic problems in, 399t
  sedatives in, 401(t)
  supplements in, 401t–402t
  topical applications in, 401(t)
Pharyngeal aspirate(s), 378
Phenobarbital, 400(t)
  ABO incompatibility and, 144
  beneficial effects of, 250
  convulsions and, 289
  intracranial hemorrhage and, 235
Phenomenon, harlequin, 336, *337*
Phentolamine, 402(t)
Phenylketonuria, 39(t), 39–40, 222
Phenytoin, 400(t)
  effects of, 248, 249(t)
Phlebotomy, 386–387
Phosphate, hypercalcemia and, 218
  hypocalcemia and, 218
Phosphorous, 494(t)
Photobilirubin, 392
Phototherapy, 392–393, *393*
  parental reactions to, 179
  rash and, 336–338
Physiologic jaundice, 136–137
Physiotherapy, chest, 392

PIE (pulmonary interstitial emphysema), 122
Pigmentation, nevus and, 338–339
  pustular melanosis and, 339
Plagiocephaly, 324–325
Plantar crease, 53(t)
Platelet(s), 358
  bleeding disorders and, 287
  normal laboratory values for, 494(t)
Plethora, 294–295
Pneumatic monitoring, 365, *366*
Pneumonia, congenital, 112–114, *114*
  neonatal, 114–115
Pneumomediastinum, 119–121, *120, 121*
  shifting of, 360
Pneumothorax, 119–121, *120, 121*
  emergency and, 283
  tension, 120, *120*, 306
pO₂. See *Oxygen tension (pO₂).*
Polydactyly, 80, *81*
Ponderal index, 209
Positive end-expiratory presssure (PEEP), 110
Positive-pressure respirator, 390
Postnatal history, 20
Potassium, metabolic disorder and, 218
  normal laboratory values for, 494(t)
  parenteral feeding and, 158
Potter's facies, 326–327, *328*
Potter's syndrome, 354
Prader-Willi syndrome, 101–102, 351
Preconceptual history, 19
Prednisone, 399t
Pregnancy, hypertension in, 7
  multiple, 170–173, *171, 172,* 172(t)
  teenage, 262
Premature labor. See also *Prematurity.*
  arresting of, 8
Premature rupture of membrane, 260
Prematurity, 163–168, 164(t), *165*
  anemia of, 238–240
  bilirubin metabolism and, 139
  breast feeding and, 164
  criteria for discharge in, 167–168
  edema and, 346
  labor and, arresting of, 8
    drugs in, 249–250
    perinatal mortality and, 260
  low-birth-weight infant and, 164, 164(t)
  lung diseases of, 164
  neonatal death and, 257
  premature rupture of membrane and, 260
  prevention of, 262
  skin mottling and, 343
  thermoregulation and, 161, 166
Prenatal history, 19–20
Pressure-limited respirator, 390

Priscoline, 402(t)
Progestin(s), 249(t)
Prolapsed cord, 17
Prong(s), nasal, 389–390, *389*
Prophylaxis, eye, 36–37
   vitamin K, 37
Propranolol, 402(t)
Prostaglandin E₁, 402(t)
Prostin, 402(t)
Protein(s), normal laboratory values for,
   494(t)–495(t)
   total, 359
   urine and, 378–379
Prothrombin time, 495(t)
Provera. See *Progestin(s)*.
Prune belly syndrome, 315, *316*
Pulmonary. See also *Lung(s); Respiratory*
   entries.
Pulmonary interstitial emphysema (PIE),
   122
Pupil(s), 332, 334
Purpura, 342
Pustule(s), 339, *340*
   erythema toxicum and, 336
   melanosis and, 339
Pyridoxine, 399t
   deficiency of, 224

Quinine, 249(t)

Radial artery, 374
Radiograph(s), of chest, 307
   of imperforate anus, 88
   of tracheoesophageal fistula, 90
   techniques for, 371–372, *370, 371, 372,*
      373
Rash. See also under *Skin*.
   phototherapy, 336–338
RBCs. See *Red blood cells (RBCs)*.
RDS. See *Respiratory distress syndrome*
   (RDS).
Rectovaginal fistula, 88
Red blood cells (RBCs), normal laboratory
   values for, 493(t)
   nucleated, 210, 357
   sedimentation rate and, 369
Red color disorder(s), 294–295
Red urine, 379
Red-purple color disorder(s), 294–295
Reducing substance(s), 379
Regitine, 402(t)
Regionalized care, 63–67, *65*, 259–260
Renal disease(s), hematuria and, 354
   oliguria and, 354–355

Renal vein thrombosis, 206
Reserpine, 248, 249(t)
Respiration(s), absence of, 298–299
   monitoring of, 365, *366*
   rate and pattern of, 35
Respirator(s), 390
Respiratory disorder(s), 107–133
   acidosis and, 358
   apnea and, monitoring of, 365, *366*
   aspiration syndromes and, 115–117
   chronic lung disease and, 125–128,
      126(t), *127*
   congenital, cystic adenomatoid malfor-
      mation and, 129
   glossoptosis and, 129
   hemorrhage and, 200
   hyaline membrane disease and, 259
   hypoplasia and, 124–125
   interstitial emphysema and, 122
   micrognathia and, 129
   persistent pulmonary hypertension and,
      122–124
   pneumomediastinum and, 119–121, *120,*
      121
   pneumonia and, 112–115, *114*
   pneumothorax and, 119–121, *120, 121*
   respiratory distress syndrome and. See
      Respiratory distress syndrome (RDS).
   retained lung fluid and, 117–118
   surgery and, 128–129
   tuberculosis and, 192
   ventilation and, assisted, 283, *389*, 390–
      391, *391*, 491
      bag-and-mask, 388
      bag-to-tube, 15
Respiratory distress syndrome (RDS),
   107–112, *108, 109*, 299–301
   death and, 259
   pharyngeal aspirate and, 378
   prevention of, 260
   type II, 118
Respiratory evaluation, 374–378
   blood gases in, 358–359
   pharyngeal aspirate and, 378
   respirograph in, 376
   transcutaneous oxygen tension in, 375–
      376
   transillumination of chest wall in, 376–
      378, *377*
Respiratory sign(s), 298–303
   apnea as, 298–299
   breathing difficulty as, 299–301
   coughing as, 303
   dyspnea as, 299–301
   hyperviscosity syndrome as, 242
   sneezing as, 302
   stridor as, 301–302
   stuffy/runny nose as, 302

Respiratory sign(s) *(Continued)*
 tachypnea as, 301
Respiratory support, 387–392. See also
 Ventilation.
 chest physiotherapy in, 392
 endotracheal intubation in, 388–389
 face mask in, 389–390
 headbox in, 387–388
 nasal catheter in, 390
 nasal prong in, 389–390, *389*
 oxygen in, 387
Respiratory syncytial virus, 198–199
Respirography, 376
Resuscitation, in delivery room, 14–16
Retained lung fluid syndrome, 117–118
Retardation, intrauterine growth. See
 Intrauterine growth retardation (IUGR).
 mental, 71
Reticulocyte(s), 495(t)
Retina, 335
Retinoic acid, 247
Retinopathy of prematurity, 167, 335
Rhesus incompatibility, 140–143, *142,*
 143(t)
 exchange transfusion and, 386
 phototherapy and, 393
 presenting signs of, 346, *347*
RhoGAM, 140
Rocker-bottom foot, 72, *74*
Rotation of staff, 64
Rubella, 326
Runny nose, 302
Runting syndrome. See *Intrauterine growth
 retardation (IUGR).*

Sampling, chorionic villus, 4
 fetal scalp, 5
 urinary catheter, 479–480, *481*
Scalp. See also *Head.*
 defects of, 340, *341*
 electrode and, 17
 sampling of, 5
Scaphoid abdomen, 313
Sclerema neonatorum, 343
Screening, maternal, 6
 techniques of, 38–40, 39t–40t
Scrotum, hematoma of, 26–27, *28*
 swelling of, neonatal emergency and,
 290
 presenting signs and, 350, *351*
Sebaceous nevus, 339, *339*
Sedatives, 401(t)
Sedimentation rate, 369, 495(t)
Seizure(s). See *Convulsion(s).*
Sepsis, 182–187, 386
Septal defect(s), atrial, 70–71, 99(t)

Septal defect(s) *(Continued)*
 ventricular, 97
Servocontrol device(s), 46–47
Sex chromosome(s), 74–76
Shock, 283–285
Shunt, ventriculoperitoneal, 86
Sickle cell disease, 39(t)
Silver nitrate, 401(t)
Single umbilical artery, 309
Skin, 336–343
 absence of, 340, *341*
 birthmark on, 338–339, *338, 339*
 blisters on, 340
 bruising of, 342–343
 cutis aplasia and, 340, *341*
 cutis marmorata and, 343
 Dubowitz score and, 53(t)
 epidermolysis bullosa of, 341
 erythema toxicum in, 336, *337*
 firm, 343
 harlequin phenomenon in, 336, *337*
 indurated, 343
 mottling of, 343
 nevus and, 338–339, *338, 339*
 peeling of, 340–342, *341*
 petechiae in, 342
 phototherapy rash in, 336–338
 purpura and, 342
 pustule and, 339, *340*
 scalp and, 340, *341*
 staphylococcal infection of, 339
 sweating and, 343
 vesicle in, 339–340
Skull, defect of, 328
 odd-shaped, 324
 transillumination of, 370
Slanting eyes, 68
Small-for-dates infant. See *Intrauterine
 growth retardation (IUGR).*
Small-for-gestational-age infant, 58, *59, 60,
 61*
Smell, abnormal, 355
Smoking, effects of, 248, 249(t)
 perinatal mortality and, 262
Sneezing, 302
Socioeconomic status, 258
Sodium, 495(t)
Sodium bicarbonate, 399t
 acidosis and, 219–220
 cardiopulmonary arrest and, 286
 emergency equipment as, 65
 meningitis and, 188
 resuscitation and, 15
Specific gravity, of urine, 379
Spina bifida, 81–85, *82, 83, 84*
Spinal fluid tap, 369–370
Spine, disorders of, 81–85, *82, 83, 84*
Spironolactone, 400(t)

Splint(s), 95–96
Stabilization, for transport, 66–67
Staff, burnout among, 64
Staphylococal infection, 183
  skin lesions and, 339
Stenosis, aortic, 99(t)
Sternomastoid muscle, hematoma of, 24
Steroid(s), 218
Stillbirth, 257. See also *Mortality.*
Stool, blood in, 311–312
  enteritis and, 379
  evaluation of, 379
  reducing substance in, 379
Strawberry hemangioma(s), 338
Streptococcus, group B, 114
Stress, cold, 45, 47
Stress test, 5
Stridor, 301–302
Stuffy nose, 302
Sturge-Weber syndrome, 338
Subarachnoid hemorrhage, 233
Subconjunctival hemorrhage, 333–334
Subcutaneous fat necrosis, 325
Subdural hemorrhage, 233
Subdural tap, 370
Subgaleal hemorrhage, 325
Subluxable hip, 95–96
Sugar. See *Glucose.*
Sulfonamide(s), bilirubin and, effects of,
  248, 249(t)
Supplement(s), vitamin, 160, 401(t)–402(t)
Supraventricular tachycardia, 286
Surfactant(s), inducers of, 110–111, 250
  treatment of RDS and, 107–112
Surgery, fetal, 9
  necrotizing enterocolitis and, 231
  respiratory disorders and, 128–129
Sweating, 343
Swelling(s). See *Edema.*
β-Sympathomimetic agent, 8
Syndactyly, 80, *81*
Syphilis, congenital, 348(t)
Systolic blood pressure, 488(t)

Tachycardia, 306
  supraventricular, 286
Tachypnea, 118, 301
  transient, of newborn, 118
Talipes equinovarus, 28–29, 79–80, *79, 80*
Tanning, 296
Tay-Sachs disease, 39(t)
Teenage pregnancy, 262
Teeth, natal, 23–24, *24*
Temperature, abnormal, 352
  body, 47
  incubator, 45–46, 46t

Temperature *(Continued)*
  monitoring of, 365–366, *367*
  regulation of, 44–48
Temporal artery, 374
Tension pneumothorax, 120, *120*
Teratogenic effects of drugs, 246–248
Tetanus, 192
Tetracycline, 248, 249(t)
Tetralogy of Fallot, 97
β-Thalassemia, 39(t)
Theophylline, 250, 399(t), 400(t)
Therapeutic technique(s), 385–394. See
  also *Diagnostic technique(s).*
  blood in, 385–387
  circumcision in, 393–394
  paracentesis in, 394
  respiratory support in, 387–392
  phototherapy in, 392–393, *393*
Thermogenesis, nonshivering, 45
Thermoregulation, 44–48. See also
  Temperature.
  intrauterine growth retardation and,
  44–45
  monitoring and, 365–366, *367*
  prematurity and, 164
Thiazides, 248–249
Thrombocytopenia, 342
  immune-mediated, 287
Thrombosis, 206
Thrush, 199, *200*
Thyroid, metabolic disorder of, 223
Ticarcillin/piperacillin, 398(t)
Tilted head, 329–330
Tocolytic agent(s), 8
Toe(s), extra, 80, *81*
  fusion of, 80, *81*
Tolazoline, 402(t)
Tomography, computed, *370, 371,* 371–372
  hydrocephalus and, 85
Tongue, abnormalities of, 129
Tooth, natal, 23–24, *24*
Topical medications, 401(t)
TORCH syndrome, 192–196, *193, 194,*
  195(t)
Toxemia, 7
Toxicity, bilirubin, 145–146, *146*
  chloramphenicol, 249(t)
Toxoplasmosis, 348(t)
Tracheoesophageal fistula(s), 89–90
Transcutaneous bilirubinometry, 380–381
Transcutaneous tension, carbon dioxide,
  376
  oxygen, 375–376, 494(t)
Transfusion(s), anemia and, 239
  exchange. See *Exchange transfusion(s).*
  simple, 385
  twin-twin, 171, *172*
Transient tachycardia, of newborn, 118

Transillumination, of chest wall, 376–378, *377*
  of skull, 370–371
Transport, 64–67, *65*
  stabilization prior to, 66–67
Tricuspid atresia, 97, 98(t)
Trimethadione, effects of, 249(t)
  teratogenesis and, 247
Trisomy, autosomal, 71–74
Trisomy 13, 71, 72, *73*
Trisomy 18, 71–72, *72, 73, 74,* 75(t), 348(t)
Trisomy 21, 6, 39(t), 68–71, *69, 70,* 348(t)
Trisomy D, 71–72
Trisomy E, 71–72, *72, 73, 74,* 75(t)
Truncus arteriosus, 98(t)
Tube(s). See specific type, e.g., *Orogastric tube(s).*
Tuberculosis, 192
Tumor(s), Wilms', 334
Turner's syndrome, 74–76
Twin pregnancy, 170–173, *171, 172,* 172(t)
Twin-twin transfusion, 171, *172*
Twin-twin transfusion syndrome, 348
Twisted head, 329–330
Two-way transport, 64–65

Ultrasonography, cephalic, 372, *372, 373*
  genetic counseling and, 101
  hydrocephalus and, 85–86
  intracranial hemorrhage and, 235
  neural tube defect and, 84
  prior to delivery, 3–4
Umbilical artery, single, 309
Umbilical artery catheter(s), placement of, 477–480, *478, 479, 480*
  sampling from, 479–480, *481*
  transport to regional center with, 66
Umbilical cord, blood sampling from, 6
  care of, 37–38
  drainage from, 317
  omphalitis and, 189
  prolapsed, problems associated with, 17
Umbilical hernia, 165
Unconjugated bilirubin, 134–135, *135,* 147–148
Undernutrition. See *Intrauterine growth retardation (IUGR).*
Undescended testes, presenting signs of, 350–351
Urea nitrogen, 495(t)
Urethra, hypospadias and, 26–27, *27*
Urinary tract, infection of, 190–191
  obstruction of, 39(t)
Urine, bloody, 354
  culture of, 368
  decreased output of, 354–355

Urine *(Continued)*
  delayed passage of, 354
  evaluation of, 378–379
  glucose in, 378
  pH of, 379
  protein in, 378–379
  red, 379
  specific gravity in, 379

VACTERL, 88
Vacuum-extractor delivery, 17
Vagina, cyst of, 26, *27*
  discharge from, 26
  retrovaginal fistula of, 88
Valium. See *Diazepam.*
Valproic acid, 247
Vancomycin, 398(t)
Varicella-zoster virus, 197
VATER association, imperforate anus and, 88–89
Ventilation. See also *Respiratory disorder(s); Respiratory support.*
  assisted, 283, *389,* 390–391, *391,* 491
  bag-and-mask, 388
  bag-to-tube, 15
Ventricular arrhythmia, 287
Ventricular hemorrhage, 233
Ventricular septal defect, 97
Ventriculoperitoneal shunt, 86
Ventriculostomy, 86
Vesicle(s), 339–340
Villus, chorionic, 4, 101
Viral infection, 197–199
Viscosity, of blood, excessive, 242–243
Vision screening, 40(t)
Vital signs, 34–35
Vitamin(s), deficiency of, 224–225
  supplemental, 160, 401(t)
Vitamin B_6, 399t
Vitamin B_{12}, 224
Vitamin D, 224
Vitamin E, 224
Vitamin K, beneficial effects of, 250
  deficiency of, 224
  hemorrhagic diseases of newborn and, 240–241
Volume-limited respirator, 390
Vomitus, 289, 309–310
Von Rosen splint, 95–96
Vulnerable child syndrome, 138

Warfarin, 249(t)
Warmed heel, blood gases and, 374–375
Washing, of hands, 33

WBCs. See *White blood cells (WBCs)*.
Weight, conversion table for, 485(t)
    determination of, at delivery, 35
    mortality risk and, 258
    prematurity and, 165–167
Well-being, fetal, test of, 5
White blood cells (WBCs), 357–358, 369
    normal laboratory values for, 493(t)
White color disorder(s), 294
WHO (World Health Organization), 257
Whole blood transfusion(s), 385
Wilms' tumor, 334
Wilson-Mikity syndrome (W-MS), 125–128,
    126(t), *127*

Witch's milk, 24, *25*
Withdrawal, drug, 252–253
W-MS. See *Wilson-Mikity syndrome
    (W-MS)*.
World Health Organization (WHO), 257

X-linked disorder(s), 101
X-ray(s), 381. See also specific organs.

Yellow-orange color disorder(s), 293–294